New Frontiers in Otolaryngology

New Frontiers in Otolaryngology

Edited by Stephanie Madison

hayle
medical

New York

Hayle Medical,
750 Third Avenue, 9th Floor,
New York, NY 10017, USA

Visit us on the World Wide Web at:
www.haylemedical.com

ISBN: 978-1-63241-725-1

Cataloging-in-Publication Data

New frontiers in otolaryngology / edited by Stephanie Madison.
    p. cm.
Includes bibliographical references and index.
ISBN 978-1-63241-725-1
1. Otolaryngology. 2. Otolaryngology--Diagnosis. 3. Ear--Diseases. 4. Nose--Diseases.
5. Throat--Diseases. I. Madison, Stephanie.
RF46 .N49 2019
617.51--dc23

Table of Contents

Preface..IX

Chapter 1   Radiological findings in patients undergoing revision endoscopic sinus surgery 1
Hisham S Khalil, Ahmed Z Eweiss and Nicholas Clifton

Chapter 2   Prognostic impact of standard laboratory values on outcome in patients with
sudden sensorineural hearing loss..7
Julia Wittig, Claus Wittekindt, Michael Kiehntopf and Orlando Guntinas-Lichius

Chapter 3   Mastoiditis and Gradenigo's Syndrome with anaerobic bacteria 14
Chris Ladefoged Jacobsen, Mikkel Attermann Bruhn, Yousef Yavarian and
Michael L Gaihede

Chapter 4   Hearing screening for school children: utility of noise-cancelling headphones......................19
Ada Hiu Chong Lo and Bradley McPherson

Chapter 5   Bacterial isolates and drug susceptibility patterns of ear discharge from
patients with ear infection at Gondar University Hospital, Northwest Ethiopia.......................29
Dagnachew Muluye, Yitayih Wondimeneh, Getachew Ferede, Feleke Moges and
Tesfaye Nega

Chapter 6   Etiological profile and treatment outcome of epistaxis at a tertiary care hospital in
Northwestern Tanzania...34
Japhet M Gilyoma and Phillipo L Chalya

Chapter 7   An observational cohort study of the effects of septoplasty with or without
inferior turbinate reduction in patients with obstructive sleep apnea..................................40
Mads Henrik Strand Moxness and Ståle Nordgård

Chapter 8   Hidden consequences of olfactory dysfunction: a patient report series 45
Andreas Keller and Dolores Malaspina

Chapter 9   Reappraisal of the glycerol test in patients with suspected Menière's disease 65
Bernd Lütkenhöner and Türker Basel

Chapter 10   Allergic rhinitis and its associated co-morbidities at Bugando Medical Centre in
Northwestern Tanzania...78
Said A Said, Mabula D Mchembe, Phillipo L Chalya, Peter Rambau and
Japhet M Gilyoma

Chapter 11   Prevalence and psychopathological characteristics of depression in consecutive
otorhinolaryngologic inpatients...87
Thomas Forkmann, Christine Norra, Markus Wirtz, Thomas Vehren,
Eftychia Volz-Sidiropoulou, Martin Westhofen, Siegfried Gauggel and
Maren Boecker

Chapter 12   **Incidental findings in MRI of the paranasal sinuses in adults: a population-based study (HUNT MRI)** 94
Aleksander Grande Hansen, Anne-Sofie Helvik, Ståle Nordgård, Vegard Bugten, Lars Jacob Stovner, Asta K Håberg, Mari Gårseth and Heidi Beate Eggesbø

Chapter 13   **Ear, nose and throat injuries at Bugando Medical Centre in northwestern Tanzania: a five-year prospective review of 456 cases** 101
Japhet M Gilyoma and Phillipo L Chalya

Chapter 14   **Cortisol suppression and hearing thresholds in tinnitus after low-dose dexamethasone challenge** 107
Veerle L Simoens and Sylvie Hébert

Chapter 15   **Posterior laryngitis: a disease with different aetiologies affecting health-related quality of life: a prospective case–control study** 117
Hillevi Pendleton, Marianne Ahlner-Elmqvist, Rolf Olsson, Ola Thorsson, Oskar Hammar, Magnus Jannert and Bodil Ohlsson

Chapter 16   **Association of the 4 g/5 g polymorphism of plasminogen activator inhibitor-1 gene with sudden sensorineural hearing loss** 125
Seong Ho Cho, Haimei Chen, Il Soo Kim, Chio Yokose, Joseph Kang, David Cho, Chun Cai, Silvia Palma, Micol Busi, Alessandro Martini and Tae J Yoo

Chapter 17   **Laryngopharyngeal reflux disease in the Greek general population, prevalence and risk factors** 131
Nikolaos Spantideas, Eirini Drosou, Anastasia Bougea and Dimitrios Assimakopoulos

Chapter 18   **Frequency of mitochondrial m.1555A > G mutation in Syrian patients with non-syndromic hearing impairment** 138
Hazem Kaheel, Andreas Breß, Mohamed A. Hassan, Aftab Ali Shah, Mutaz Amin, Yousuf H. Y. Bakhit and Marlies Kniper

Chapter 19   **Knowledge and care seeking practices for ear infections among parents of under five children** 142
Kaitesi Batamuliza Mukara, Peter Waiswa, Richard Lilford and Debara Lyn Tucci

Chapter 20   **Hibernoma: a rare case of adipocytic tumor in head and neck** 150
Alexandra Rodriguez Ruiz, Sven Saussez, Thibaut Demaesschalck and Jérôme R. Lechien

Chapter 21   **Generic quality of life in persons with hearing loss** 154
Øyvind Nordvik, Peder O. Laugen Heggda, Jonas Brännström, Flemming Vassbotn, Anne Kari Aarstad and Hans Jørgen Aarstad

Chapter 22   **Three year experience with the cochlear BAHA attract implant** 167
Panagiotis A. Dimitriadis, Matthew R. Farr, Ahmed Allam and Jaydip Ray

Chapter 23   **A questionnaire using vocal symptoms in quality control of phonosurgery: vocal surgical questionnaire** 175
Aleksander Grande Hansen, Chi Zhang, Jens Øyvind Loven, Hanne Berdal-Sørensen, Magnus TarAngen and Rolf Haye

Chapter 24   The role of tonsillectomy in the Periodic Fever, Aphthous stomatitis,
Pharyngitis and cervical Adenitis syndrome 182
Jostein Førsvoll and Knut Øymar

Chapter 25   The burden of chronic rhinosinusitis and its effect on quality of life among
patients re-attending an otolaryngology clinic.. 189
Victoria Nyaiteera, Doreen Nakku, Esther Nakasagga, Evelyn Llovet,
Elijah Kakande, Gladys Nakalema, Richard Byaruhanga and Francis Bajunirwe

Chapter 26   Glomangiomyoma of the neck in a child.. 198
Bishow Tulachan and Buddha Nath Borgohain

Chapter 27   A retrospective study of long-term treatment outcomes for reduced vocal
intensity in hypokinetic dysarthria 203
Christopher R. Watts

Chapter 28   Survival in sinonasal and middle ear malignancies: a population-based study
using the SEER 1973–2015 database... 210
Mitchell R. Gore

Chapter 29   An abrupt bleeding of the anteriorly-displaced sigmoid sinus: a rare
complication of myringoplasty.. 221
Sarah Zaher Addeen and Mohammad Al- Mohammad

Permissions

List of Contributors

Index

Preface

The purpose of the book is to provide a glimpse into the dynamics and to present opinions and studies of some of the scientists engaged in the development of new ideas in the field from very different standpoints. This book will prove useful to students and researchers owing to its high content quality.

The surgical sub-speciality of medicine concerned with the conditions related to the ear, nose, throat, and the structures of the neck and head is known as otolaryngology. A specialist in this field is called an otolaryngologist, head and neck surgeon, or ENT surgeon. They deal with the surgical management of tumors and cancers related to the neck and head. Otology and neurotology are two significant sub-fields of otolaryngology. Otology deals with the anatomy and physiology of the ear, and its diseases, along with their diagnosis and treatment. Neurotology focuses on the disorders of the inner ear. This book is a compilation of chapters that discuss the most vital concepts and emerging trends in the field of otolaryngology. The various studies that are constantly contributing towards advancing technologies and evolution of this field are examined in detail in this book. Those in search of information to further their knowledge will be greatly assisted by this book. It attempts to understand the multiple branches that fall under the discipline of otolaryngology and how such concepts have practical applications.

At the end, I would like to appreciate all the efforts made by the authors in completing their chapters professionally. I express my deepest gratitude to all of them for contributing to this book by sharing their valuable works. A special thanks to my family and friends for their constant support in this journey.

Editor

Radiological findings in patients undergoing revision endoscopic sinus surgery: a retrospective case series study

Hisham S Khalil[1*], Ahmed Z Eweiss[1] and Nicholas Clifton[2]

Abstract

Background: Functional endoscopic sinus surgery (FESS) is now a well-established strategy for the treatment of chronic rhinosinusitis which has not responded to medical treatment. There is a wide variation in the practice of FESS by various surgeons within the UK and in other countries.

Objectives: To identify anatomic factors that may predispose to persistent or recurrent disease in patients undergoing revision FESS.

Methods: Retrospective review of axial and coronal CT scans of patients undergoing revision FESS between January 2005 and November 2008 in a tertiary referral centre in South West of England.

Results: The CT scans of 63 patients undergoing revision FESS were reviewed. Among the patients studied, 15.9% had significant deviation of the nasal septum. Lateralised middle turbinates were present in 11.1% of the studied sides, and residual uncinate processes were identified in 57.1% of the studied sides. There were residual cells in the frontal recess in 96% of the studied sides. There were persistent other anterior and posterior ethmoidal cells in 92.1% and 96% of the studied sides respectively.

Conclusions: Analysis of CT scans of patients undergoing revision FESS shows persistent structures and non-dissected cells that may be responsible for persistence or recurrence of rhinosinusitis symptoms. Trials comparing the outcome of conservative FESS techniques with more radical sinus dissections are required.

Keywords: Functional endoscopic sinus surgery rhinosinusitis, revision FESS, sinus C.T scan, uncinate process

Background

Functional endoscopic sinus surgery (FESS) has become a well established strategy for the treatment of rhinosinusitis not responding to medical treatment [1]. Published success rates for FESS vary from 76% to 98% [2]. However, there remains a group of patients in whom FESS does not provide symptomatic relief [3]. Some of these patients may require revision FESS. In a national audit of the sinonasal surgery in the UK, it was shown that 11.4% of patients had revision surgery within 3 years of the primary procedure [4].

Revision endoscopic sinus surgery represents a challenge to all who practise sinus surgery. Among the most important considerations in revision sinus surgery is the identification of the anatomy that is contributing to the patient's symptoms and the disease process [5].

A patient with persistent chronic sinusitis or recurrent infections after primary sinus surgery needs aggressive treatment with antibiotics and steroids. If, despite sufficient medical treatment, the patient's symptoms persist, a C.T scan is obtained to identify the source of infection. Once an anatomic aetiology of the primary surgical failure is identified, revision surgery is usually indicated [6].

Several anatomic findings have been identified in revision sinus surgery including a remnant of the uncinate process obstructing the maxillary ostium, residual ethmoidal partitions, lateralised middle turbinate and scarring of the frontal recess [5]. In the current study we have attempted to identify the anatomic factors that

* Correspondence: hisham.khalil@phnt.swest.nhs.uk
[1]Department of Otolaryngology, Derriford Hospital, Plymouth, U.K. and Faculty of Medicine, University of Alexandria, Egypt
Full list of author information is available at the end of the article

may be related to residual or recurrent sinus disease, as reflected on the C.T scans of patients admitted for revision FESS.

Methods

The axial and coronal C.T scans of 63 patients admitted for revision FESS between January 2005 and November 2008 under care of the senior author (HSK) were retrospectively reviewed as a part of an audit of the outcomes of FESS. Some of the primary procedures had been performed in the authors' hospital, a tertiary referral centre in South West England, and some had been performed in other U.K hospitals and were referred to the senior author for revision surgery. All patients presented with symptoms and endoscopic findings of recurrent sinusitis that did not respond to medical treatment. All patients had had bilateral FESS and were all listed for bilateral revision FESS. The data collated included identification of significant septal deviation, middle turbinate lateralisation, residual uncinate process, residual Haller (infraorbital) cells, residual cells in the frontal recess, residual other anterior or posterior ethmoidal cells and condition of the sphenoid sinus ostium. The nasal septum was considered to be significantly deviated when the distance between the summit of the convex part of the septum and the lateral nasal wall was less than the distance between the summit of the convexity and the midline (figure 1). The middle turbinate was considered lateralised when it was close enough to the lamina papyracea to interfere with the sinus drainage pathways in the middle meatus (figure 2).

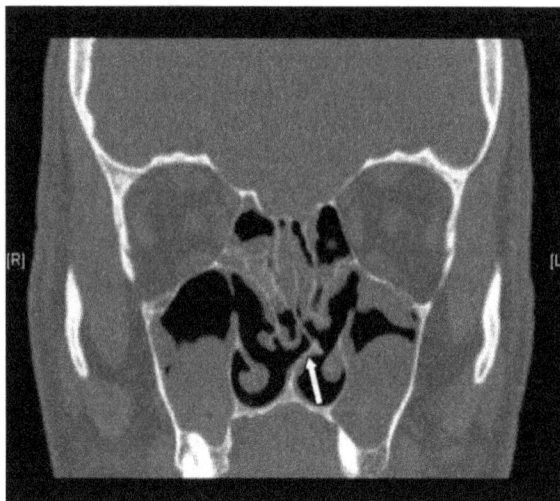

Figure 1 Residual septal deviation. A coronal C.T scan of a patient admitted for revision FESS showing a residual significant septal deviation (arrow).

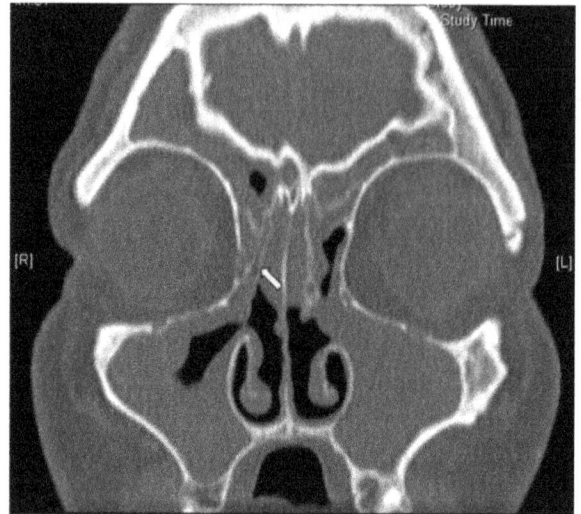

Figure 2 Lateralised right middle turbinate. A coronal C.T scan of a patient admitted for revision FESS showing a lateralised right middle turbinate (arrow).

The mucosal disease of the paranasal sinuses and the ostiomeatal complex status were scored according to the Lund - Mackay staging system [7], where a sinus with no opacification is given a score of zero, a sinus with partial opacification is given a score of 1 and a sinus with full opacification is given a score of 2. A patent ostiomeatal complex is given a score of zero, while a blocked one is given a score of 2.

This study was registered as an audit in our hospital audit department, and thus no approval was required from the ethics committee.

Results

The patients' ages ranged from 20 to 76 years, with a mean age of 50.3 years (+/- 12.1). There were 45 males and 18 females. As all patients had bilateral surgery, a total of 126 sides of paranasal sinuses were studied on the scans. The following results were identified:

The septums were significantly deviated in 10 patients (15.9%).

The middle turbinates were lateralised in 14 sides (11.1%).

Residual uncinate processes were identified in 72 sides (57.1%)

Residual Haller cells were identified in 29 sides (23%).

Residual frontal recess cells (Agger nasi and/or frontoethmoidal cells) were identified in 121 sides (96%).

Residual other anterior ethmoidal cells were identified in 116 sides (92.1%).

Residual posterior ethmoidal cells were identified in 121 sides (96%).

Blocked sphenoid sinus ostia were identified in 83 sides (65.9%).

The anterior ethmoidal and the frontal were the sinuses most frequently showing total opacification on the scans. Each of these 2 sinuses was totally opacified in 67 of the studied sides (53.2%).

The maxillary was the sinus least frequently showing total opacification, being totally opacified in 41 of the studied sides (32.5%).

The sphenoid was the most frequent sinus to show no opacification. This was detected in 36 of the studied sides (28.6%).

The maxillary was the least frequent sinus to show no opacification. This was found in only 3 of the studied sides (2.4%).

The ostiomeatal complex was patent in 21 of the studied sides (16.7%), and was blocked in 105 sides (83.3%).

Table 1 summarises the incidence of anatomical abnormalities identified on the CT scans of the paranasal sinuses. Figures 1, 2, 3, 4, 5 and 6 demonstrate the abnormalities identified on the CT scans.

Table 2 summarises the mucosal status of the paranasal sinuses as assessed from the C.T scans.

Discussion

Several reasons have been identified for failure of primary FESS. Kennedy [8] noted that patients with bilateral ethmoid disease and additional disease in 2 or more dependant sinuses on each side, as well as patients with diffuse polyps, had significantly worse outcome after FESS than patients with less severe sinus disease. Lazar et al [9] found that fibrosis and adhesion formation, particularly between the middle turbinate and the lateral nasal wall, was the most common intraoperative findings in revision FESS. This was found in 43% of their patients. Recurrence of polyps was the second commonest finding, occurring in 22% of patients. Other causes for failure of primary FESS include lateralisation of the middle turbinate, frontal recess obstruction, recirculation between the natural ostium of the maxillary sinus

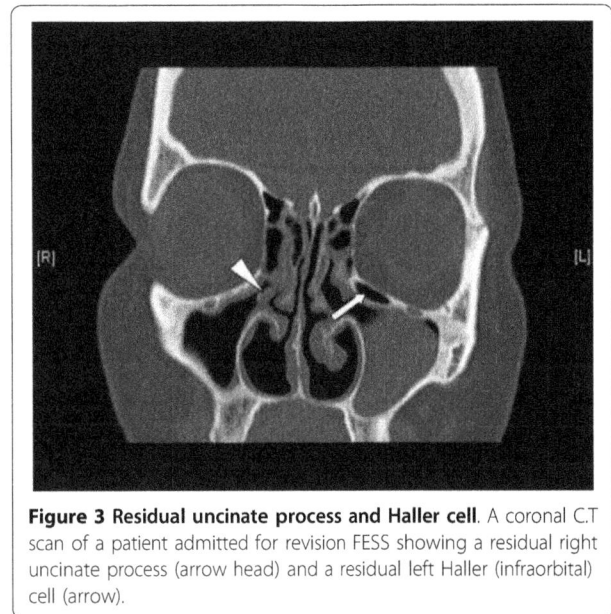

Figure 3 **Residual uncinate process and Haller cell**. A coronal C.T scan of a patient admitted for revision FESS showing a residual right uncinate process (arrow head) and a residual left Haller (infraorbital) cell (arrow).

and the antrostomy, persistent uncinate process, persistent agger nasi cells, severe septal deviations and devitalised bone [6].

Very few articles attempted to identify the incidence of the various anatomic findings in patients undergoing revision FESS. Musy and Kountakis [2] found that the most common anatomic factor associated with primary sinus surgical failure was lateralisation of the middle turbinate, occurring in 78% of their patients. Their results also showed residual anterior ethmoidal cells in 64% of patients. Scarred frontal recesses were found in 50% of patients. Residual posterior ethmoidal cells were present in 41% of patients. Residual agger nasi cells were present in 49% of patients. Residual uncinate processes were present in 37% of patients. Finally, middle meatal antrostomy stenosis was present in 39% of patients. In another study by Ramadan [10], the most common anatomic finding during revision FESS was adhesions, often involving a lateralised middle turbinate.

Table 1 Anatomical abnormalities

Anatomical Abnormality	Incidence in 63 patients	Incidence in 126 studied sides
Septal Deviation	10 (15.9%)	
Lateralized Middle Turbinate	11 (17.5%)	14 (11.1%)
Residual Uncinate Process	38 (60.3%)	72 (57.1%)
Residual Haller Cells	16 (25.4%)	29 (23%)
Residual Frontal Recess Cells	61 (96.8%)	121 (96%)
Residual Anterior Ethmoidal Cells	58 (92.1%)	116 (92.1%)
Residual Posterior Ethmoidal Cells	61 (96.8%)	121 (96%)
Obstructed Sphenoid Sinus Ostium	43 (68.3%)	83 (65.9%)

Anatomical abnormalities in the CT scans of the paranasal sinuses of 63 patients admitted for bilateral revision FESS.

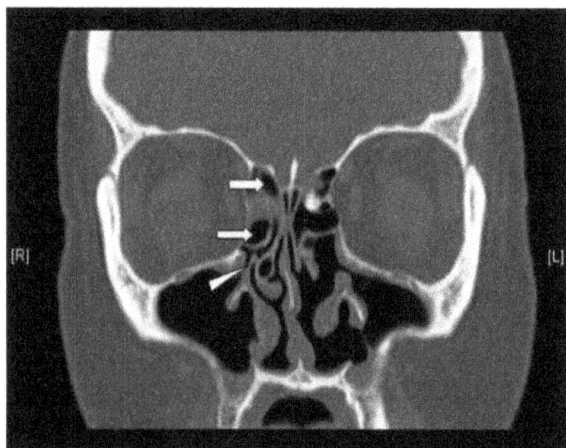

Figure 4 Residual uncinate process and anterior ethmoidal cells. A coronal C.T scan of a patient admitted for revision FESS showing a residual right uncinate process (arrow head) and residual anterior ethmoid cells (arrows).

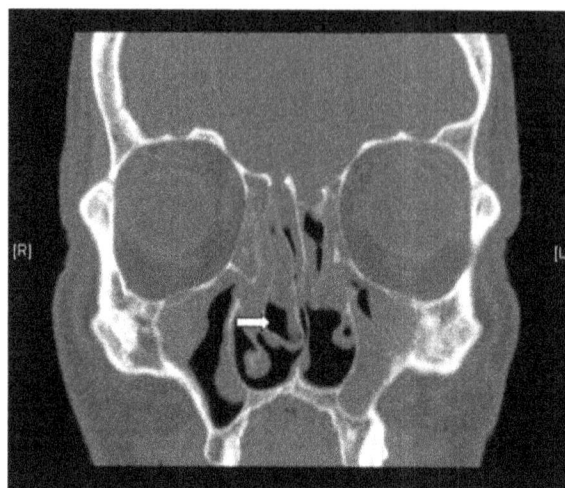

Figure 6 Residual large right concha bullosa. A coronal C.T scan of a patient admitted for revision FESS showing a residual large right concha bullosa (arrow).

This occurred in 56% of patients. This investigator also detected residual ethmoidal cells in 31%, middle meatal antrostomy stenosis in 27% and frontal sinus ostium stenosis in 25% of patients undergoing revision FESS.

In comparison with Musy and Kountakis' findings [2], the current study showed a noticeably higher incidence of residual cells. Our data show that 96% of the studied

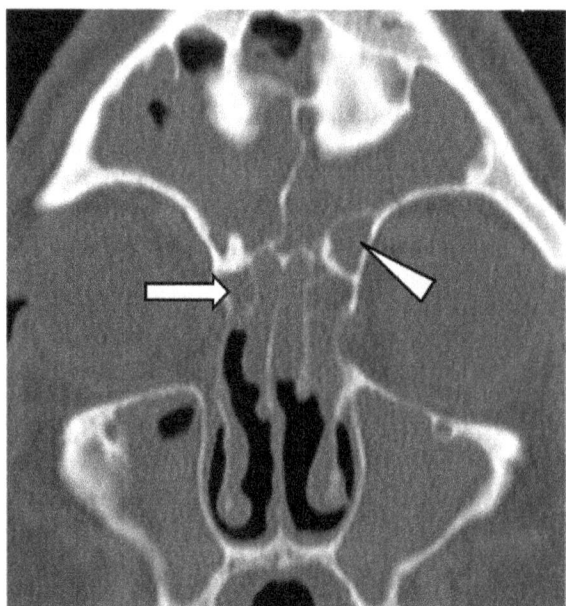

Figure 5 Residual frontal recess cells. A coronal C.T scan of a patient admitted for revision FESS showing a residual right agger nasi cell (arrow) pneumatising within right frontal recess and a residual left type III frontal cell (arrow head) pneumatising from the left frontal recess into the frontal sinus and partly obstructing the frontal sinus ostium.

sides (96.8% of patients) had residual posterior ethmoidal cells, 96% of the sides (95.2% of patients) had residual frontal recess cells and 92.1% of the sides (92.1% of patients) had residual other anterior ethmoidal cells. On the contrary, lateralisation of the middle turbinate was only detected in 11.1% of the sides (17.5% of patients), which was significantly less than Musy and Kountakis' figure of 78% [2]. These results may reflect the more conservative FESS techniques practised by the majority of the surgeons in the U.K, in comparison with the practice in the U.S. It is of course to be argued that removal of all cells is not required in the majority of FESS procedures, and that the procedure has to be tailored to the extent of the pathology. However, the majority of the patients in the current study had pansinusitis, as can be seen from the Lund-Mackay [7] scoring of the involved sinuses, where only 2.4% of the maxillary sinuses, 7.1% of the anterior and posterior ethmoids and 22.2% of the frontal sinuses were non opacified. It is therefore reasonable to assume that the majority of these patients needed more aggressive surgical dissections than what they had during the primary surgery.

The current study showed that 57.1% of the sides (60.3% of the patients) had a residual uncinate process. Chiu and Kennedy [5] advised that identifying an uncinate process remnant was the most critical step in revising a middle meatal antrostomy. They also commented that residual Haller (infraorbital) cells could be a source of persistent obstruction of the maxillary sinus. The latter cells were found in 23% of the sides (25.4% of the patients) in the current study. However, recently some studies have advocated preservation of the uncinate

Table 2 Mucosal status of the paranasal sinuses

Sinus involved	Number of sides with no opacification	Number of sides with partial opacification	Number of sides with total opacification
Anterior ethmoids	9 (7.1%)	50 (39.7%)	67 (53.2%)
Posterior ethmoids	9 (7.1%)	61 (48.4%)	56 (44.4%)
Maxillary	3 (2.4%)	82 (65.1%)	41 (32.5%)
Frontal	28 (22.2%)	31 (24.6%)	67 (53.2%)
Sphenoid	36 (28.6%)	41 (32.5%)	49 (38.9%)
Ostiomeatal complex	21 (16.7%)		105 (83.3%)

The mucosal status of the paranasal sinuses of 63 patients admitted for bilateral revision FESS as evident on their C.T scans.

process due to its role in protecting the sinuses from allergens and contaminated inspired air [11,12].

The above discussion highlights the fact that there is a wide variation in the practice of endoscopic sinus surgery. Some surgeons prefer more conservative techniques. Recently, the principle of minimally invasive sinus technique (MIST) has been introduced [13,14]. It is claimed that this entails a standardised conservative endoscopic technique that can be applied to all patients requiring sinus surgery, regardless of the extent of their pathology. Other authors, however, have disapproved of the principles of MIST [15]. On the other extreme, some surgeons prefer radical endoscopic surgical techniques to treat advanced inflammatory sinus pathology. Such techniques may involve total sphenoethmoidectomies with extensive mucosal resection [16], and may even involve middle turbinate resection as well [17-19].

We have not attempted in our study to investigate the clinical outcome after revision surgery as the aim of the study was to identify the residual anatomic factors that may result in recurrent rhinosinusitis after primary surgery, and to reflect on the practice of FESS in the U.K. We hope, however, that this work will stimulate further studies to compare conservative versus more aggressive sinus surgery techniques, and to answer the question of how extensive sinus surgery should be.

Conclusions

Analysis of C.T scans of patients undergoing revision FESS demonstrates persistent anatomic structures and non dissected cells that may be responsible for persistence or recurrence of rhinosinusitis. Trials comparing the outcome of conservative FESS techniques with more radical sinus dissections are required.

Acknowledgements
This article was presented as an oral presentation by the first author in the IFOS meeting in Sao Paolo in June 2009, and presented as a poster in BACO meeting in Liverpool in July 2009.

Author details
[1]Department of Otolaryngology, Derriford Hospital, Plymouth, U.K. and Faculty of Medicine, University of Alexandria, Egypt. [2]Department of Otolaryngology, Derriford Hospital, Plymouth, UK.

Authors' contributions
The first author (HSK) initiated the idea of the study. All patients were treated under his care. Both the first and the second authors reviewed the patients' scans and collated the data. The second author (AE) reviewed the literature and prepared the manuscript, which was revised by the first author. The third author (NC) reviewed the scans and helped making the revisions recommended by the reviewers. All authors have reviewed and approved the final manuscript.

Competing interests
The authors declare that they have no competing interests.

References
1. Khalil h, Nunez DA: **Functional endoscopic sinus surgery for chronic rhinosinusitis.** *Cochrane Database of Systematic Reviews* 2006, , **3**: CD004458.
2. Musy PY, Kountakis SE: **Anatomic findings in patients undergoing revision functional endoscopic sinus surgery.** *Am J Otolaryngol* 2004, **25**:418-422.
3. King JM, Caldarelli DD, Pigato JB: **A review of revision functional endoscopic sinus surgery.** *Laryngoscope* 1994, **104**:404-408.
4. Hopkins C, Browne JP, Slack R, Lund V, Topham J, Reeves B, Copley L, Brown P, Vander Meulen J: **The national comparative audit of surgery for nasal polyposis and chronic rhinosinusitis.** *Clin Otol* 2006, **31**:390-398.
5. Chiu AG, Kennedy DW: **Tips and pearls in revision sinus surgery.** In *Revision sinus surgery.* Edited by: Kountakis SE, Jacobs J, Gosepath J. Verlag Berlin Heidelberg: Springer; 2008:79-89.
6. Stankiewicz JA, Donzelli JJ, Chow JM: **Failures of functional endoscopic sinus surgery and their surgical correction.** *Oper Tech Otolaryngol Head Neck Surg* 1996, **7**:297-304.
7. Lund V, Mackay I: **Staging in rhinosinusitis.** *Rhinology* 1993, **31**:183-184.
8. Kennedy DW: **Prognostic factors, outcomes and staging in ethmoids sinus surgery.** *Laryngoscope* 1992, **102**:1-18.
9. Lazar RH, Younis RT, Long TE, Gross CW: **Revision functional endonasal sinus surgery.** *Ear Nose Throat J* 1992, **71**:131-133.
10. Ramadan HH: **Surgical causes of failure in endoscopic sinus surgery.** *Laryngoscope* 1999, **109**:27-29.
11. Nayak DR, Balakrishnan R, Murty KD: **Functional anatomy of the uncinate process and its role in endoscopic sinus surgery.** *Indian J Otolaryngol Head Neck Surg* 2001, **53**:27-31.
12. Nayak DR, Balakrishnan R, Murty KD: **Endoscopic physiologic approach to allergy associated chronic rhinosinusitis: A preliminary study.** *Ear Nose Throat J* 2001, **80**:390-403.
13. Catalano PJ: **Minimally invasive sinus technique: What is it? Should we consider it?** *Curr Opin Otolaryngol Head Neck Surg* 2004, **12**:34-37.
14. Catalano PJ, Strouch M: **The minimally invasive sinus technique: theory and practice.** *Otolaryngol Clin North Am* 2004, **37**:401-409.

15. Chiu AG, Kennedy DW: **Disadvantages of minimal techniques for surgical management of chronic rhinosinusitis.** *Curr Opin Otolaryngol Head Neck Surg* 2004, **12**:38-42.

16. Klossek JM, Peloquin L, Friedman WH, Ferrier JC, Fontanel JP: **Diffuse nasal polyposis: postoperative long term results after endoscopic sinus surgery and frontal irrigation.** *Otolaryngol Head Neck Surg* 1997, **117**:355-361.

17. Jankowski R, Pigret D, Decroocq F: **Comparison of functional results after ethmoidectomy and nasalization for diffuse and severe nasal polyposis.** *Acta Otolaryngol* 1997, **117**:601-608.

18. Jankowski R, Bodino C: **Olfaction in patients with nasal polyposis: effect of systemic steroids and radical ethmoidectomy with middle turbinate resection (nasalization).** *Rhinology* 2003, **41**:220-230.

19. Marchioni D, Alicandri-Ciufelli M, Mattioli F, Marchetti A, Jovic G, Massone F, Presutti L: **Middle turbinate preservation versus middle turbinate resection in endoscopic surgical treatment of nasal polyposis.** *Acta Otolaryngol* 2008, **128**:1019-1026.

Prognostic impact of standard laboratory values on outcome in patients with sudden sensorineural hearing loss

Julia Wittig[1], Claus Wittekindt[1,2], Michael Kiehntopf[3] and Orlando Guntinas-Lichius[1*]

Abstract

Background: Aim of the present study was to evaluate prognostic factors, in particular standard laboratory parameters, for better outcome after idiopathic sudden sensorineural hearing loss (SSNHL).

Methods: Using a retrospective review, 173 patients were included presenting between 2006 and 2009 with unilateral SSNHL, $\geq$30 dB bone conduction in three succeeding frequencies between 0.125 to 8 kHz in pure tone audiometry (PTA), and a time interval between first symptoms and diagnostics $\leq$ 4 weeks. Hearing gain of <10 dB versus $\geq$10 dB in the affected ear in 6PTA values was the primary outcome criterion. Univariate and multivariate statistical tests were used to analyze predictors for better outcome.

Results: The initial hearing loss was 50.6 $\pm$ 27.2 dB. The absolute hearing gain was 15.6 $\pm$ 20.1 dB. Eighty-one patients (47%) had a final hearing gain of $\geq$10 dB. Low-frequency hearing loss (p <0.0001); start of inpatient treatment <4 days after onset ($p = 0.018$); first SSNHL (versus recurrent SSNHL, $p = 0.001$); initial hearing loss $\geq$ 60 dB ($p < 0.0001$); an initial quick value lower than the reference values ($p = 0.040$); and a pretherapeutic hyperfibrinogenemia ($p = 0.007$) were significantly correlated to better outcome ($\geq$10 dB absolute hearing gain). Multivariate analysis revealed that first SSNHL ($p = 0.004$), start of treatment <4 days after onset ($p = 0.015$), initial hearing loss $\geq$ 60 dB ($p = 0.001$), and hyperfibrinogenemia ($p = 0.032$) were independent prognostic factors for better hearing recovery.

Conclusion: Better hearing gain in patients with hyperfibrinogenemia might be explained by the rheological properties of the applied therapy and supports the hypothesis that SSNHL is caused in part by vascular factors.

Keywords: Serology, Blood value, Outcome, Prognostic marker, Hearing loss

Background

Idiopathic sudden sensorineural hearing loss [SSNHL) is defined as unexplained unilateral sensorineural hearing loss of 30 dB HL or greater over 3 continuous frequencies with onset over a period of less than 72 hours and with no marked vestibular symptoms [1]. SSNHL has an estimated incidence between 160 and 400 per 100,000 persons per year, i.e. much higher than assumed in older studies [2,3]. The causes of SSNHL are speculative and probably multifactorial [4]. Cardiovascular disease, cigarette smoking, and hypertension appear to be the most common risk factors associated with SSNHL [2,4].

Advanced age, severe hearing loss, heredity, audiogram shape, and presence of vertigo seem to be significant negative prognostic factors [4,5]. Most studies analyzing prognostic factors do not evaluate if the therapy itself applied to the patients with SSNHL has an influence on these prognostic factors. Furthermore, most studies include a variety of therapy regimes and sometimes also patients who did not receive any therapy. This makes it difficult to interpret the concrete role of the discovered risk factors. In a recent study using a uniform standardized therapy consisting of carbogen inhalation and oral prednisone, the prognostic factors for better recovery were severity of initial hearing loss, presence of vertigo, time between onset and treatment, the hearing of the other ear, and the audiogram shape [5].

* Correspondence: orlando.guntinas@med.uni-jena.de
[1]Department of Otorhinolaryngology, Jena University Hospital, Lessingstrasse 2, Jena D-07740, Germany
Full list of author information is available at the end of the article

Although especially vascular factors are constantly discussed to be related to the etiology of SSNHL, it is surprising that so far the prognostic impact of the entire range of routine laboratory values has not been evaluated systematically. Therefore, the present study investigated whether patients with SSNHL and its comorbidity also influence routine pretherapeutic laboratory values and whether these values have prognostic influence on hearing recovery after a standardized combined glucocorticoid and rheological therapeutic regime.

Methods

Patients

A standardized retrospective analysis was performed in the Department of Otorhinolaryngology of the University Hospital Jena in Germany. The study protocol was approved by the institutional ethics committee of the Friedrich-Schiller University, Jena, Germany. All adult patients who were treated for unilateral idiopathic sudden sensorineural hearing loss between 2006 and 2009 were included in the database for this study. Prerequisite was a differential diagnostic evaluation excluding a specific etiology (like head trauma, vestibular schwannoma) explaining the sudden hearing loss. All patients received a brainstem electrical response audiometry (BERA). If the BERA was pathologic, a magnetic resonance imaging (MRI) of the head and cerebellopontine angle was performed. Further inclusion criterion was that at least 2 pure-tone audiograms were available: the first at presentation prior to initiation of therapy, and a second after therapy. If more than one follow-up audiogram was available, the last audiogram was taken for analysis. Follow-up audiometry was stopped when no further hearing improvement was seen. Exclusion criteria were: Hearing loss <30 dB bone conduction in three succeeding frequencies between 0.125 to 8 kHz as revealed by pure tone audiometry; time interval between first symptoms and diagnostics > 4 weeks; acute bilateral hearing loss; combination with acute vestibular hypofunction (excluded by caloric vestibular testing); history of chronic ear disease (like otosclerosis, chronic otitis media, Menière's disease). A search of the patients' electronic charts was performed, and the following variables were obtained: age, sex, smoking behavior (yes/no), Charlson comorbidity index [6], presentation of a metabolic syndrome (if patient had ≥3 of the following diseases: diabetes mellitus, hypertension, adiposity, atherosclerosis, gout, hyperlipidemia), presentation of cardiovascular risk factors (if patients had at least 1 of the following diseases/history of diseases: vein thrombosis, apoplexy, cardiac infarction, diabetes mellitus, hypertension, hyperlipidemia) and tinnitus (yes/no).

All patients were hospitalized. Treatment followed the German guideline for sudden idiopathic sensorineural hearing loss as 1-week combination of glucocorticoid and rheological therapy with pentoxifyllin [6,7]. Mainly, a tapered course of oral corticosteroids is regarded as standard treatment [1].

Audiometric assessment

Audiometric evaluation included air conduction and bone conduction thresholds on the affected and the contralateral side revealed by pure tone audiometry. The pure tone average (PTA) was calculated from the results of bone conduction at 0.25, 0.5, 1, 2, 4, and 6 kHz (6PTA). The severity of the hearing loss was described exactly according to Cvorovic et al. [5] as 1) mild, PTA of 15 to 39 dB; 2) moderate, PTA of 40 to 59 dB; 3) severe, PTA of 60 to 79 dB; 4) profound, PTA of 80 to 100 dB; and 5) deaf, PTA of greater than 100 dB [5]. Furthermore, the pattern of the initial audiogram was categorized into 1 of 4 types [5]: Low frequencies were defined as 0.5 kHz or less, midfrequencies as greater than 0.5 and 2 kHz or greater, and high frequencies as greater than 2 and 8 kHz or less. The following types of audiograms were defined: 1) low frequency, ascending, greater than 15 dB HL from the poorer low-frequency thresholds to the higher frequencies; 2) midfrequency, U-shaped, greater than 15 dB HL difference between the poorest thresholds in the midfrequencies and those at higher and lower frequencies; 3) high frequency, descending, greater than 15 dB HL difference between the mean of 0.5 and 1 kHz and the mean of 4 and 8 kHz; 4) flat, less than 15 dB HL difference between the mean of 0.25-, 0.5-kHz thresholds, the mean of 1 and 2 kHz, and the mean of 4 and 8 kHz; and 5) total deafness, hearing loss of 100 dB or more in 0.5, 1, 2, and 4 kHz.

Hearing gain was expressed as absolute hearing gain (Δ6PTA; dB values) from initial PTA minus dB values from final PTA. If a negative value was calculated, the hearing gain was set to zero. For calculation of the relative hearing gain, the absolute gain ΔPTA was divided by the initial PTA. In order to calculate the relative hearing gain in relation to the contralateral ear, ΔPTA was divided by the initial PTA minus PTA on the contralateral side [8].

Laboratory values

The assessment of pretreatment laboratory values included: Hematologic profile with red blood cells, hemoglobin, mean corpuscular volume (MCV), mean corpuscular hemoglobin (MCH), mean corpuscular hemoglobin concentration (MCHC), white blood cells, and platelets; glucose; electrolytes covered sodium, potassium, calcium, urea and creatinine values; the inflammation parameter C-reactive protein (CRP); lipid metabolism with cholesterol, low density lipoprotein (LDL), high density lipoprotein (HDL), LDL/HDL index, and finally the coagulation parameters Quick value, activated partial thromboplastin time (aPTT), and fibrinogen. The blood samples were taken before start of treatment to rule out an influence of the treatment on the laboratory values. The normal reference values for all laboratory parameters are given in Table 1. Most parameters are pathological if lower or higher than the reference range, but some are only pathological if lower than normal range (e.g. Quick value) or higher than the normal range (e.g. CRP).

Statistical analysis

If not indicated otherwise, data are presented with mean values ± standard deviation (SD). All statistical analyses were performed using IBM SPSS, version 20.0. Primary outcome criterion was absolute hearing gain (Δ6PTA) dichotomized into two groups of patients (<10 dB versus ≥10 dB).

The chi-square test was used to compare subgroups for ordinal parameters (e.g. gender, side, laboratory parameters dichotomized into normal versus pathologic values. The non-parametric Mann-Whitney U-test was used to compare subgroups for continuous parameters (e.g. age). Prognostic factors associated with higher frequency of hearing gain ≥10 dB with a probability value of $p < 0.05$ were included in a binary (<10 dB versus ≥10 dB hearing gain) logistic regression analysis. Nominal p values of two-tailed tests are reported. The significance level was set at $p < 0.05$.

Results

Patients' and disease characteristics

One hundred and seventy-three (173) patients were included into the study and constituted the database for this study. Patients' characteristics and details on SSNHL are given in Table 2. The median age was 64 years. The

Table 1 Blood values at time of diagnosis (n = 173)

Parameter	Mean (SD)	Median	Min.	Max.	Normal range	Patients outside normal range (%)
aPTT (sec)	30.3 (5.8)	29	20	56	26-36	39 (23)
Quick (%)	95.4 (24.7)	100.5	9	128	70-130	17 (10)
Fibrinogen (g/l)	3.1 (1)	3	1.3	8.7	1.8-3.5	43 (25)
Red-cell count (Tptl/l) women	4.6 (0.3)	4.6	3.5	5.5	4.1-5.1	9 (5)
Red-cell count (Tptl/l) men	4.9 (0.5)	4.9	3.7	7.2	4.5-5.9	19 (11)
Hemoglobin (mmol/l) women	8.5 (0.6)	8.5	7	10	7.6-9.5	8 (5)
Hemoglobin (mmol/l) men	9.1 (0.8)	9.2	6.1	10.7	8.7-10.9	21 (12)
Hematocrit women	0.41 (0.03)	0.4	0.34	0.48	0.35-0.45	5 (3)
Hematocrit men	0.43 (0.03)	0.43	0.32	0.49	0.36-0.48	4 (2)
White-cell count (/µl)	8462.4 (3102.6)	7600	1100	20900	4400-11300	28 (16)
Platelet count (Gpt/l)	250 (65.7)	245	89	610	150-360	9 (5)
MCH	1.86 (0.1)	1.9	1.2	2.12	1.74-2.05	21 (21)
MCHC	21.1 (0.6)	21.1	18.7	22.5	19.7-22.1	7 (4)
MCV	88.2 (4.8)	88	63	99	80-96	8 (5)
Glucose (mmol/l)	6.7 (2.3)	5.9	3.6	17.4	3.9-5.8	91 (53)
Sodium (mmol/l)	140.8 (2.7)	141	130	149	135-145	10 (6)
Potassium (mmol/l)	3.9 (0.4)	3.9	2.6	5.3	3.3-4.5	23 (13)
Calcium (mmol/l)	2.4 (0.1)	2.4	2	2.9	2.2-2.6	10 (6)
Urea (mmol/l)	6.1 (2.1)	5.8	2.2	17.4	2.6-7.5	32 (19)
Creatinine (lmol/l) women	80 (17.4)	78	50	189	58-96	6 (4)
Creatinine (lmol/l) men	96.3 (21.3)	92	57	182	72-127	14 (8)
C-reactive protein (mg/l)	4.7 (15.3)	1.9	1.9	188.2	≦ 7.5	12 (7)
Cholesterol (mmol/l)	5.6 (1.1)	5.6	3.1	9.3	≦ 5.2	65 (38)
LDL (mmol/l)	3.3 (1)	3.3	1.2	6.1	≦ 4.1	22 (13)
HDL (mmol/l)	1.4 (0.4)	1.3	0.8	2.8	≧ 1.0	8 (5)
LDL/HDL	2.5 (0.9)	2.4	0.6	5.3	≦ 4.1	4 (2)
Triglycerides (mmol/l)	1.81 (1.1)	1.4	0.4	7	≦ 1.7	39 (23)

SD = standard deviation; Min = Minimum; Max = Maximum; PPT = partial thromboplastin time Tpt/l = 10^3 cells per liter; Gpt/l = 10^9 cells per liter; MCV = mean corpuscular volume, MCH = mean corpuscular hemoglobin, MCHC = mean corpuscular hemoglobin concentration; LDL = low-density lipoprotein; HDL = high-density lipoprotein.

Table 2 Patients' characteristics (n = 173)

	Number of patients (%)
Gender	
Female	82 (47)
Male	91 (53)
Affected side	
Left	91 (53)
Right	82 (47)
First SSNHL	124 (72)
Recurrent SSNHL	49 (28)
Audiogram pattern	
Low-frequency	9 (5)
Mid-frequency	12 (7)
High-frequency	63 (36)
Flat	55 (32)
Total deafness	34 (20)
Contralateral ear	
Normal hearing	97 (56)
Abnormal hearing	40 (44)
Tinnitus, additionally	
Yes	139 (80)
No	34 (20)
Vertigo	
Yes	33 (19)
No	140 (81)
Smoking	
Yes	24 (14)
No	149 (86)
Charlson Comorbidity Index	
Index = 0	121 (70)
Index = 1	27 (16)
Index = 2	19 (11)
Index ≥ 3	6 (4)
Vascular risk profile	
Yes	93 (54)
No	80 (46)
Metabolic syndrome	
Yes	4 (2)
No	169 (98)
Final absolute hearing gain (Δ6PTA)	
0 dB	24 (14)
1-19 dB	110 (64)
≥20 dB	39 (23)
	Median, range
Age (years)	64, 18-88
Interval onset to therapy (days)	3.5, 0-28

Table 2 Patients' characteristics (n = 173) *(Continued)*

Hearing loss, initial (6PTA; dB)	42.5, 14.2-110
Hearing loss, final (6 PTA; dB)	30, 0.8-105.8
Hearing gain, absolute (Δ6PTA; dB)	9, 0-100
Hearing loss, contralateral ear, initial (6PTA)	17.5, 0-120

gender ratio was balanced (47% female and 53% male patients, respectively). There was no side predominance (53% left and 47% right ear, respectively). Four of five patients complained also of tinnitus in the affected ear. Only 14% of patients were smokers. About two of three patients (70%) had no relevant comorbidity according to Charlson comorbidity index but half of the patients showed cardiovascular risk factors.

Due to the 6PTA, the initial hearing loss was 50.6 ± 27.2 dB. The contralateral ear had a 6PTA of 21.2 ± 15.7 dB. The contralateral ear had a 6PTA of <20 dB, i.e. a normal hearing result, in 56% of the cases. Three patients were deaf on the contralateral ear. The interval between onset of hearing loss and begin of in-patient therapy was 5.7 ± 6.1 days. The average follow-up period, i.e. the time from first to last audiogram without further hearing improvement, was 51.0 ± 44.9 days (range: 10 – 280 days).

Overall recovery

The absolute hearing gain between the initial audiogram and the final audiogram was 15.6 ± 20.1 dB. The mean relative hearing gain was 27.6 ± 23.7%. The mean relative hearing gain in relation to the contralateral side was 49.4 ± 45.6%. Eighty-one patients (47%) had a final hearing gain of ≥10 dB. Twenty-nine patients (17%) had a relative hearing gain of ≥50%. Seventy-two patients (42%) had a relative hearing gain in relation to the contralateral side of ≥50%.

Prognostic impact of clinical and laboratory parameter

An overview about the serology results at time of diagnosis is presented in Table 1. Blood parameters were very variable in the study sample. About half of the patients had elevated glucose values. About one third had elevated cholesterol and a about quarter elevated triglyceride values. One quarter showed a hyperfibrinogenemia.

The univariate analysis on prognostic factors for better outcome is summarized in Table 3. The following clinical parameters were significantly correlated to better outcome (≥10 dB absolute hearing gain): Low-frequency hearing loss had a better outcome than other audiogram patterns (p <0.0001). Start of inpatient treatment <4 days after onset was better than a delayed treatment ≥4 days after onset (p = 0.018). First SSNHL had a better outcome than recurrent SSNHL (p = 0.001), and initial hearing loss ≥ 60 dB had a better outcome than an initial

Table 3 Prognostic influence of clinical and serologic parameters on hearing gain (Δ6PTA) ≥10 dB absolute hearing gain

Parameter	Δ6PTA <>10 dB p
Gender	0.160
Age	0.176
Side	0.624
Tinnitus	0.133
Vertigo	0.574
Smoker	0.586
Comorbidity (Charlson Index ≥1)	0.435
Vascular risk factor	0.402
Low-frequency hearing loss	**<0.0001**
Start of inpatient treatment <4 days after onset	**0.018**
Interval between first and last audiogram	0.065
First SSNHL	**0.001**
Contralateral ear with normal hearing	0.159
Initial hearing loss ≥ 60 dB	**<0.0001**
aPTT, normal	0.905
Quick, lower than normal	**0.040**
Fibrinogen (g/l), high (hyperfibrinogenemia)	**0.007**
Red-cell count (Tptl/l) women	0.611
Red-cell count (Tptl/l) men	0.593
Hemoglobin (mmol/l) women	0.901
Hemoglobin (mmol/l) men	0.946
Hematocrit women	0.727
Hematocrit men	0.086
White-cell count (/µl)	0.433
Platelet count (Gpt/l)	0.749
MCH	0.456
MCHC	0.445
MCV	0.582
Glucose (mmol/l)	0.078
Sodium (mmol/l)	0.656
Potassium (mmol/l)	0.164
Calcium (mmol/l)	0.273
Urea (mmol/l)	0.694
Creatinine (lmol/l) women	0.116
Creatinine (lmol/l) men	0.497
C-reactive protein (mg/l)	0.380
Cholesterol (mmol/l)	0.088
LDL (mmol/l)	0.131
HDL (mmol/l)	0.922
LDL/HDL	0.367
Triglycerides (mmol/l)	0.970

p values in bold are p values below 0.05, i.e. significant p values.

loss < 60 dB ($p < 0.0001$). Two laboratory parameters had influence on the outcome: a quick value lower than the reference values ($p = 0.040$); and a hyperfibrinogenemia ($p = 0.007$).

Multivariate analysis revealed that first SSNHL ($p = 0.004$), start of inpatient treatment <4 days after onset ($p = 0.015$), initial hearing loss ≥ 60 dB ($p = 0.001$), and hyperfibrinogenemia ($p = 0.032$) were independent prognostic factors for better hearing gain (Table 4).

Discussion

We analyzed 173 patients with unilateral SSNHL treated within four years with a standardized treatment protocol. Interested in predictors of the prognosis, we focused not only on clinical and audiological data like in several previous studies, but included also all laboratory values of clinical routine into the univariate and multivariate analysis. Interestingly, two serologic markers with influence on the rheology of the blood, a lower quick value (<70%) and a hyperfibrinogenemia (fibrinogen > 3 g/l), were associated with better outcome.

In comparison to other studies, the observed median initial hearing loss was high with 42.5 dB. Absolute median hearing gain after combined prednisolone plus pentoxiphylline therapy was low with 9 dB. The relative hearing was 49%. Including also only SSNHL of ≥30 dB and using carbogen inhalation and prednisone orally, Cvorovic et al. recently reported for 541 patients a 15.1 dB absolute hearing gain and a relative hearing gain of 47%, i.e. in the range of the present study [5]. Using a comparable treatment regime in one study arm, a recent prospective trial reported an equivalent relative hearing gain of 43% [9]. A spontaneous hearing recovery rate without treatment for SSNHL of more than 25 dB and a relative hearing gain of 47-63% is reported [10-12]. We hypothesize that a negative selection bias is responsible for high initial hearing loss and the relative less pronounced hearing gain in the present study. First, only patients with sudden hearing loss of ≥30 dB were included. Second, inpatient treatment is mainly intended (and only covered by health insurance) in Germany if outpatient treatment fails to improve hearing within the first days after onset of SSNHL or if other symptoms like vertigo or severe hearing impairment on the contralateral side are existent. In the present study sample half of the patients had unsuccessful outpatient treatment before admission for inpatient treatment.

The two clinical factors: start of inpatient treatment <4 days after onset and first SSNHL were associated with better outcome. Furthermore, two audiological factors: low-frequency hearing loss and initial hearing loss ≥60 dB were related to better outcome. These results are partly in accordance to previous studies. It has been shown that hearing recovery is greatest when corticosteroid treatment is

Table 4 Multivariate binary logistic regression analysis on independent prognostic factors for better outcome measured as absolute hearing gain ≥ 10 dB

Parameter	B	S.E.	Wald	p	Odds ratio	95% CI lower	95% CI upper
First SSNHL	-1.280	0.445	8.291	**0.004**	3.597	1.506	8.621
Low-frequency type	1.238	0.692	3.205	0.073	3.450	0.889	13.389
Quick lower than reference value	0.388	0.669	0.337	0.562	1.474	0.397	5.469
Fibrinogen high (hyperfibrinogenemia)	-0.967	0.451	4.595	**0.032**	2.631	1.086	6,369
Interval between onset and therapy begin <4 days	0.912	0.375	5.915	**0.015**	2.489	1.194	5.191
Initial hearing loss ≥60 dB	-1.482	0.463	10.243	**0.001**	4.406	1.776	10.869

p values in bold are p values below 0.05, i.e. significant p values.

started within the first 1-2 weeks after onset of SSNHL [1,2,5,10]. Many studies revealed that low-frequency losses do better than high-frequency losses [5,10,13,14]. More severe initial hearing loss has higher probability of improvement in some studies but in other studies a lower probability [2,5,15]. In contrast to others, in present study vertigo or impaired hearing on the contralateral ear had no negative prognostic influence [2,5,3]. The reason why vertigo had no influence in the present study might be that patients with acute vestibular deficits elicited by caloric testing were strictly excluded.

If at all of interest, laboratory investigations were mainly analyzed on their role as risk factors for SSNHL. For instance, hypercholesterolemia and hyperglycemia were observed more frequently in SSNHL patients than in control populations [16,17]. Consistent to that, we found a hypercholesterolemia in 38% and a hyperglycemia in 53% of the patients at the time of diagnosis (cf. Table 1). Only a few studies have analyzed the prognostic role of laboratory values on treatment outcome of SSNHL. In two older studies, in times when CRP was not yet part of routine blood examinations, an elevated erythrocyte sedimentation rate was correlated to better outcome [2,10]. In the present study CRP values had no influence on outcome. As CRP is accepted to be more sensitive and specific for acute inflammatory reactions [18], and observing increased CRP values only for 7% of the study sample, we state that acute inflammatory reaction or an underlying inflammatory disease, respectively, is not related to at least most cases of SSNHL and therefore does not play a prognostic role.

Univariate statistical analysis exposed that a decreased Quick test value (<70%) at time of diagnosis was related to better hearing gain. The Quick prothrombin time test still is the basis for monitoring anticoagulant therapy in many countries worldwide [19]. Unfortunately, International normalized ratio (INR) values were not available for the majority of patients. INR values would have the advantage that the data would have been directly comparable to data from other laboratories. Seventeen (10%) of the patients with SSNHL (initial hearing loss of these patients was 65.4 ± 30.1 dB; 7 patients with initial loss ≥60 dB) had

a decreased Quick value because of anticoagulant therapy in accordance to anticoagulation guidelines for cardiac diseases, history of stroke, peripheral arterial disease, or venous thromboembolism. Only patients under anticoagulant therapy showed decreased Quick values. The anticoagulant therapy was sustained during treatment of SSNHL holding Quick values in the therapeutic range (data not shown). The antithrombotic effects of the anticoagulants decrease the viscosity of the plasma. We speculate that the combination of the SSNHL therapy with the anticoagulant therapy significantly improved the microcirculatory blood flow of the inner ear. In turn, this supports the theory that a vascular impairment with disturbance of the inner ear microcirculation is at least in some patients with SSNHL a causative factor [20,21].

Even more striking was the prognostic effect of fibrinogen at time of diagnosis on the hearing gain as this parameter remained also significantly relevant in the multivariate analysis. A quarter of patients had elevated fibrinogen values at time of SSNHL diagnosis. It has been widely accepted that hyperfibrinogenemia is an independent risk factor for cardiovascular diseases [2]. Fibrinogen is the substrate for thrombin and represents the final step in the coagulation cascade and is essential for platelet aggregation [22]. Furthermore, hyperfibrinogenemia seems to be a risk factor for SSNHL [23,24]. This was the basis to introduce fibrinogen apheresis as treatment option for SSNHL [9]. Recently, it has been shown in guinea pigs that acute hyperfibrinogenemia has a direct negative impact on the cochlear microcirculation [25]. We hypothesize that patients with hyperfibrinogenemia in the present study sample had a better outcome because a vascular factor/event triggered the SSNHL. The treatment regime used primarily was designed to improve the rheological blood performance with the aim to improve the cochlear microcirculation [26].

If fibrinogen is qualified to be a biomarker for treatment selection has to be proven by further prospective trials. In deployment of the assumption that SSNHL is an umbrella term for a disease with several causative factors, such biomarkers are needed at least to select patients with vascular origin of SSNHL as only these patients can profit optimally from vascular therapy regimes.

Conclusion

The presented cohort study on 173 patients with SSNHL revealed that beside clinical and audiological factors also the laboratory markers: decreased Quick test value and a hyperfibrinogenemia were positive prognostic markers for better outcome using a treatment regime mainly intending to improve the cochlear microcirculation. Therefore, hyperfibrinogenemia is not only a risk factor for SSNHL but also a positive prognostic marker of outcome when using a rheological regime to treat SSNHL. Especially fibrinogen seems to be an interesting candidate as biomarker for better patient selection for treatment regimens of SSNHL focusing on the refinement of cochlear microcirculation.

Abbreviations

SSNHL: Sudden sensorineural hearing loss; PTA: Pure tone audiometry; MCV: Mean corpuscular volume; MCH: Mean corpuscular hemoglobin; MCHC: Mean corpuscular hemoglobin concentration; CRP: C-reactive protein; LDL: Low density lipoprotein; HDL: High density lipoprotein; aPTT: Activated partial thromboplastin time; SD: Standard deviation; Min: Minimum; Max: Maximum; PPT: Partial thromboplastin time; Tpt/l: 10^3 cells per liter; Gpt/l: 10^9 cells per liter; BERA: Brainstem electrical response audiometry; MRI: Magnetic resonance imaging.

Competing interests

There is no competing interest. The authors confirm that they do not have any financial relationship concerning this research.
The authors indicate that they have no a financial relationship with any organization or company mentioned in the manuscript. The research was not sponsored by a third party.

Authors' contribution

OGL and CW had the idea for the study. OGL and MK drafted the manuscript. JW performed the data collection. OGL and JW performed the statistical analysis. OGL designed tables and figures. All authors read and approved the final manuscript.

Author details

[1]Department of Otorhinolaryngology, Jena University Hospital, Lessingstrasse 2, Jena D-07740, Germany. [2]Present address: Department of Otorhinolaryngology, University Giessen, Giessen, Germany. [3]Institute of Clinical Chemistry and Laboratory Diagnostics, Jena University Hospital, Jena, Germany.

References

1. Stachler RJ, Chandrasekhar SS, Archer SM, Rosenfeld RM, Schwartz SR, Barrs DM, Brown SR, Fife TD, Ford P, Ganiats TG, Hollingsworth DB, Lewandowski CA, Montano JJ, Saunders JE, Tucci DL, Valente M, Warren BE, Yaremchuk KL, Robertson PJ: Clinical practice guideline: sudden hearing loss. *Otolaryngol Head Neck Surg* 2012, **146**(Suppl):S1–S35.
2. Byl FM Jr: Sudden hearing loss: eight years' experience and suggested prognostic table. *Laryngoscope* 1984, **94**:647–661.
3. Egli Gallo D, Khojasteh E, Gloor M, Hegemann SC: Effectiveness of systemic high-dose dexamethasone therapy for idiopathic sudden sensorineural hearing loss. *Audiol Neurootol* 2013, **18**:161–170.
4. Chau JK, Lin JR, Atashband S, Irvine RA, Westerberg BD: Systematic review of the evidence for the etiology of adult sudden sensorineural hearing loss. *Laryngoscope* 2010, **120**:1011–1021.
5. Cvorovic L, Deric D, Probst R, Hegemann S: Prognostic model for predicting hearing recovery in idiopathic sudden sensorineural hearing loss. *Otol Neurotol* 2008, **29**:464–469.
6. D'Hoore W, Sicotte C, Tilquin C: Risk adjustment in outcome assessment: the Charlson comorbidity index. *Meth Inf Med* 1993, **32**:382–387.
7. Michel O: [The revised version of the german guidelines "sudden idiopathic sensorineural hearing loss"]. *Laryngorhinootologie* 2011, **90**:290–293.
8. Plontke SK, Bauer M, Meisner C: Comparison of pure-tone audiometry analysis in sudden hearing loss studies: lack of agreement for different outcome measures. *Otol Neurotol* 2007, **28**:753–763.
9. Suckfull M: Fibrinogen and LDL apheresis in treatment of sudden hearing loss: a randomised multicentre trial. *Lancet* 2002, **360**:1811–1817.
10. Mattox DE, Simmons FB: Natural history of sudden sensorineural hearing loss. *Ann Otol Rhinol Laryngol* 1977, **86**:463–480.
11. Probst R, Tschopp K, Ludin E, Kellerhals B, Podvinec M, Pfaltz CR: A randomized, double-blind, placebo-controlled study of dextran/pentoxifylline medication in acute acoustic trauma and sudden hearing loss. *Acta Otolaryngol* 1992, **112**:435–443.
12. Weinaug P: [How high is the rate of spontaneous healing of sudden deafness? Comments on the contribution "Spontaneous healing of sudden deafness"]. *HNO* 2001, **49**:431–432. discussion 3.
13. Shaia FT, Sheehy JL: Sudden sensori-neural hearing impairment: a report of 1,220 cases. *Laryngoscope* 1976, **86**:389–398.
14. Jun HJ, Chang J, Im GJ, Kwon SY, Jung H, Choi J: Analysis of frequency loss as a prognostic factor in idiopathic sensorineural hearing loss. *Acta Otolaryngol* 2012, **132**:590–596.
15. Fetterman BL, Saunders JE, Luxford WM: Prognosis and treatment of sudden sensorineural hearing loss. *American J Otol* 1996, **17**:529–536.
16. Aimoni C, Bianchini C, Borin M, Ciorba A, Fellin R, Martini A, Scanelli G, Volpato S: Diabetes, cardiovascular risk factors and idiopathic sudden sensorineural hearing loss: a case-control study. *Audiol Neurootol* 2010, **15**:111–115.
17. Cadoni G, Scorpecci A, Cianfrone F, Giannantonio S, Paludetti G, Lippa S: Serum fatty acids and cardiovascular risk factors in sudden sensorineural hearing loss: a case-control study. *Ann Otol Rhinol Laryngol* 2010, **119**:82–88.
18. Osei-Bimpong A, Meek JH, Lewis SM: ESR or CRP? A comparison of their clinical utility. *Hematol* 2007, **12**:353–357.
19. Jackson CM, Esnouf MP: Has the time arrived to replace the quick prothrombin time test for monitoring oral anticoagulant therapy? *Clin Chem* 2005, **51**:483–485.
20. Lin RJ, Krall R, Westerberg BD, Chadha NK, Chau JK: Systematic review and meta-analysis of the risk factors for sudden sensorineural hearing loss in adults. *Laryngoscope* 2012, **122**:624–635.
21. Ballesteros F, Tassies D, Reverter JC, Alobid I, Bernal-Sprekelsen M: Idiopathic sudden sensorineural hearing loss: classic cardiovascular and new genetic risk factors. *Audiol Neurootol* 2012, **17**:400–408.
22. Koenig W: Fibrin(ogen) in cardiovascular disease: an update. *Thromb Haemost* 2003, **89**:601–609.
23. Suckfull M, Wimmer C, Reichel O, Mees K, Schorn K: Hyperfibrinogenemia as a risk factor for sudden hearing loss. *Otol Neurotol* 2002, **23**:309–311.
24. Rudack C, Langer C, Stoll W, Rust S, Walter M: Vascular risk factors in sudden hearing loss. *Thromb Haemost* 2006, **95**:454–461.
25. Ihler F, Strieth S, Pieri N, Göhring P, Canis M: Acute hyperfibrinogenemia impairs cochlear blood flow and hearing function in guinea pigs in vivo. *Int J Audiol* 2012, **51**:210–215.
26. Michel O, Jahns T, Joost-Enneking M, Neugebauer P, Streppel M, Stennert E: [The Stennert antiphlogistic-rheologic infusion schema in treatment of cochleovestibular disorders]. *HNO* 2000, **48**:182–188.

Mastoiditis and Gradenigo's Syndrome with anaerobic bacteria

Chris Ladefoged Jacobsen[1*], Mikkel Attermann Bruhn[1], Yousef Yavarian[2] and Michael L Gaihede[1]

Abstract

Background: Gradenigo's syndrome is a rare disease, which is characterized by the triad of the following conditions: suppurative otitis media, pain in the distribution of the first and the second division of trigeminal nerve, and abducens nerve palsy. The full triad may often not be present, but can develop if the condition is not treated correctly.

Case presentation: We report a case of a 3-year-old girl, who presented with fever and left-sided acute otitis media. She developed acute mastoiditis, which was initially treated by intravenous antibiotics, ventilation tube insertion and cortical mastoidectomy. After 6 days the clinical picture was complicated by development of left-sided abducens palsy. MRI-scanning showed osteomyelitis within the petro-mastoid complex, and a hyper intense signal of the adjacent meninges. Microbiological investigations showed Staphylococcus aureus and Fusobacterium necrophorum. She was treated successfully with intravenous broad-spectrum antibiotic therapy with anaerobic coverage. After 8 weeks of follow-up there was no sign of recurrent infection or abducens palsy.

Conclusion: Gradenigo's syndrome is a rare, but life-threatening complication to middle ear infection. It is most commonly caused by aerobic microorganisms, but anaerobic microorganisms may also be found why anaerobic coverage should be considered when determining the antibiotic treatment.

Keywords: Gradenigo's syndrome, Acute mastoiditis, Apical petrositis, Acute otitis media, Abducens palsy, Fusobacterium necrophorum

Background

Gradenigo's Syndrome (GS) is a clinical triad of the following conditions; otitis media, pain in the distribution of the first and second division of the trigeminal nerve and ipsilateral abducens palsy. It was originally described in 1907 by Guiseppe Gradenigo [1]. Before the antibiotic era it was not uncommonly seen as a complication to acute otitis media (AOM) and mastoiditis. The symptoms occur as the infection spreads to the petrous apex of the temporal bone, where the sixth cranial nerve and the trigeminal ganglion are in close proximity only separated by the dura mater. The involvement of the sixth cranial nerve is seen as a reaction caused by the adjacent inflammation, as the nerve passes through Dorello´s canal under the petroclinoid ligament [2].

The full triad of symptoms in GS may not always be present. For instance, the absence of abducens palsy does not rule out apical petrositis. Radiologic evaluation by computed tomography (CT) and magnetic resonance imaging (MRI) are helpful tools in the diagnosis and management of GS, as well as they may exclude differential diagnoses like septic sinus thrombosis or other non-infectious entities [3,4]. With the widespread use of antibiotics the incidence of apical petrositis is now rare, reportedly two per 100,000 children with acute otitis media [5].

We report a case of AOM complicated by mastoiditis and apical petrositis presenting as Gradenigo's syndrome.

Case presentation

A 3-year-old healthy girl with no prior medical history was admitted to the pediatric department after 4 days with a high fever (39–40.4°C; 102.9-104°F) and left-sided otorrhea. Upon admission the child was in poor condition, dehydrated, pyretic and pale. Physical examination showed

---

* Correspondence: chlaj@rn.dk
[1]Department of Otolaryngology, Head and Neck Surgery, Aalborg Hospital - Aarhus University Hospital, Aalborg, Denmark
Full list of author information is available at the end of the article

left mastoid tenderness with retroauricular erythema, edema and fluctuation. Furthermore, examination of the eyes revealed normal movements and reflexes; there were no meningeal signs, changes in consciousness or other neurological findings. No cervical lymph nodes were enlarged. Initial blood samples showed a C-reactive protein of 256 mg/L and intravenous antibiotic treatment with benzyl penicillin was initiated.

The child was transferred to our ORL department, where otomicroscopy showed edema of the external auditory canal and a bulging, hyperemic tympanic membrane. These findings led to surgical drainage of the abscess under general anesthesia and insertion of a ventilation tube into the left tympanic membrane. Mucopurulent material from the abscess and the middle ear was sent for microbiological examination. The day after the operation the child showed signs of improvement with remission of fever as well as the retroauricular edema and erythema, and the anorexia diminished. However, later the same day, fever relapsed (39.0°C; 102,2°F), as well as progression of the erythema and swelling around the incision. Because of the rapid deterioration acute mastoidectomy and drainage were performed.

During the following days continuous clinical improvement was registered. Six days after the operation the child had problems maintaining balance, and the parents noticed that she had developed a slight strabismus. No headache or involvement of the trigeminal nerve were found. Physical examination showed normal visus on both eyes, but discrete left-sided papillar edema and abducens palsy (Figure 1).

In order to exclude the possibility of sinus thrombosis, an MRI scanning was performed. This demonstrated osteomyelitis within the petro-mastoid complex (Figures 2 and 3); further, thickening and enhancement of the adjacent meninges were demonstrated (Figure 4), whereas there were no signs of sinus thrombosis. Finally, no intracranial abscesses were found after contrast injection.

The pus culture isolated from the mastoid abscess revealed growth of Staphylococcus aureus sensitive for dicloxacillin and cefuroxime, but resistant to penicillin and Fusobacterium necrophorum was demonstrated sensitive to metronidazole and penicillin. The child was discharged after a total of 20 days of intravenous antibiotics as a combination of cefuroxime and metronidazole. By the time of 8 weeks clinical follow-up examination there were no signs of recurrent infection or abducens palsy.

Conclusions

GS as a result of petrositis is rarely seen after the introduction and widespread use of antibiotics. It remains, however, a serious and potentially fatal complication to AOM and acute mastoiditis.

Whereas the pneumatisation of the mastoid cells of the temporal bone is almost universal, the pneumatisation of the petrous apex varies and is only found in one third of adult patients; in such cases it may provide a path for AOM to spread also medially causing apical petrositis [4]. In addition, this condition may also be a result of direct extension of the infection through bony destruction or hematologically through venous channels causing true osteomyelitis in the non-pneumatized areas of the petrous bone [6]. Due to the central location of the petrous apex, apical petrositis may rapidly develop into severe and life threatening complications like meningitis, brain abscess, lateral sinus thrombosis, empyema

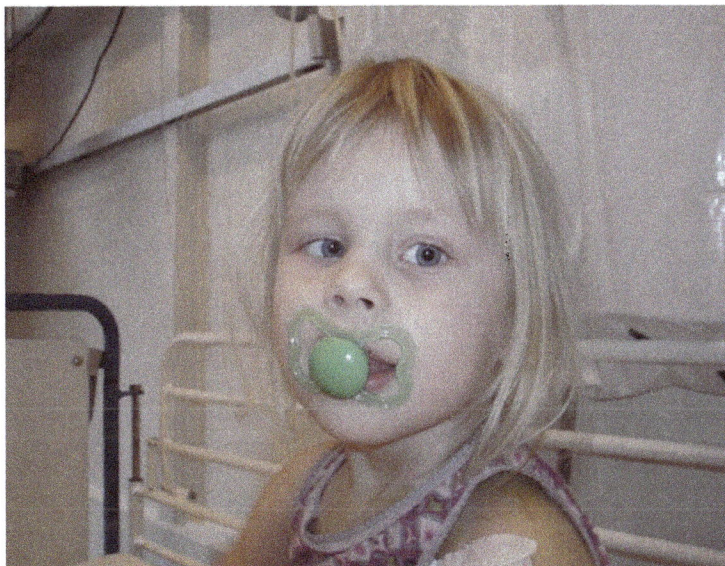

Figure 1 Left-sided abducens palsy at its onset 6 days after mastoidectomy.

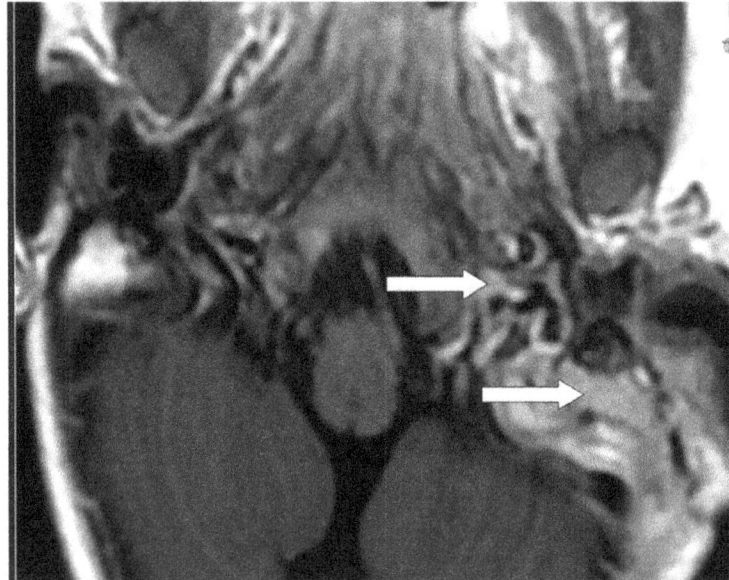

Figure 2 MRI horizontal section T1 + Gadolinium. Arrows show areas with enhancement in left pars petrosa.

and cranial nerve palsies [4-6]. The delay between otologic symptoms and cranial nerve involvement varies from 1 week to 2–3 months [7]. In our case, the time between the onset of the initial symptoms and the registration of the abducens palsy was two weeks.

We found the causative pathogens to be Staphylococcus aureus in combination with Fusobacterium necroforum found in both the middle ear and the mastoid cavity. Staphylococcus aureus are frequently found in acute mastoiditis (8.6 %), only surpassed by Pseudomonas aeruginosa (11.8 %), Streptococcus pneumoniae (9.9 %) and Streptococcus pyogenes (9.2 %) [8]. It has been argued that S. aureus has a greater tendency to invade bone, since it has been found in more cases with osteomyolitis [8].

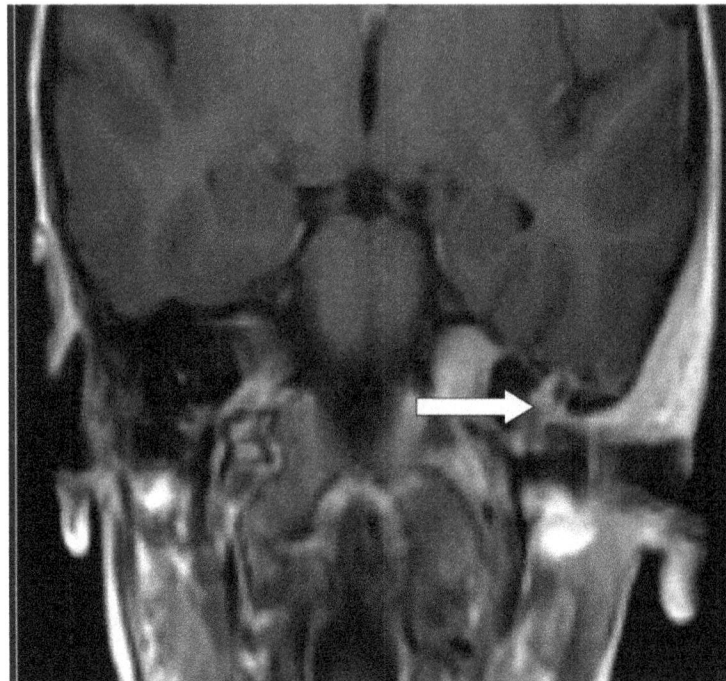

Figure 3 MRI coronal section T1 + Gadolinium. Arrow shows area with enhancement in left pars petrosa.

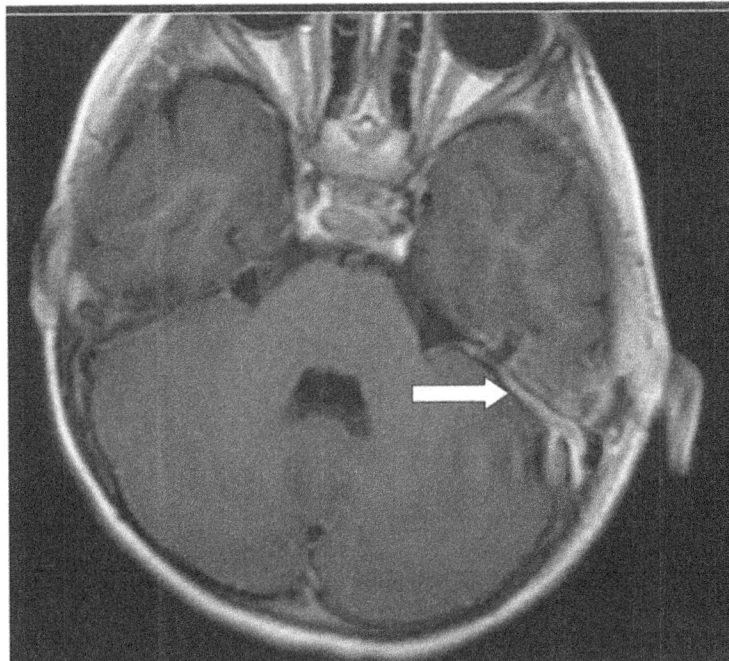

Figure 4 MRI horizontal section T1 + Gadolinium. Arrow shows local thickening and enhancement of the dura.

The demonstration of Fusobacterium necrophorum in GS is more unusual, and to our knowledge this has only been reported in two cases previously [9,10]. Fusobacterium necrophorum is an anaerobic, non-motile Gram-negative rod, usually found in the oral flora, the gastro-intestinal tract as well as the genito-urinary tract in females. It usually does not invade mucosal surfaces in healthy individuals, but if the host's defence system is compromised it has been known to cause a variety of rapidly progressing serious infections including bacteremia; these clinical conditions are known as necrobacillosis [11].

The demonstration of Fusobacterium necrophorum is difficult, since the cultivation is complex and depends on a prolonged incubation period; this may cause an under-estimation of its clinical demonstration [12] however the cultivation of anaerobic microorganism should be con-sidered. Thus, when empiric antibiotical treatment is started, it can be recommended to include both a potent anti-staphylococcal agent as well as metronidazole to cover anaerobic organisms.

CT scan is the first choice of imaging, since it is widely available and has a high sensitivity for detection of changes in bone structures including lesions in the pet-rous apex where GS in most cases will appear [4]. Fur-thermore it may detect the presence of intercranial abscesses, though it is less sensitive than MRI. An MRI is useful in evaluating the extent of the lesion of the pet-rous apex localised on the CT scan, as well as demon-strating meningeal involvement. Moreover, MRI is superior in detecting intracranial complications [3,4,13].

An MRI angiography may be performed to rule out signs of sinus thrombosis.

GS is a rare, but life-threatening complication to mid-dle ear infection that should be taken into consideration when atypical symptoms develop after AOM. Radio-logical modalities such as CT and MRI should not be delayed and CT should be regarded as first choice of im-aging when GS is suspected. Treatment should include drainage of the middle ear and mastoidectomy as well as intravenous broad spectrum antibiotics. GS is most com-monly caused by aerobic microorganisms, but it may also be found in interaction with anaerobic microorganisms. Due to the severity of related complications we suggest that antibiotic treatments include anaerobic coverage.

Abbreviations
GS: Gradenigo's Syndrome; AOM: Acute otitis media; CT: Computed tomography; MRI: Magnetic resonance imaging.

Competing interests
The authors declare that they have no competing interests.

Authors' contributions
CJ carried out the writing of the manuscript, acquisition of informed consent and literature research and approval of all images in the case report. MB helped in outlining and modification of the manuscript as well as selection and acquisition of photographs used in the case report. YY carried out the

radiological evaluation, selection and description of the MRI images and modification and approval of the imaging section. MG supervised, commented and helped in the revision and final approval of the manuscript. All authors have read and approved the final manuscript.

Financial and non-financial disclosure
None.

Author details
[1]Department of Otolaryngology, Head and Neck Surgery, Aalborg Hospital - Aarhus University Hospital, Aalborg, Denmark. [2]Department of Radiology, Aalborg Hospital - Aarhus University Hospital, Aalborg, Denmark.

References
1. Gradenigo G: **Uber die paralyse des n. Abduzens bei otitis.** *Arch F Ohrenheilk* 1907, **74:**149–158.
2. Gillanders DA: **Gradenigos Syndrome revisited.** *J Otolaryngol* 1983, **12:**169–174.
3. Murakami T, Tsubaki J, Tahara Y, Nagashima T: **Gradenigo's syndrome: CT and MRI findings.** *Pediatric radiol* 1996, **26**(9):684–685.
4. Jackler RK, Parker DA: **Radiographic differential diagnosis of petrous apex lesion.** *Am J Otol* 1992, **13:**561–574.
5. Goldstein NA, Casselbrant ML, Bluestone CD, Kurs-Lasky M: **Intratemporal complications of acute otitis media in infants and children.** *Otolaryngol Head Neck Surg* 1998, **119:**444–454.
6. Contrucci RB, Sataloff RT, Myers DL: **Petrous apicitis.** *Ear Nose Throat J* 1985, **64**(9):427–431.
7. Marianowski R, Rocton S, Ait-Amer JL, Morisseau-Durand MP, Manach Y: **Conservative management of Gradenigo syndrome in a child.** *Int J Pediatr Otorhinolaryngol* 2001, **57**(1):79–83.
8. Luntz M, Brodsky A, Nusem S, Kronenberg J, Keren G, Migirov L, *et al*: **Acute mastoiditis.** *Int J Pediatr Otorhinolaryngol* 2001, **57**(1):1–9.
9. Piron K, Gordts F, Herzeel R: **Gradenigo Syndrome a case report.** *Bull Soc Belge Ophtalmol* 2003, **290:**43–47.
10. Hananya S, Horowitz Y: **Gradenigo syndrome and cavernous sinus thrombosis in fusobacterial acute otitis media.** *Harefuah* 1997, **133**(7–8):284–286.
11. Pace-Balzan A, Keith AO, Curley JW, Ramsden RT, Lewis H: **Otogenic Fusobacterium necrophorum meningitis.** *J Laryngol Otol* 1991, **105:**119–120.
12. Bank S, Nielsen HM, Mathiasen BH, Leth DC, Kristensen LH, Prag J: **Fusobacterium necrophorum- detection and identification on a selective agar.** *APMIS* 2010, **118**(12):994–999. 2010 Oct 11.
13. Hardjasudarma M, Edwards RL, Ganley JP, Aarstad RF: **Magnetic resonance imaging features of Gradenigo's syndrome.** *Am J Otolaryngol* 1995, **16**(4):247–250.

Hearing screening for school children: utility of noise-cancelling headphones

Ada Hiu Chong Lo and Bradley McPherson[*]

Abstract

Background: Excessive ambient noise in school settings is a major concern for school hearing screening as it typically masks pure tone test stimuli (particularly 500 Hz and below). This results in false positive findings and subsequent unnecessary follow-up. With advances in technology, noise-cancelling headphones have been developed that reduce low frequency noise by superimposing an anti-phase signal onto the primary noise. This research study examined the utility of noise-cancelling headphone technology in a school hearing screening environment.

Methods: The present study compared the audiometric screening results obtained from two air-conduction transducers—Sennheiser PXC450 noise-cancelling circumaural headphones (NC headphones) and conventional TDH-39 supra-aural earphones. Pure-tone hearing screening results (500 Hz to 4000 Hz, at 30 dB HL and 25 dB HL) were obtained from 232 school children, aged 6 to 8 years, in four Hong Kong primary schools.

Results: Screening outcomes revealed significant differences in referral rates between TDH-39 earphones and NC headphones for both 30 dB HL and 25 dB HL criteria, regardless of the inclusion or exclusion of 500 Hz results. The kappa observed agreement (OA) showed that at both screening intensities, the transducers' referral agreement value for the 500 Hz inclusion group was smaller than for the 500 Hz exclusion group. Individual frequency analysis showed that the two transducers screened similarly at 1000 Hz and 2000 Hz at 25 dB HL, as well as at both 30 dB HL and 25 dB HL screening levels for 4000 Hz. Statistically significant differences were found for 500 Hz at 30 dB HL and at 25 dB HL, and for 1000 Hz and 2000 Hz at 30 dB HL. OA for individual frequencies showed weaker intra-frequency agreement between the two transducers at 500 Hz at both intensity criterion levels than at higher frequencies.

Conclusions: NC headphones screening results differed from those obtained from TDH-39 earphones, with lower referral rates at 500 Hz, particularly at the 25 dB HL criterion level. Therefore, NC headphones may be able to operate at lower screening intensities and subsequently increase pure-tone screening test sensitivity, without compromising specificity. NC headphones show some promise as possible replacements for conventional earphones in school hearing screening programs.

Keywords: Background noise, Headphones, Hearing loss, Hearing screening, School children

Background

There are two main types of audiometric screening that target children—newborn hearing screening and school hearing screening. Since between 1% and 14% of children have permanent or transient hearing loss, respectively, at school [1] and studies have shown that a significant proportion of these children are not detected by newborn hearing screening programs [2,3], school hearing screening is valuable even where universal newborn hearing screening has been implemented. Thus organizations such as the American Academy of Pediatrics [4] recommend periodic hearing screening for school-age children. In developing countries, where newborn hearing screening and preventive measures for childhood hearing loss are often unavailable, it is of utmost importance that all children be screened at school entry [5]. This is so that intervention can be carried out to minimize the adverse impacts of childhood hearing loss on well-being, development and future vocational opportunities [6-11]. In addition to early detection of hearing loss, routine school screening can also reduce the medical access barriers faced by families in rural areas and/or in

* Correspondence: dbmcpher@hku.hk
Division of Speech and Hearing Sciences, Faculty of Education, University of Hong Kong, Pokfulam Road, Pokfulam, Hong Kong

developing countries [12] as they do not need to travel long distances to major cities for screening services but can gain access in their local communities.

Among all school hearing screening methods, pure-tone audiometry remains the most widely performed test worldwide. Pure-tone audiometry has served as the 'gold standard' for more than 50 years [13] because of its high sensitivity and specificity [14]. A commonly used passing criterion for pure-tone screening is 25 dB HL [15], which is a standard fence for normal hearing. Some screening protocols use a 20 dB HL criterion to better detect minimal hearing loss [16-19]. Nevertheless, both of these criteria are often not feasible in screening programs due to the presence of excessive ambient noise in the test setting. In usual practice, a higher cutoff value from 30 dB HL to 40 dB HL is adopted [20-23]. School hearing screening usually takes place in an enclosed, un-occupied, furnished classroom where ambient noise ranges from 30 to 64 dB A [23-30], often far exceeding the 35 dB A standard recommended by the American National Standards Institute (ANSI) [31] and the American Speech-Language-Hearing Association (ASHA) [32] for unoccupied, furnished classroom environments. Classroom noise originates from lighting and HVAC (heating, ventilation and air conditioning) systems, adjacent classrooms and external traffic noise [27,29]. Lack of acoustic treatments such as acoustic ceiling tiles, acoustically modified furniture, carpets, and double-glazed windows in most school settings further aggravates classroom background noise [33,34]. Classroom acoustics in developing countries are often particularly poor. The mean ambient noise in a public school in Brazil may be as high as 63.3 dB A [30], more than 10 dB A greater than levels reported from studies in Britain, Hong Kong and the USA. Schools in developing countries are more vulnerable to ambient noise because more basic infrastructure, such as concrete walls and bare floors [35] with the absence of a roof or walls in some cases [36], provides poor acoustic isolation. Furthermore, opening windows and doors for better ventilation allows external urban noise to easily enter [33,35,37].

Classroom ambient noise is concentrated at low frequencies (500 Hz and below) [23,29,38,39] and masks test tones, which may leave them undetected in pure-tone audiometry. This leads to high false positive findings and subsequent unnecessary diagnostic assessments. Masking, in particular of lower frequency test tones, remains a great problem for pure-tone screening in schools. Conventional TDH-39 supra-aural earphones used in pure-tone hearing screening [40] fail to eliminate low frequency (500 Hz and below) ambient noise [38,39] despite good noise attenuation ability at high frequency regions. This is because noise penetrates into the headset via cable passageways and splits between the receivers and ear cushions [41]. The low frequency region has the lowest

suggested permissible noise level [42] for pure-tone hearing assessment (Table 1).

With advances in technology, an active noise control (ANC) technique can now be applied to headphones and this may help mitigate the problems created by low frequency noise. The resultant noise-cancelling (NC) headphones have built-in microphones outside the headset that input external ambient noise and inside the headset that input residual noise leaking into the ear cups through cable passageways and gaps between headphones and ear cushions. Such a 'duo microphones' system can capture most surrounding noise and send the assembled signals to an ANC system which generates an anti-noise signal of equal amplitude but 180° out-of-phase to the captured noise [43,44]. This anti-noise signal is emitted via the headset speakers and is superimposed on the primary noise signal, to cancel noise near the listener's tympanic membrane [43-47]. In this way, much background noise is not perceived by listeners. NC headphones on average have higher noise reduction ability across nearly all frequencies than TDH-39 earphones (Table 1). Since noise is measured in a logarithmic scale, the 6 dB and 2 dB greater noise attenuation of NC headphones compared with TDH-39 earphones at 250 Hz and 500 Hz, respectively, suggests that less low frequency noise will be perceived by listeners when NC headphones are used. Noise attenuation below 500 Hz should lead to less masking effects on a 500 Hz test tone. Non-adaptive feedback ANC, an ANC design commonly found in commercial NC headphones, allows up to 20 dB noise attenuation for frequencies below 700 Hz [47].

Although NC headphone technology has been widely adopted in the audio and music industries, gaining a good reputation for effectiveness, no research has evaluated its efficacy in audiometric screening and this

Table 1 Comparison of noise attenuation levels of noise-cancelling headphones and TDH-39 supra-aural earphones across frequencies

Octave band frequency (Hz)	Noise attenuation of noise-cancelling headphones (dB)*	Typical attenuation of TDH-39 supra-aural earphones (dB)**	Difference in noise attenuation level (dB)
	A	B	(A − B)
125	11	3	8
250	11	5	6
500	9	7	2
1000	23	15	8
2000	23	26	−3
4000	35	32	3
8000	33	24	9

* Values of Sennheiser PXC450 noise-cancelling circumaural headphones [51].
** Values from ISO 8253–1 (1989).

potential application requires investigation. In the present study it was hypothesized that the use of NC headphones would increase the specificity of school hearing screening for children. Screening with NC headphones was expected to lead to significantly lower overall referral rates and higher passing rates at 500 Hz than screening with TDH-39 earphones, for both 30 dB HL and 25 dB HL referral criteria. Passing rates at 1000, 2000 and 4000 Hz for screening were expected to be similar using both transducer types.

Methods

Participants

246 children, aged 6 to 8 years on the day of testing, were recruited on a voluntary basis. This age range was chosen as it matches the school entry age of most children in developing countries [48], where effective new NC headphone technology may be most needed. This age group was also included in the targeted grade levels for hearing screening advised by the American Academy of Pediatrics [4]. None of the participants reported any otological problems prior to testing. All research was performed in accordance with the Declaration of Helsinki and was approved by the Human Research Ethics Committee for Non-Clinical Faculties at the University of Hong Kong prior to participant enrollment. Written consents were obtained from each participant and their parents prior to testing. The data were collected over a period of three months within the same school year.

Pilot study

14 normal hearing children (28 ears), nine male and five female, with a mean age of 6.7 years (S.D.: 0.64 years), were recruited from the local community. A GSI 17 audiometer was fitted with a pair of TDH-39 earphones and a pair of Sennheiser PXC450 NC headphones. This model of NC headphones was chosen as it had greater low frequency noise attenuation when compared to other models and brands available at the time of purchase. Since calibration data and specifications for the NC headphones were not provided, they were biologically calibrated with a group of normal hearing children using a calibrated GSI 17 portable screening audiometer equipped with a pair of TDH-39 earphones, using a protocol modified from Sliwa et al.'s study [19]. To avoid a practice effect, transducer type and right-left selection were randomized. The pilot study was conducted in a double-walled, sound-treated test booth. Participants were first conditioned to raise their hand when a sound was heard using a 1000 Hz tone at 60 dB HL, as this tone has good test-retest reliability [49]. When participants became familiar with the task, thresholds at four standard screening frequencies—1000 Hz, 2000 Hz, 4000 Hz and 500 Hz—were obtained sequentially. The

tone intensity was varied by ±5 dB HL, starting from 30 dB HL. Thresholds were determined by obtaining two positive responses out of three trials using a modified Hughson-Westlake up-down threshold determination procedure [49]. Individual frequency specific correction factors for the NC headphones were derived for both right and left channels with reference to thresholds measured using the TDH-39 earphones (Table 2), to ensure equal output intensities for each transducer type. Mean thresholds for the pediatric listeners for TDH-39 earphones at each test frequency were obtained and were compared to the same thresholds obtained for NC headphones, with the difference between the two means used as the correction factor. These values were applied in the subsequent main study screening assessments.

Main study

237 students were recruited from four mainstream primary schools in Hong Kong that agreed to take part in the study. Five participants were excluded from data analysis due to unreliable test results and/or were out of the study target age range. The final main study group was composed of 232 participants (464 ears), with 121 males and 111 females, and a mean age of 7.4 years (S.D.: 0.58 years).

All pure-tone screening audiometers (GSI 17) used in the main study were calibrated according to ANSI S3.6-1989 standards prior to use. A biological calibration check of the audiometers was also conducted by the first author before each screening session. Two calibrated GSI 17 audiometers were used to conduct hearing screening. One audiometer was fitted with NC headphones and another was equipped with TDH-39 earphones. A type 1 sound level meter (SLM) (Cesva SC-30) and Cesva Capture Studio software were used to measure and analyze the ambient noise in the test venues of the participating schools. The SLM was each day calibrated with a CB006 Class 1 acoustic calibrator with reference to IEC 60942: 2003 standards prior to measurements.

The main study was conducted in classrooms arranged by participating schools on school attendance days. All the screening test rooms were unoccupied and quiet, but not sound-treated, with all ventilation devices, windows and doors closed during testing. Visual distractions in

Table 2 Correction factors for right and left channels of Sennheiser PXC450 noise-cancelling headphones with reference to TDH-39 supra-aural earphones

Correction factor	Frequency (Hz)			
	500	1000	2000	4000
Right	0	0	+5[*]	+10[*]
Left	0	+5[*]	0	0

*A positive sign indicates additional acoustic output to obtain a hearing threshold in Sennheiser PXC450 noise-cancelling headphones to be equivalent to TDH-39 supra-aural earphones.

the rooms, if any, were minimized to reduce disturbance to participants so that they could concentrate on the screening test. Ambient noise levels in the assigned classrooms were measured and analyzed using a SLM on at least three occasions, each for 5-minute intervals with sampling rate at 1s, randomly selected during the screening session.

Each participant received two hearing screenings, one using TDH-39 earphones and one with NC headphones. To avoid order effects, transducer type and right-left ear selection were randomized. Participants were first conditioned to raise their hand when they heard a sound using a 1000 Hz tone at 60 dB HL. After a few practice trials, participants were screened at 30 dB HL and 25 dB HL at the four screening frequencies. To avoid any visual cues during testing, participants were seated at right angles to the tester in both the pilot and main studies. The passing criterion was two positive responses out of three trials at each frequency at 30 dB HL and 25 dB HL, bilaterally. Failure to respond at a particular frequency at a criterion intensity was regarded as 'did not pass' for that frequency at that presentation level. Parents of all tested participants were given a hard copy of their child's hearing screening report. Professional referral was provided to those who failed to respond at any frequency using a 30 dB HL criteria in either ear with conventional TDH-39 earphones.

Data analysis

To investigate the acoustic conditions at each testing venue, overall noise levels in dB A (slow) and dB SPL, and frequency spectrum analysis in octave bands from 31.5 Hz to 16 kHz in dB SPL, were calculated by averaging the three to five samples obtained on each school visit. Descriptive methods were applied to gather demographic data of the participants. Nonparametric analysis incorporating a Pearson chi-square test or Fisher's exact probability test was conducted to examine the overall (failed at any frequency at either ear) and frequency specific referral rates at the two screening intensities—30 dB HL and 25 dB HL—of the two transducers. Statistical tests of association between individual test results with NC headphones and TDH-39 earphones were also applied using Kappa values of agreement. Statistical significance was set at $p = 0.05$ (one-tailed).

Results

Ambient noise levels

Mean ambient noise levels in four primary schools are shown in Table 3. Data represents the average noise levels obtained from at least three samplings on each school visit. The noise levels were similar in the four schools and the average noise level for 90% of the test sessions (L_{90}) in all schools was 43.25 dB SPL.

An overall frequency spectrum analysis of ambient noise in each classroom is given in Figure 1. Unoccupied

Table 3 Mean ambient noise levels in unoccupied classrooms of four primary schools

	dB A$_{eq5min}$	L$_{50}$	L$_{90}$
School A	52	46	43
School B	46	42	40
School C	53	47	44
School D	49	49	46

classroom ambient noise level decreased with increasing octave band frequency. A clear predominance of low frequency noise was observed in all school settings. School B revealed a substantially reduced noise level at low frequencies compared with other schools, probably because the test venue was located in the basement of the school.

Comparison between TDH-39 supra-aural earphones and noise-cancelling headphones

232 school children received hearing screening with both TDH-39 earphones and NC headphones. Their demographic characteristics are shown in Table 4. Table 5 shows the overall referral rates, with all frequencies included, for both transducer types decreased as age increased for screening at 30 dB HL. Nevertheless, this relationship was not statistically significant (P = 1, d.f. = 2), as revealed by Fisher's exact test. Neither overall referral rates at 25 dB HL nor referral rates when the 500 Hz tone was excluded showed a statistically significant age effect.

Since no age effect was present, data from all age groups were combined to compare the pass/refer rates before and after excluding results of 500 Hz for both transducer types. When all frequencies were included, the referral rates for the NC headphones and the TDH-39 earphones were 3.2% and 12.9% at 30 dB HL, respectively. At 25 dB HL, referral rates of the NC headphones and the TDH-39 earphones were 13.8% and 28.2%, respectively. Results from a chi-square test or Fisher's exact probability test, as appropriate, revealed that at both 30 dB HL and 25 dB HL criteria, referral rates before and after excluding 500 Hz results for the two transducers were statistically different—before exclusion, at 30 dB HL (P< 0.05, d.f. = 1) and at 25 dB HL (χ^2 = 28.76, P < 0.05, d.f. = 1); after excluding 500 Hz, at 30 dB HL (P< 0.05, d.f. = 1) and 25 dB HL (P< 0.05, d.f. = 1) (Table 6). Kappa observed agreement (OA) of the 500 Hz inclusion group (at 30 dB HL: OA = 0.864; at 25 dB HL: OA = 0.735) was smaller than that of the 500 Hz exclusion group (at 30 dB HL: OA = 0.991; at 25 dB HL: OA = 0.946). This indicates that TDH-39 earphones and NC headphones differed in screening outcome when 500 Hz results were included. In the 500 Hz exclusion group, the discrepancies between Fisher's exact test and OA results can be attributed to the small cell size, 5 or below, when the two transducers obtained opposite results, i.e.,

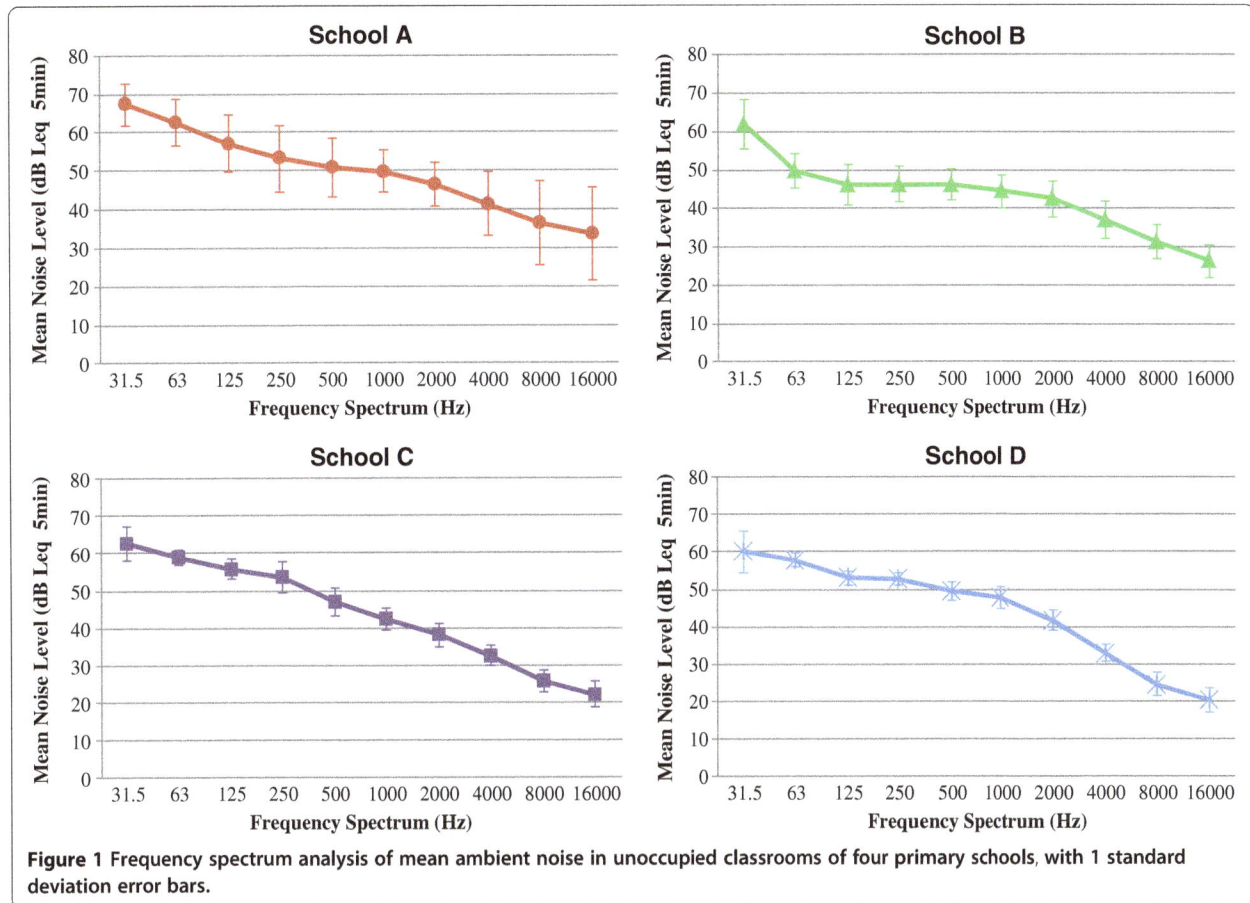

Figure 1 Frequency spectrum analysis of mean ambient noise in unoccupied classrooms of four primary schools, with 1 standard deviation error bars.

pass for one and fail for the other, as majority of participants passed with both the TDH-39 earphones and the NC headphones. This would affect Fisher's exact test analysis and therefore, OA results should be given greater weight.

In order to investigate whether NC headphones and TDH-39 earphones screen similarly, referral rates at the individual frequencies of 500 Hz, 1000 Hz, 2000 Hz and 4000 Hz were also compared using chi-square or Fisher's exact test. Results in Table 7 show that the two transducers screened similarly at 1000 Hz (P > 0.05, d.f. = 1) and 2000 Hz (P > 0.05, d.f. = 1) at 25 dB HL. No

statistical difference was found for 4000 Hz at both 30 dB HL (P > 0.05, d.f. = 1) and 25 dB HL (P > 0.05, d.f. = 1) criteria. However, statistical significant differences were observed for 500 Hz at 30 dB HL (P < 0.05, d.f. = 1) and at 25 dB HL (χ^2 = 34.86, P < 0.05, d.f. = 1), 1000 Hz (P < 0.05, d.f. = 1), and 2000 Hz (P < 0.05, d.f. =1) at 30 dB HL. When OA was considered, it showed that the two transducer types had almost perfect agreement, i.e., they screened similarly at all frequencies (e.g., 1000 Hz: OA = 0.996) except at 500 Hz (at 30 dB HL: OA = 0.873; at 25 dB HL: OA = 0.750). Larger discrepancies between Fisher's exact test and OA at 1000 Hz and 2000 Hz were again influenced by the small cell size, 5 or below, when the two transducers obtained opposite results, as previously mentioned.

Discussion

Effect of ambient noise on school screening

Unoccupied classrooms with furniture only are quieter than occupied classrooms, and are usually chosen for school hearing screening. Nevertheless, such so-called quiet venues usually fail to meet the 35 dB A upper limit recommended by ANSI [31] and ASHA [32] for unoccupied furnished classroom noise level. In the present study, mean overall ambient noise level and L_{90} measured in four

Table 4 Age, gender and grade distribution of participants

	Female (n = 111)	%	Male (n =121)	%	Total (n= 232)	%
Age (years)						
6	19	17	35	29	54	23
7	71	64	73	60	144	62
8	21	19	13	11	34	15
Grade						
Primary 1	28	25	45	37	65	28
Primary 2	83	75	76	68	167	72

Table 5 Association between age and referral rates in participants using TDH-39 supra-aural earphones and noise-cancelling headphones at 30 dB HL and 25 dB HL

Referral rates	No. of Refer (%)		x^2	p-value
	TDH-39	PXC-450		
500 Hz Included				
30 dB HL				
6 (n= 108)	15.7% (17)	3.7% (4)		
7 (n=288)	13.5% (39)	3.5% (10)	N/A[1]	1
8 (n=68)	11.8% (8)	1.5% (1)		
25 dB HL				
6 (n= 108)	29.6% (32)	15.7% (17)		
7 (n=288)	26.0% (75)	12.8% (37)	0.04	0.9802
8 (n=68)	29.4% (20)	14.7% (10)		
500 Hz Excluded				
30 dB HL				
6 (n= 108)	1.9% (2)	0.9% (1)		
7 (n=288)	0.3% (1)	1% (3)	N/A[1]	0.6786
8 (n=68)	0% (0)	1.5% (1)		
25 dB HL				
6 (n= 108)	2.8% (3)	2.8% (3)		
7 (n=288)	3.5% (10)	4.3% (12)	N/A[1]	1
8 (n=68)	2.9% (2)	2.9% (2)		

N/A[1]: Fisher's Exact Test used; d.f. = 2; α = 0.05.

urban mainstream primary schools ranged from 46 to 52 dB $LA_{eq\ 5\ min}$ and 40 – 46 dB SPL, respectively. This noise level is approximately 10 dB A above the published guidelines, and these findings were comparable to previous studies in other schools [26-29,33,37]. Spectrum analysis revealed that classroom ambient noise was predominately at low frequencies (Figure 1). The noise level at 250 Hz and 500 Hz was of most concern as this range exerts the greatest masking effect on 500 Hz test tones in screening. In this study, the average 250 Hz and 500 Hz background noise levels in the four schools were 51.25 dB $LZeq_{5min}$ and 48.5 dB $LZeq_{5min}$, respectively. Such intensity levels

are much higher than the intensity of the 25dB HL screening stimuli, leaving 500 Hz difficult to detect. This may well account for the highest referral rate—27.8%—associated with 500 Hz screening frequency when 25 dB HL was the passing criterion and TDH-39 earphones were used.

Utility of noise-cancelling headphones in school hearing screening

In order to examine the effectiveness of NC headphones in counteracting the masking effect of ambient noise during hearing screening, the overall referral rates of pure-tone screening both including and excluding 500 Hz results were compared. When a 30 dB HL passing criterion was applied, the overall referral rates of TDH-39 earphones including and excluding 500 Hz results were 12.9% and 0.6%, respectively. A large reduction in referral rate of 12.3% was revealed. However, the difference in referral rates for the NC headphones with and without 500 Hz was much smaller than that of the TDH-39 earphones, with only a 2.1% difference (from 3.2% to 1.1%). A much larger difference for the TDH-39 earphones than that of the NC headphones suggested that the former was much more susceptible to ambient noise effects. When a more stringent pass/refer criterion—25 dB HL—was adopted, it was expected that the referral rate difference before and after exclusion of 500 Hz results would widen in both transducer types as the 500 Hz tone became harder to detect as the signal to ambient noise ratio was reduced. The degree of difference between 500 Hz results included and excluded was much greater in TDH-39 earphones (25%; from 28.2% to 3.2%) than NC headphones (9.9%; from 13.8% to 3.9%). This further confirmed that the TDH-39 earphones were more affected by ambient noise, which led to higher fail counts. TDH-39 earphones are more vulnerable to background noise than NC headphones because they attenuate noise by passive shielding—maintained by contact between the MX-4I/AR rubber earphone cushion and the pinna through pressure exerted by the earphone headband. In contrast, NC headphones directly eliminate low frequency ambient noise by generating an equal amplitude

Table 6 Comparison of the overall pass and referral rates between TDH-39 supra-aural earphones and Sennheiser PXC450 noise-cancelling headphones before and after excluding screening results at 500 Hz at 30 dB HL and 25 dB HL

No. of ears (n=464)	No. of pass (%)		No. of refer (%)		Observed agreement	Kappa	x^2	p-value	Odds ratio
	TDH-39	PXC-450	TDH-39	PXC-450					
Before excluding 500 Hz									
30 dB HL	404 (87.1%)	449 (96.8%)	60 (12.9%)	15 (3.2%)	0.864	0.1142	N/A[1]	0.0072	5.88
25 dB HL	333 (71.8%)	400 (86.2%)	131 (28.2%)	64 (13.8%)	0.735	0.2257	28.76	< 0.0001	4.13
After excluding 500 Hz									
30 dB HL	461 (99.4%)	459 (98.9%)	3 (0.6%)	5 (1.1%)	0.991	0.4959	N/A[1]	0.0003	305.33
25 dB HL	449 (96.8%)	446 (96.1%)	15 (3.2%)	18 (3.9%)	0.946	0.2147	N/A[1]	0.0017	11.30

N/A[1]: Fisher's Exact Test used; d.f. =1; α = 0.05.

Table 7 Comparison of the pass and referral rates at individual frequencies for TDH-39 supra-aural earphones and Sennheiser PXC450 noise-cancelling headphones at 30 dB HL and 25 dB HL

No. of ears (n=464)	No. of pass (%)		No. of refer (%)		Observed agreement	Kappa	χ^2	p-value	Odds ratio
	TDH-39	PXC-450	TDH-39	PXC-450					
500 Hz									
30 dB HL	406 (87.5%)	453 (97.6%)	58 (12.5%)	11 (2.4%)	0.873	0.109	N/A[1]	0.0066	6.29
25 dB HL	335 (72.2%)	413 (89%)	129 (27.8%)	51 (11%)	0.750	0.245	34.86	<0.0001	5.49
1000 Hz									
30 dB HL	463 (99.8%)	462 (99.6%)	1 (0.2%)	2 (0.4%)	0.996	0.004	N/A[1]	0.0043	∞
25 dB HL	450 (97%)	451 (97.2%)	14 (3%)	13 (2.8%)	0.950	0.123	N/A[1]	0.0546	6.65
2000 Hz									
30 dB HL	461 (99.4%)	462 (99.6%)	3 (0.6%)	2 (0.4%)	0.998	0.80	N/A[1]	0.0000	∞
25 dB HL	461 (99.4%)	461 (99.4%)	3 (0.6%)	3 (0.6%)	0.996	0.75	N/A[1]	6.0452	∞
4000 Hz									
30 dB HL	464 (100%)	462 (99.6%)	0 (0%)	2 (0.4%)	0.994	1	N/A[1]	1	N/A
25 dB HL	464 (100%)	459 (98.9%)	0 (0%)	5 (1.1%)	0.987	1	N/A[1]	1	N/A

N/A[1]: Fisher's Exact Test used; d.f. = 1; α = 0.05.

but completely out of phase signal to cancel the primary noise signal. This approach allows NC headphones to effectively eliminate steady noise types as the anti-phase signal is locked to the noise source by real-time noise capture and analysis via the 'duo microphones' and ANC system.

When 500 Hz results were included, a smaller OA between the two transducers was found for the 25 dB HL criterion (OA = 0.735) when compared to 30 dB HL (OA = 0.864). Similar findings were observed when 500 Hz results were analyzed alone—smaller OA with 25 dB HL criterion (OA = 0.75) than 30 dB HL screening level (OA = 0.873). This indicates that differences in referral rates for the two transducers in this study were greater with lower screening intensity. Evidence that NC headphones screened more effectively at the more stringent passing criterion than TDH-39 earphones when a low frequency pure-tone was included in the protocol supports the use of NC headphones if a screening program includes a 500 Hz test tone at 25 dB HL. The capability of NC headphones to operate at lower screening intensities gives higher screening sensitivity with test specificity maintained. ASHA modified its screening 1997 guidelines by excluding a 500 Hz test tone, which was previously included in its 1990 guidelines, because of ambient noise considerations [15,50]. This has also been routinely done in many school screening programs outside North America due to the high false positive findings generated as a consequence of the masking effect of ambient noise [5,51-53]. However, this practice is not preferred as it may leave otitis media or other conductive loss undetected since low frequency acuity is a good indicator of middle ear integrity [54]. Otitis media is a common cause of hearing loss in young children [55], particularly in developing countries. A prevalence rate of 9.4% to 25.5% has been noted in a range of developing

nations [22,56-62]. With the use of NC headphones, it may be feasible to include a 500 Hz test tone in school settings even with the presence of low frequency background noise.

Identification of mild hearing loss may also be more practicable when NC headphones are used as they allow screening protocols to adopt a lower screening intensity level. Research suggests that mild hearing loss in children may lead to substantial difficulties in auditory perception—including speech discrimination, recognition and hearing in noise difficulties [63,64], as well as speech and language disorders [8,65]. Early detection of mild hearing loss allows implementation of remedial strategies to facilitate a child's learning. Even in developing countries where amplification systems are unavailable, measures as simple as preferential seating in the classroom may benefit identified children a great deal. Results in this study favor the possible use of NC headphones at the more stringent criterion—25 dB HL. Future studies could explore the possibility of lowering the intensity to 20 dB HL as this level can further increase screening sensitivity and more effectively identify slight to mild hearing loss.

A shortcoming of NC headphones is that there is a lack of calibration specifications, which makes psychoacoustic calibration with a group of normal hearing individuals necessary prior to audiometric use. Specific calibration information that readily enabled NC headphone output to be compared to that of TDH-39 earphones, at audiometric test frequencies, would be valuable. Also, provision of frequency response curves for NC headphones and noise-attenuation information at a wide range of frequencies (e.g., octave band frequencies from 31.5 Hz to 16000 Hz) would make comparison of noise reduction capabilities amongst different NC headphones more convenient. If specific calibration is not available then improved biological calibration is important. The present study developed individual frequency specific correction factors for the NC headphones based on a small sample only of paediatric listeners with normal hearing.

Noise attenuation of noise-excluding headphones, TDH-39 supra-aural earphones and noise-cancelling circumaural headphones

Some hearing screening protocols have used noise-excluding headphones, i.e., TDH-39 earphones mounted inside circumaural audiocups (TDH-39/A headphones) instead of TDH-39 earphones alone, for extra attenuation [18,23,38,55,60]. TDH-39/A headphones provide greater noise attenuation as the audiocups thoroughly enclose the entire pinna with a soft plastic cushion [66,67] to reduce the chances of pure-tone leakage and noise entry. The principle used to achieve noise attenuation with audiocups is, however, similar to that of TDH-39 earphones and is based on the assumption that the cushion completely seals the ear while in reality, due to anatomical differences of the head and pinna among listeners, gaps can hardly be avoided. Therefore, it is expected that TDH-39/A headphone noise-attenuation ability will be poorer than that of noise-cancelling headphones. An early study comparing the attenuation characteristics of noise-excluding headphones ('Otocups' Mark III) and TDH-39 earphones showed that the former had approximately 10 dB greater mean noise attenuation than the TDH-39 earphones across frequencies [67]. The measured mean attenuation values at 500 Hz for TDH-39 earphones enclosed in 'Otocups' shells and TDH-39 earphones alone were 15 dB and 7 dB, respectively. Such attenuation data pointed to a large attenuation gain with noise-excluding circumaural headphones compared with conventional headphones at low frequencies. However, when the standard deviations at 500 Hz for this early study are taken into account (7.5 dB for 'Otocups' and 9.2 dB for TDH-39 earphones) there was not a great difference in noise attenuation between the two transducers. The large intrasubject variation observed in mean attenuation values with audiocups and TDH-39 earphones might be due to headphone positioning effects. In a recent study, it was pointed out that a headset that physically excludes noise does not automatically guarantee accurate hearing threshold measurement, due to calibration issues. Calibration of TDH-style earphones using a 6cc coupler is based on the assumption that the receiver and its ear cushion is in close contact with the pinna. However, it is hard to mount TDH-style earphones that are inside audiocups in an optimal position, so that when placed on listeners the earphones seal the ears well but loosely cover the pinna [41]. Due to this issue, TDH-39/A headphones and TDH-39 earphones may in practice show similar noise attenuation capabilities. However, further research that explicitly compares the noise attenuation performance of TDH-39 earphones,

TDH-39/A earphones and NC headphones in a school hearing screening environment is needed before a truly informed choice of optimal school hearing screening headphones can be made. When comfort factors are considered, TDH-39/A headphones are less optimal than NC headphones as the latter (315 g, battery included) are approximately half the weight of the 620 g TDH-39/A headphones, due to the absence of the bulky noise-excluding shells. Also, NC headphones do not need to be positioned as tightly as noise-excluding headphones on a child's head, and thus may cause less discomfort to young children. This is because NC headphones do not rely on a tight seal between the cushion and ear to exclude noise but rather create a quiet listening environment around the listener ear by phase cancellation.

Potential value of noise-cancelling headphones in developing countries

Environmental test conditions as well as tester and equipment availability are important factors for effective implementation of hearing screening programs in developing countries [21]. School hearing screening usually takes place in far from ideal conditions which are affected by a considerable amount of ambient noise, predominately at low frequencies. Since the environment is usually hard to modify, selection of appropriate screening technology is a practical way to tackle the noise problem. NC headphones have potential to replace TDH-39 earphones in school screening because they actively eliminate ambient noise. Alternatively, one could choose insert earphones to replace conventional headphones for school screening as they have better noise attenuation [68]. Nonetheless, the foam tips used in insert earphones are disposable and this recurrent expenditure is expensive in both developing and developed economies. In addition, large concentrations of cerumen are common in school children, particularly in developing countries where rates for impacted cerumen can be as high as 52.6% [69]. The small diameter sound bore in insert earphones is prone to blockage by even minor amounts of cerumen, leading to false positive screening outcomes. For these reasons insert earphones are not advised for use in school hearing screening programs [70].

For selection of screening tools, cost is an important consideration particularly for health workers in developing countries. Results from a Google search showed that the retail price of new set of TDH-39/A headphones offered by medical equipment vendors is at least $US 355 (shipping excluded). The price of TDH-39 earphones was not determined as they are usually provided with purchase of a screening audiometer. The NC headphones (Sennheiser PXC450) used in this study had the highest specification among all available models and brands in the market at the time of purchase and cost $US 410. There were other brands of NC headphones with lesser noise attenuation specifications which were much more affordable. Although the current cost of NC headphones is higher than that of TDH-39/A headphones, the price of NC headphones is expected to decrease in future due to keen competition in the commercial market and the wide application of noise-cancelling technology.

Although a standard AAA battery is needed to drive NC headphones, this type of battery can be easily obtained in most developing countries. NC headphones require little power to function and frequent battery replacement is not necessary. In this study, only two alkaline cells were used to screen more than 200 students. The use of rechargeable batteries to replace alkaline cells could reduce the ongoing cost of battery replacement.

Conclusions

NC headphones had significantly lower overall referral rates (with 500 Hz results included) than the TDH-39 earphones at both 30 dB HL and 25 dB HL criteria. Similar results were found for referral rates at exclusively 500 Hz. When mid and high frequencies (1000 Hz to 4000 Hz) were considered, both NC headphones and TDH-39 earphones had comparable referral rates. This suggests that NC headphones may be a promising alternative to TDH-39 earphones for hearing screening in schools due to their higher resistance to low frequency ambient noise and light weight. With NC headphones, audiologists or screening professionals may not need to adopt loose screening criteria because of the unfavorable noise screening conditions often found in school settings. Screening at lower intensity levels becomes possible with NC headphones without compromising screening specificity. Future large scale studies that compare the noise attenuation of NC headphones and TDH-39/A equipment, as well research on the implications of a further reduced pass /refer criteria of 20 dB HL, will provide more information on appropriate headphone selection for optimal school hearing screening test accuracy.

Competing interests
The authors declare that they have no competing interests.

Authors' contributions
AL undertook the data collection, statistical analysis and drafted the original manuscript. BM developed the initial study design and supported data analysis. Both authors read and approved the final manuscript.

Acknowledgements
The authors wish to thank all the children who participated in this study, and their parents, for their support and cooperation during hearing screening, as well as express our gratitude to the four primary schools (including Lok Sin Tong Primary School) involved in the study. We also wish to thank Loretta Ho, Cherry Li, Chris Li, Gloria Ng, Jessie Poon and Annabelle Wong, who assisted in data collection and Felix Lam, Kit-ting Lau, Elco Wong, Sing-wan Wong and Tin-wai Wong, who provided administrative support during school screening visits. This project was supported by the Faculty of Education Research Fund, University of Hong Kong.

References
1. White K: *Twenty years of early hearing detection and intervention (EHDI): where we've been and what we've learned*, Paper presented at the American speech-language-hearing association audiology virtual conference. American Speech-Language-Hearing Association: Rockville MD; 2010.
2. Fortnum H, Summerfield A, Marshall D, Davis A, Bamford J, Yoshinaga-Itano C, Hind S: Prevalence of permanent childhood hearing impairment in the United Kingdom and implications for universal neonatal hearing screening: Questionnaire based ascertainment study. *Br Med J* 2001, **323**(7312):536–542.
3. Grote J: Neonatal screening for hearing impairment. *Lancet* 2000, **355**(9203):513–514.
4. American Academy of Pediatrics: Recommendations for preventive pediatric health care. *Pediatrics* 2007, **120**:1376.
5. Rao RS, Subramanyam MA, Nair NS, Rajashekhar B: Hearing impairment and ear diseases among children of school entry age in rural South India. *Int J Ped Otorhinolaryngol* 2002, **64**:105–110.
6. Carney A, Moeller M: Treatment efficacy: hearing loss in children. *J Speech Lang Hear Res* 1998, **41**:S61–S64.
7. Downs MP: Contribution of mild hearing loss to auditory learning problems. In *Auditory disorders in school children: the Law, identification, remediation*. 4th edition. Edited by Roeser RJ, Downs MP. New York: Thieme; 2004:233–248.
8. Kennedy CR, McCann DC, Campbell MJ, Law CM, Mullee M, Petrou S, Watkin P, Worsfold S, Yuen HM, Stevenson J: Language ability after early detection of permanent childhood hearing impairment. *New Eng J Med* 2006, **354**:2131–2141.
9. Olusanya BO: Addressing the global neglect of childhood hearing impairment in developing countries. *PLoS Med* 2007, **4**(4):e74.
10. Olusanya BO, Newton VE: Global burden of childhood hearing impairment and disease control priorities for developing countries. *Lancet* 2007, **369**:1314–1317.
11. Yoshinaga-Itano C, Sedey A, Coulter D, Mehl A: Language of early- and later-identified children with hearing loss. *Pediatrics* 1998, **102**:1161–1171.
12. Wang CN, Bovaird S, Ford-Jones E, Bender R, Parsonage C, Yau M, Ferguson B: Vision and hearing screening in school settings: reducing barriers to children's achievement. *Paediatr Child Health* 2011, **16**:271–272.
13. Sabo MP, Winston R, Macias JD: Comparison of pure tone and transient otoacoustic emissions screening in a grade school population. *Am J Otol* 2000, **21**:88–89.
14. Sideris I, Glattke TJ: A comparison of two methods of hearing screening in the preschool population. *J Commun Disord* 2006, **39**:391–401.
15. American Speech-Language-Hearing Association: Guidelines for screening for hearing impairments and middle ear disorders. *ASHA* 1990, **32**:17–24.
16. Flanary VA, Flanary CJ, Colombo J, Kloss D: Mass hearing screening in kindergarten students. *Int J Ped Otorhinolaryngol* 1999, **50**:93–98.
17. Olusanya BO, Okolo AA, Adeosun AA: Predictors of hearing loss in school entrants in a developing country. *J Postgrad Med* 2004, **50**:173–179.
18. Sarafraz M, Ahmadi K: A practical screening model for hearing loss in Iranian school-aged children. *World J Pediatr* 2009, **5**:46–50.
19. Sliwa L, Hatzopoulos S, Kochanek K, Pilka A, Senderski A, Skarzynski PH: A comparison of audiometric and objective methods in hearing screening of school children. A preliminary study. *Int J Ped Otorhinolaryngol* 2011, **75**:483–488.
20. Bento RF, Albernaz PLM, Di Francesco RC, Wiikmann C, Frizzarini R, Castilho AM: Detection of hearing loss in elementary schools: a national campaign. *Int Congr Ser* 2003, **1240**:225–229.
21. Gell PM, White E, Newell K, Mackenzie I, Smith A, Thompson S, Hatcher J: Practical screening priorities for hearing impairment among children in developing countries. *Bull World Health Organ* 1992, **70**:645–655.
22. Jacob A, Rupa V, Job A, Joseph A: Hearing impairment and otitis media in a rural primary school in South India. *Int J Ped Otorhinolaryngol* 1997, **39**:133–138.
23. McPherson B, Law MMS, Wong MSM: Hearing screening for school children: comparison of low-cost, computer-based and conventional audiometry. *Child Care Health Dev* 2010, **36**:323–331.
24. Bess FH, Sinclair JS, Riggs DE: Group amplification in schools for the hearing impaired. *Ear Hear* 1984, **5**(3):138–144.

25. Crandell C, Bess F: **Speech recognition of children in a "typical" classroom setting.** *ASHA* 1986, **29:**87.

26. Hay B: **A pilot study of classroom noise levels and teacher' reactions.** *Voice+* 1995, **4:**127–134.

27. Knecht HA, Nelson PB, Whitelaw GM, Feth LL: **Background noise levels and reverberation times in unoccupied classrooms: predictions and measurements.** *Am J Audiol* 2002, **11:**65–71.

28. Moodley A: **Acoustic conditions in mainstream classrooms.** *J Brit Assoc Teachers Deaf* 1989, **13:**48–54.

29. Shield B, Dockrell JE: **External and internal noise surveys of London primary schools.** *J Acoust Soc Am* 2004, **115:**730–738.

30. Zannin PHT, Marcon CR: **Objective and subjective evaluation of the acoustic comfort in classrooms.** *Appl Ergon* 2007, **38:**675–680.

31. Institute ANS: *Acoustical performance criteria, design requirements and guidelines for schools (Standard S12.60-2002).* American National Standards Institute: Washington, DC; 2002.

32. American Speech-Language-Hearing Association: *Acoustics in educational settings: technical report.* http://www.asha.org/docs/html/TR2005-00042.html.

33. Choi CY, McPherson B: **Noise levels in Hong Kong primary schools: implications for classroom listening.** *Int J Disabil Dev Ed* 2005, **52:**345–360.

34. Shield B, Greenland E, Dockrell J: **Noise in open plan classrooms in primary schools: a review.** *Noise Health* 2010, **12:**225–234.

35. Olusanya BO: **Classification of childhood hearing impairment: Implications for rehabilitation in developing countries.** *Disabil Rehabil* 2004, **26:**1221–1228.

36. Benavot A, Gad L: **Actual instructional time in African primary schools: factors that reduced school quality in developing countries.** *Prospects* 2004, **34**(3):291–310.

37. Lepore SJ, Shejwal B, Kim BH, Evans GW: **Associations between chronic community noise exposure and blood pressure at rest and during acute noise and non-noise stressors among urban school children in India.** *Int J Environ Res Public Health* 2010, **7:**3457–3466.

38. Hallett CP, Gibbs AC: **The effect of ambient noise and other variables on pure tone threshold screening in a population of primary school entrants.** *Brit J Audiol* 1983, **17**(3):183–190.

39. McPherson B, Knox E: **Test-retest variability using the Liverpool screening audiometer in a field environment.** *Brit J Audiol* 1992, **26:**139–141.

40. American Academy of Audiology: *Childhood hearing screeening guidelines.* 2011. http://www.cdc.gov/ncbddd/hearingloss/recommendations.html.

41. Williams W: **The calculation of maximum permissible ambient noise levels for audiometric testing to a given threshold level with a specified uncertainty.** *National Acoustic Laboratories Report* 2010, **133:**1–11.

42. International Organization for Standardization (ISO): *ISO 8253-1 Acoustics-Audiometric test methods, part 1: Basic pure tone air and bone conduction audiometry.* Geneva: International Organization for Standardization; 1989.

43. Gan WS, Kuo SM: **An integrated audio and active noise control headset.** *IEEE Trans Consumer Electronics* 2002, **48**(2):242–247.

44. Krüger H, Jeub M, Schumacher T, Vary P, Beaugeant C: *Investigation and development of digital active noise control headsets.* Tel Aviv, Israel: Proceedings of International Workshop on Acoustic Echo and Noise Control (IWAENC); 2010.

45. Kuo SM, Gan WS: **Active noise control system for headphone applications.** *IEEE Trans Control Systems Technol* 2006, **14:**331–335.

46. Sauert B, Vary P: *Near end listening enhancement optimized with respect to speech intelligibility index and audio power limitations.* Aalborg, Denmark: Proceedings of European Signal Processing Conference (EUSIPCO); 2010:1919–1923.

47. Schumacher T, Kruger H, Jeub M, Vary P, Beaugeant C: *Active noise control in headsets: A new approach for broadband feedback ANC.* Prague, Czech Republic: Proceedings of the IEEE International Conference on Acoustics, Speech and Signal Processing (ICASSP); 2011:417–420.

48. Bommier A, Lamber S: **Education demand and age at school enrollment in Tanzania.** *J Hum Resour* 2000, **35:**177–203.

49. Schlauch RS, Nelson P: **Puretone evaluation.** In *Handbook of clinical audiology.* 6th edition. Edited by Katz J, Medwetsky L, Burkard R, Hood LJ. Baltimore: Lippincott Williams & Wilkins; 2009:30–49.

50. American Speech-Language-Hearing Association: *Guidelines for audiologic screening.* http://www.asha.org/policy/GL1997-00199.htm.

51. Bamford J, Fortnum H, Bristow K, Smith J, Vamvakas G, Davies L, Taylor R, Watking P, Fonseca S, Davis A, Hind S: **Current practice, accuracy,**

effectiveness and cost-effectiveness of the school entry hearing screen. *Health Technol Assess* 2007, **11**(32):1–168.

52. Mathers C, Smith A, Concha M: *Global burden of hearing loss in the year 2000,* Global burden of disease 2000. Geneva: World Health Organization; 2003:1–30.

53. Saunders JK, Vaz S, Greinwald JH, Lai J, Morin L, Mojica K: **Prevalence and etiology of hearing loss in rural Nicaraguan children.** *Laryngoscope* 2007, **117:**387–398.

54. Silman S, Silverman CA, Arick DS: **Pure-tone assessment and screening of children with middle-ear effusion.** *J Am Acad Audiol* 1994, **5:**173–182.

55. Seely DR, Gloyd SS, Wright AD, Norton SJ: **Hearing loss prevalence and risk factors among Sierra Leonean children.** *Arch Otolaryngol Head Neck Surg* 1995, **121:**853–858.

56. McPherson B, Holborow CA: **A study of deafness in west Africa: the Gambian hearing health project.** *Int J Ped Otorhinolaryngol* 1985, **10:**115–135.

57. McPherson B, Swart SM: **Childhood hearing loss in sub-Saharan Africa: a review and recommendations.** *Int J Ped Otorhinolaryngol* 1997, **40:**1–18.

58. Miller SA, Omeme JA, Bluestone CD, Torkelson DW: **A point prevalence of otitis media in a Nigerian village.** *Int J Ped Otorhinolaryngol* 1983, **5:**19–29.

59. Minja BM, Machemba A: **Prevalence of otitis media, hearing impairment and cerumen impaction among school children in rural and urban Dar es Salaam, Tanzania.** *Int J Ped Otorhinolaryngol* 1996, **37:**29–34.

60. Olusanya BO, Okolo AA, Ijaduola GTA: **The hearing profile of Nigerian school children.** *Int J Ped Otorhinolaryngol* 2000, **55:**173–179.

61. Saim A, Saim L, Saim S, Ruszymah BHI, Sani A: **Prevalence of otitis media with effusion amongst pre-school children in Malaysia.** *Int J Ped Otorhinolaryngol* 1997, **41:**21–28.

62. Zakzouk SM: **Epidemiology and etiology of hearing impairment among infants and children in a developing country: Part II.** *J Otolaryngol* 1997, **26:**402–410.

63. Wake M, Poulakis Z: **Slight and mild hearing loss in primary school children.** *J Paediatr Child Health* 2004, **40:**11–13.

64. Davis A, Reeve K, Hind S, Bamford J: **Children with mild and unilateral hearing impairment.** In *A sound foundation through early amplification 2001. Proceedings of the second international conference.* Edited by Seewald RC, Gravel JS. Chicago: Phonak AG; 2002:179–186.

65. Briscoe J, Bishop DV, Norbury CF: **Phonological processing, language, and literacy: a comparison of children with mild-to-moderate sensorineural hearing loss and those with specific language impairment.** *J Child Psychol Psychiatry* 2001, **42:**329–340.

66. Amplivox Limited: *Amplivox audiocups.* http://sonici.com.au/wp-content/uploads/AMPLIVOX-Audiocups-Brochure.pdf.

67. Coles RRA: **A noise-attenuating enclosure for audiometer earphones.** *Brit J Ind Med* 1967, **24:**41–51.

68. Wright DC, Frank T: **Attenuation values for a supra-aural earphone for children and insert earphone for children and adults.** *Ear Hear* 1992, **13:**454–459.

69. Olusanya BO: **Hearing impairment in children with impacted cerumen.** *Ann Trop Paediatr* 2003, **23:**121–128.

70. McPherson B, Olusanya BO: **Screening for hearing loss in developing countries.** In *Audiology in developing countries.* Edited by McPherson B, Brouillette R. Hauppauge, NY: Nova Publishers; 2008:75–105.

Bacterial isolates and drug susceptibility patterns of ear discharge from patients with ear infection at Gondar University Hospital, Northwest Ethiopia

Dagnachew Muluye[1], Yitayih Wondimeneh[1*], Getachew Ferede[1], Feleke Moges[1] and Tesfaye Nega[2]

Abstract

Background: Ear infection is a common problem for both children and adults especially in developing countries. However in Ethiopia particularly in the study area, there is no recent data that shows the magnitude of the problem. The aim of this study was to determine the bacterial isolates and their drug susceptibility patterns from patients who had ear infection.

Method: A retrospective study was conducted from September, 2009 to August, 2012 at Gondar University Hospital, Northwest Ethiopia. Ear discharge samples were cultured on MacConkey agar, blood agar and chocolate agar plates. A standard biochemical procedure was used for full identification of bacterial isolates. Antimicrobial susceptibility tests were done on Mueller-Hinton agar by using disk diffusion method. Data were entered and analyzed by using SPSS version 20 software and P-value of < 0.05 was considered statistically significant.

Result: A total of 228 ear discharge samples were tested for bacterial isolation and 204 (89.5%) cases were found to have bacterial isolates. From the total bacterial isolates, 115 (56.4%) were gram negative bacteria and the predominant isolate was *proteus species* (27.5%). Of individuals who had ear infection, 185 (90.7%) had single bacterial infection while 19 (9.3%) had mixed infections. Under five children were more affected by ear infection. The prevalence of ear infection was significantly high in males (63.7 vs 36.3%) (P = 0.017). Of all bacterial isolates, 192 (94.1%) had multiple antibiotic resistant pattern. Non Lactose Fermenter Gram Negative Rods (46.0%), *Klebsella species* (47.7%) and *Pseudomonas species* (48.5%) were resistant against the commonly used antibiotics.

Conclusion: The prevalence of ear infection was very high in the study area. Majority of the bacterial isolates were resistant to multiple antibiotics. Hence antibiotics susceptibility test is mandatory before prescribing any antibiotics.

Keywords: Ear infection, Bacterial isolates, Drug susceptibility, Gondar university hospital

Background

Ear infection is an inflammation of the ear and ear discharge is one of the commonest symptoms of ear infection [1]. About 65-330 million people suffer from ear infection worldwide and 60% of them had significant hearing impairment [2]. The health-economic burden of ear infection is also severe especially in Africa and other developing nations where the disease prevalence is estimated as high as 11% [3].

Ear infection is a common problem for both children and adults but the magnitude is different in different countries. Anatomically the children's Eustachian tube is shorter, more horizontal with a more flaccid cartilage which can easily impair its opening and hence ear infection is a major health problem of them especially in those with poor socioeconomic status [4].

The etiologies and prevalence of ear infection is different indifferent geographical areas [5,6]. According to World Health Organization (WHO) survey, countries can be clustered into those having low ear infection when a prevalence rate of ear infection among children is between 1-2% and high when it is 3-6% and Ethiopia belongs to the latter category [7]. Though ear infection

* Correspondence: yitayihlab@gmail.com
[1]School of Biomedical and Laboratory Sciences, College of Medicine and Health Sciences, University of Gondar, P.O. Box 196, Gondar, Ethiopia
Full list of author information is available at the end of the article

can be caused by viruses and fungi infections, the major causes of ear infection are bacterial isolates such as *Pseudomonas aeruginosa, Staphylococcus aureus, Proteus mirabilis, Klebsiella pneumonia* and *Escherichia coli* which are found in the skin of the external ear and enter into the middle ear through a chronic perforation [8,9].

In addition, antimicrobial resistance profile of bacteria varies among population because of the difference in geography, local antimicrobial prescribing practices and prevalence of resistant bacterial strains in a given area [10]. So there should be up to date information on microbial resistance pattern at national and local levels to guide the rational use of the existing antimicrobial drugs.

In Ethiopia particularly in the study area, there is no such type of recent data that shows the magnitude of the problem. Therefore, the aim of this study was to determine the bacterial isolates and their drug susceptibility patterns from patients who gave ear discharge samples at Gondar University Hospital.

Methods

Study design, area and period
A retrospective study was conducted from September, 2009 to August, 2012 at Gondar University Hospital, Northwest Ethiopia. This University Hospital provides inpatient and outpatient services for more than 5 million populations surrounding it.

Study participants and data collection
The study participants were all individuals who had complain of ear infection and those who provide ear discharge sample at Gondar University Hospital during the study period. Socio-demographic and laboratory results which contain different bacterial isolates and drug susceptibility patterns of patients who had ear discharges were collected from the University Hospital Microbiology Laboratory unit registration books by using standard data collection format.

Culture and identification
According to the standard operation procedures, the ear discharge samples were collected aseptically by using cotton swab techniques from different OPDs and wards of the University Hospital and transported to microbiology laboratory. Ear discharge samples were cultured on MacConkey agar, blood agar and chocolate agar plates and then incubated aerobically at 37°C for 24 hours. The swarming feature of proteus species were managed by sub culturing mixed colonies in to MacConkey agar that contains bile salt and by adding 90% ethanol. Pure isolates of bacterial pathogen were preliminary characterized by colony morphology, gram-stain and catalase test. Bacterial species were identified as per the standard microbiological methods [11].

Antimicrobial susceptibility testing
Antimicrobial susceptibility tests were done on Mueller-Hinton agar (Oxoid, England) using disk diffusion method [12]. The antimicrobial agents tested were tetracycline (30 μg), penicilin G (10 μg), erythromycin (15 μg), chloramphenicol (30 μg), gentamicin (10 μg), ciprofloxacin (5 μg), norfloxacillin (10 μg), cotrimoxazole (25 μg), ceftriaxone (30 μg), ampicillin (10 μg) and amoxycillin (10 μg) (Oxoid, England). The drug susceptibility pattern was interpreted according to Clinical and Laboratory Standards Institute (CLSI, 2006) (formerly known as National Committee for Clinical Laboratory Standards/NCCLS) [13]. Reference strains of *E. coli* ATCC 25922 and *S. aureus* ATCC 25923 were used for quality control for antimicrobial susceptibility tests [13].

Statistical analysis
Data were cleaned manually and entered and analyzed by using SPSS version 20 software. Chi-square test was employed to compare the proportion of bacterial isolates with patients' demographic information and comparison of antimicrobial resistances. P-value < 0.05 was considered statistically significant.

Ethical considerations
Ethical clearance was obtained from the Institutional Review Board of University of Gondar. A supportive letter was also obtained from College of Medicine and Health Sciences and the University Hospital clinical director before collecting the data.

Result
A total of 250 ear discharge samples were analyzed at the University Hospital Microbiology Laboratory unit during the study period but only 228 (91.2%) of them had complete information for this analysis. Majority of the study participants were males (66.2% vs 33.8%). The mean age of the study participants was 18 (18 ±16) years with the minimum and maximum age of 10 months and 84 years old respectively. Majority of the study participants 58 (25.4%) were under five age groups.

The overall prevalence of bacterial isolates was 204 (89.5%). From the total bacterial isolates, 115 (56.4%) were gram negative bacteria. Of individuals who had bacterial isolates, 185 (90.7%) had single bacterial infection while 19 (9.3%) had mixed bacterial infections.

In this study, the predominant bacterial isolates were *proteus species* 56 (27.5%) followed by *S. aureus* 54 (26.5%). Majority (51 (25.0%)) of the bacterial isolates were found in under five age groups (P = 0.057). Males were more affected than females with significant difference (63.7 vs 36.3%) (P = 0.017) (Table 1).

From 2,248 antibiotics which have been tested against the bacterial isolates, 871 (38.9%) had resistant pattern.

Table 1 The distribution of bacterial isolates from ear discharge in different sex and age categories of study participants at Gondar University Hospital, Northwest Ethiopia (2009-2012)

Age and sex	Bacterial isolates No (%)									P-value
	S. aureus	NLF GNR	E.coli	Pseud. spps	CNStaph spps	Strep. spps	Prot. spps	Kleb. spps	Total	
Age in years										
0–5	12 (23.5)	5 (9.8)	5 (9.8)	4 (7.8)	5 (9.8)	3 (5.9)	16 (31.4)	1 (2.0)	51 (25.0)	0.057
6–10	9 (29.0)	3 (9.7)	2 (6.5)	2 (6.5)	5 (16.1)	2 (6.5)	7 (22.6)	1 (3.2)	31 (15.2)	
11–15	5 (29.4)	0	0	1 (5.9)	1 (5.9)	2 (11.8)	8 (47.1)	0	17 (8.3)	
16–20	3 (13.6)	2 (9.1)	3 (13.6)	2 (9.1)	0	0	11 (50.0)	0	21 (10.3)	
21–30	14 (31.1)	3 (6.7)	0	3 (6.7)	6 (13.3)	3 (6.7)	8 (17.8)	8 (17.8)	45 (22.1)	
31–40	8 (38.1)	1 (4.8)	3 (14.3)	4 (19.0)	2 (9.5)	0	1 (4.8)	2 (9.5)	21 (10.3)	
≥41	3 (16.7)	1 (5.6)	1 (5.6)	2 (11.1)	4 (22.2)	2 (11.1)	5 (27.8)	0	18 (8.8)	
Total	54 (26.5)	15 (7.4)	14 (6.9)	18 (8.8)	23 (11.3)	12 (5.9)	56 (27.5)	12 (5.9)	204 (89.5)	
Sex										
Male	32 (24.6)	6 (4.6)	8 (6.2)	12 (9.2)	16 (12.3)	7 (5.4)	44 (33.8)	5 (3.8)	130 (63.7)	0.017
Female	22 (29.7)	9 (12.2)	6 (8.1)	6 (8.1)	7 (9.5)	5 (6.8)	12 (16.2)	7 (9.5)	74 (36.3)	

S. aureus Staphylococcus aureus, NLF GNR Non Lactose Fermenter Gram Negative rods, Pseud. spps Pseudomonas species, CN Staph spps Coagulase Negative Staphylococcus species, Strep. spps Streptococcus species, Prot. spps Proteus species, Kleb. Spps Klebsella species.

Of these, 71.4% of E.coli was resistant for both ampicillin and amoxicillin, 75% of streptococcus species were resistant for tetracycline, 77.8% of the pseudomonas species were resistant for ampicillin and tetracycline, and 83.3% of the Klebsella species were resistant to ampicillin (Table 2). From the total bacterial isolates, 192 (94.1%) had multiple antibiotic resistant pattern (resistant to two or more antibiotics) and 10 (4.9%) of the isolates were resistant for at least one antibiotic. Only 2 (1.0%) bacterial isolates were susceptible to all antibiotics.

Discussion

Ear discharge is one of the most frequently ordered samples for microbiological analysis in the study area. This indicates that ear infection is a common problem in the given area. In this study, 89.5% cases of ear discharges were found to be positive for bacteria, which is in agreement with other studies in Ethiopia [9] and Nigeria [14].

Majority of the ear infection (56.4%) in the present study were caused by gram negative bacteria which is similar to previous studies that have been conducted in Ethiopia [9,15] and Nigeria [16]. In the present study, majority of the patients 185 (90.7%) had single bacterial infections which is similar to the other studies in Ethiopia [9] and Nigeria [14].

According to this study, majority of the bacterial isolates were found in under five years old children. A similar finding was also documented in previous studies [9,16,17]. This indicates that under five children were more affected by ear infections. This may be due to different factors such as anatomy of Eustachian tubes, the nutritional status of the children and other health problems like upper respiratory tract infections which are common in children [18].

There was significant difference on the prevalence of ear infections in genders. Males were more affected by

Table 2 Antimicrobial resistance pattern of bacterial isolates from ear discharge samples of study participants at Gondar University Hospital, Northwest Ethiopia (2009-2012)

Bacterial isolates	Total NO	Resistance pattern of antimicrobial agents (R %)										
		AMP	AMX	CRO	CAF	CIP	ERY	CN	NOR	PG	SXT	TTC
S. aureus	54	26 (48.1)	34 (63.0)	13 (24.1)	14 (25.9)	10 (18.2)	17 (31.5)	16 (29.6)	16 (29.6)	27 (50.0)	22 (40.7)	25 (46.3)
NLF GNR	15	9 (60.0)	10 (66.7)	4 (26.7)	11 (73.3)	4 (26.7)	6 (40.0)	5 (33.3)	2 (13.3)	6 (40.0)	9 (60.0)	10 (66.7)
E.coli	14	10 (71.4)	10 (71.4)	12 (50.0)	1 (7.1)	2 (14.3)	6 (42.9)	2 (14.3)	1 (7.1)	4 (28.6)	9 (64.3)	8 (57.1)
Pseud. spps	18	14 (77.8)	13 (72.2)	6 (33.3)	14 (77.8)	3 (16.7)	5 (27.8)	6 (33.3)	3 (16.7)	6 (33.3)	12 (66.7)	14 (77.8)
CN staph spps	23	9 (39.1)	3 (13.0)	5 (21.7)	7 (30.4)	5 (21.7)	5 (21.7)	5 (21.7)	6 (26.1)	6 (26.1)	11 (47.8)	11 (47.8)
Strep.spps	12	6 (50.0)	4 (33.3)	1 (8.3)	2 (16.7)	3 (25.0)	3 (25.0)	4 (33.3)	4 (33.3)	5 (41.7)	6 (50.0)	9 (75.0)
Prot. spps	56	31 (55.4)	24 (42.9)	17 (30.4)	32 (57.1)	10 (17.9)	13 (23.2)	12 (21.4)	12 (21.4)	19 (33.9)	23 (41.1)	44 (78.6)
Kleb. spps	12	10 (83.3)	8 (66.7)	7 (58.3)	5 (41.7)	4 (33.3)	4 (33.3)	4 (33.3)	3 (25.0)	7 (58.3)	6 (50.0)	5 (41.7)

AMP Ampicillin, AMX Amoxacillin, CRO Ceftriaxone, CAF Chloramphenicol, CIP Ciprofloxacin, ERY Erythromycin, CN Gentamycin, NOR Norfluxaciline, PG Penicillin G, SXT Co-trimoxazole, TTC Tetracycline.

ear infections than females (63.7 vs 36.3%) (P = 0.017). A similar finding was also reported by Egbe *et al* [19] but according to Hassan *et al* report [20], females were more affected by ear infections. This may be due to the difference between ear cleaning habit of the males and females. In some tradition, females use cotton swabs to clean their ear and this may contribute for the introduction of microorganisms from the external surface to the middle ear. However in some other studies [14,21], there is no difference on the prevalence of ear infections between males and females.

In this study, the predominant bacterial isolates were proteus species 56 (27.5%) followed by s. aureus 54 (26.5%) which is similar to previous study in Ethiopia [9]. However, in other studies [14,22], the predominant isolates were *Pseudomonas aeruginosa* and *s. aureus*. This may be due to the difference in climate and geographical variations in different countries. The other organisms which have been isolated in the present study in descending order were coagulase negative *staphylococcus species, pseudomonas species, Non lactose fermenter gram negative rods, E.coli, streptococcus species and Klebsella species.*

In the present study, different bacterial species had high level of resistance pattern to different antibiotics. For example, 71.4% of E.coli was resistant for both ampicillin and amoxicillin, 75% of streptococcus species were resistant for tetracycline, 77.8% of the pseudomonas species were resistant for ampicillin and tetracycline, and 83.3% of the Klebsella species were resistant to ampicillin. Similar finding were also reported in other studies [9,23-25]. Prescription of antibiotics without laboratory guidance and over sales of antibiotics without proper drug prescription may be some of the different factors that can contribute for this high level drug resistant pattern. Therefore, drug prescription for patients should be laboratory evidence based.

Conclusion

In conclusion, the overall prevalence of bacterial isolates was high and majority of the isolates were gram negative bacteria. The predominant isolates were *Proteus species* and *S.aureus*. The bacteria which have been isolated from otitis media have shown high level of antibiotics resistance in the study area. Majority of the bacterial isolates had multiple antibiotic resistant patterns. Hence antibiotics susceptibility test is mandatory before prescribing any antibiotics.

Limitation of the study

Due to the nature of the study, ear diagnosis is not clearly indicated and it is difficult to show whether the ear infection is acute otitis media with perforation, chronic suppurative otitis media, or otitis external. We are also unable correlate the bacterial findings with the severity of the infection. Some of the bacterial isolates were reported as non-lactose fermenting Gram negative rods and CN Staphylococci which are not specific. The isolated bacterial species were tested only for few antibiotics. In addition, there was no data about anaerobic bacteria and other fungal ear infections.

Competing interest
The authors declared that no competing interest with respect to the authorship and/or publication of this research paper.

Authors' contributions
DM: participated in conception and design of the study, data collection and analysis, interpretation of the findings. YW: Participated in the design of the study, analysis and interpretations of the findings, drafting the manuscript and write up. GF: Participated in conception and design of the study, data analysis and interpretations of the findings. FM: Participated in conception and design of the study, data analysis and interpretations of the findings. TN: Participated in conception and design of the study and data collection. All authors reviewed and approved the final manuscript.

Acknowledgement
We acknowledge the staff of Gondar University Hospital Bacteriology laboratory staffs for their cooperation during data collection.

Author details
[1]School of Biomedical and Laboratory Sciences, College of Medicine and Health Sciences, University of Gondar, P.O. Box 196, Gondar, Ethiopia. [2]Unit of Bacteriology, Gondar University Hospital, P.O. Box 196, Gondar, Ethiopia.

References
1. Variya A, Tainwala S, Mathur S: **Bacteriology of acute otitis media in children.** *Indian J Med Microbiol* 2002, **20**:54–55.
2. Woodfield G, Dugdale A, Evidence behind the WHO guidelines: hospital care for children: **What is the most effective antibiotic regime for chronic suppurative otitis media in children?** *J Tropical Pediatric* 2008, **54**(3):151–156.
3. Akinpelu OV, Amusa YB, Komolafe EO, Adeolu AA, Oladele AO, Ameye SA: **Challenges in management of chronic suppurative otitis media in a developing country.** *J Laryngol Otol* 2008, **122**(1):16–20.
4. Bluestone CD, Klein JO: **Microbiology.** In *Otitis media in infants and children.* 3rd edition. Edited by Bluestone CD, Klein JO. Philadelphia: P A W B. Saunders; 2001:79–1014.
5. Brook I, Frazier E: **Microbial dynamics of persistent purulent otitis media in children.** *J Pediatrician* 1996, **128**(2):237–240.
6. Kenna M: **Etiology and pathogenesis of chronic suppurative otitis media.** *Arch Otolaryngol Head Neck Surg* 1988, **97**(2):16–17.
7. World Health Organization: *Chronic suppurative otitis media, burden of illness and management option.* Geneva: WHO; 2004:10–47.
8. Bluestone CD: **Otitis media; to treat or not to treat.** *Consultant* 1998:1421–1433.
9. Abera B, Kibret M: **Bacteriology and antimicrobial susceptibility of otitis media at dessie regional health research laboratory, Ethiopia.** *Ethiopian J Health Develop* 2011, **25**(2):161–167.
10. Noh KT, Kim CS: **The changing pattern of otitis media in Korea.** *Int J Pediatrician Otorhinolaryngol* 1985, **9**:77–87.
11. Cheesbourgh M: *Medical laboratory manual for tropical countries.* Part 2: 2nd edition. England: Butterworthr-Heineman LTD; 2006:45–70.
12. Bauer AW, Kirby WMM, Sherris JC, Turck M: **Antibiotic susceptibility testing by standard single disc method.** *Am J Clin Pathol* 1966, **45**:493–496.
13. Clinical and Laboratory Standards Institute: *Performance standards for antimicrobial susceptibility testing; seventeenth information supplement.* CLSI document M100-S17, Clinical and Laboratory Standards Institute Wayne Pennsylvania; 2006.
14. Osazuwa F, Osazuwa E, Osime C, Igharo EA, Imade PE, Lofor P, Momoh M, Omoregie R, Dirisu J: **Aetiologic agents of otitis media in Benin city, Nigeria.** *North Am J Med Sci* 2011, **3**:95–98.

15. Tesfaye G, Asrat D, Woldeamanuel Y, Gizaw M: **Microbiology of discharging ears in Ethiopia.** *Asian Pacific J Tropical Med* 2009, **2**(1):60–67.

16. Iseh KR, Adegbite T: **Pattern and bacteriology of acute suppurative otitis media in Sokoto, Nigeria.** *Ann Afri Med* 2004, **3**(4):164–166.

17. Ferede D, Geyid A, Lulseged S, *et al*: **Drug susceptibility pattern of bacterial isolates from children with chronic suppurative otitis media.** *Ethiopian J Health Develop* 2001, **15**(2):89–96.

18. Melaku A, Lulseged S: **Chronic suppurative otitis media in children hospital in Addis Ababa, Ethiopia.** *Ethiopian Med J* 1999, **37**(4):237–246.

19. Egbe CA, Mordi R, Omoregie R, Enabulele O: **Prevalence of Otitis media in Okada Community, Edo State, Nigeria.** *Macedonian J Med Sci* 2010, **3**(3):299–302.

20. Hassan O, Adeyemi A: **A study of bacterial isolates in cases of otitis media in patients attending oauthc, Ile-Ife.** *African j Clin Exper Microbiol* 2007, **8**(3):130–136.

21. Parry D, Roland D: **Middle Ear chronic suppurative otitis media.** *Med treat* 2002:12–15.

22. Nwabuisi C, Ologe FE: **Pathogenic agents of chronic suppurative otitis media in Ilorin, Nigeria.** *East Africa Med J* 2002, **79**(4):202–205.

23. Okeke IN, Lamikara A, Edelman R: **Socio-economic and behavioural Factors leading to acquired bacterial resistance to antibiotics in developing countries.** *Emerg Infect Dis* 1999, **5**:18–27.

24. Gerhard G: **Challenges in reducing the burden of otitis media disease: an ENT perspective on improving management and prospects for prevention.** *Int J Pediatric Otorhinolaryngol* 2010, **74**(6):572–577.

25. Gebre-Selassie S: **Antimicrobial resistance of clinical bacterial isolates in Southern Ethiopia.** *Ethiopian Med J* 2007, **45**(4):363–375.

Etiological profile and treatment outcome of epistaxis at a tertiary care hospital in Northwestern Tanzania: a prospective review of 104 cases

Japhet M Gilyoma[*] and Phillipo L Chalya[†]

Abstract

Background: Epistaxis is the commonest otolaryngological emergency affecting up to 60% of the population in their lifetime, with 6% requiring medical attention. There is paucity of published data regarding the management of epistaxis in Tanzania, especially the study area. This study was conducted to describe the etiological profile and treatment outcome of epistaxis at Bugando Medical Centre, a tertiary care hospital in Northwestern Tanzania.

Methods: This was a prospective descriptive study of the cases of epistaxis managed at Bugando Medical Centre from January 2008 to December 2010. Data collected were analyzed using SPSS computer software version 15.

Results: A total of 104 patients with epistaxis were studied. Males were affected twice more than the females (2.7:1). Their mean age was 32.24 ± 12.54 years (range 4 to 82 years). The modal age group was 31-40 years. The commonest cause of epistaxis was trauma (30.8%) followed by idiopathic (26.9%) and hypertension (17.3%). Anterior nasal bleeding was noted in majority of the patients (88.7%). Non surgical measures such as observation alone (40.4%) and anterior nasal packing (38.5%) were the main intervention methods in 98.1% of cases. Surgical measures mainly intranasal tumor resection was carried out in 1.9% of cases. Arterial ligation and endovascular embolization were not performed. Complication rate was 3.8%. The overall mean of hospital stay was 7.2 ± 1.6 days (range 1 to 24 days). Five patients died giving a mortality rate of 4.8%.

Conclusion: Trauma resulting from road traffic crush (RTC) remains the most common etiological factor for epistaxis in our setting. Most cases were successfully managed with conservative (non-surgical) treatment alone and surgical intervention with its potential complications may not be necessary in most cases and should be the last resort. Reducing the incidence of trauma from RTC will reduce the incidence of emergency epistaxis in our centre.

Keywords: Epistaxis, etiology, treatment outcome, Tanzania

Background

Epistaxis or nasal bleeding is recognized as one of the most common otorhinolaryngological emergencies worldwide and presents a challenge in resource-poor centres where facilities for caring of these patients are limited [1]. Epistaxis is a problem frequently encountered in general practice and may present as an emergency, as a chronic problem of recurrent bleeds or may be a symptom of a generalized disorder [2]. It cannot only affect the hemodynamic but may cause great anxiety to patients and their relatives.

Epistaxis is estimated to occur in 60% of persons worldwide during their lifetime, and approximately 6% of those with nosebleeds seek medical treatment [1-4]. The prevalence is increased for children less than 10 years of age and then rises again after the age of 35 years [5]. Generally, males are slightly affected than

* Correspondence: drgilyoma2@yahoo.com
† Contributed equally
Department of Surgery, Weill- Bugando University College of Health Sciences, Mwanza, Tanzania

females until the age of 50, but after 50 no deference between sexes as reported [2,4,5].

Epistaxis is commonly divided into anterior and posterior epistaxis, depending on the site of origin [5]. Anterior nosebleeds arise from damage to Kiesselbach's plexus on the lower portion of the anterior nasal septum, known as the Little's area, whereas posterior nosebleeds arise from damage to the posterior nasal septal artery [4,6]. Anterior epistaxis is far more common than posterior epistaxis, accounting for more than 80% of cases [4,6,7].

The aetiology of epistaxis can be broadly divided into the local or systemic causes, although even this distinction is difficult to make and the term "Idiopathic Epistaxis" is ultimately used in about 80-90% of the cases [4,8]. The etiological profile of epistaxis has been reported to vary with age and anatomical location [4-8]. Traumatic epistaxis is more common in younger individuals (under age 35 years) and is most often due to digital trauma, facial injury, or a foreign body in the nasal cavity [6-8]. Non-traumatic epistaxis is more characteristic of older patients (over age 50 years) and may be due to organ failure, neoplastic conditions, inflammation, or environmental factors (temperature, humidity, altitude) [7,8]. Epistaxis that occurs in children younger than 10 years usually is mild and originates in the anterior nose, whereas epistaxis that occurs in individuals older than 50 years is more likely to be severe and to originate posteriorly [9]. Epistaxis poses a greater risk in elderly people in whom clinical deterioration may progress rapidly if the blood loss is significant [7].

The treatment of epistaxis requires a systematic and methodical approach, and options vary according to the cause, location, and severity of the hemorrhage [4,6,7,9]. Both conservative and surgical treatment modalities have been used in the treatment of epistaxis [2,6]. However, their outcome has never been evaluated in our setting partly because of paucity of local data.

Most of the underlying causes of epistaxis are preventable [8,9]. A clearer understanding of the causes, treatment and outcome of these patients is essential for establishment of preventive strategies as well as treatment guidelines [1,7,8]. Such data is lacking in our environment as there is no local study which has been done on the subject. This study was conducted in our setting to identify the etiological profile and to determine the outcome of treatment of these patients. The results of this study will provide basis for planning of preventive strategies and establishment of treatment guidelines.

Methods

Study design and setting

This was a prospective descriptive study of patients who presented with nasal bleeding (epistaxis) at Bugando

Medical Centre (BMC) over a three-year period from January 2008 to December 2010. BMC is a consultant, tertiary care and teaching hospital for Weill- Bugando University College of Health Sciences (WBUCHS) and has a bed capacity of 1000.

Study subjects

The study subjects included all patients who presented with epistaxis at BMC during the period under study. These patients were received through Accident & Emergency department, ENT clinic and as referral from other departments. Patients who died before initial assessment and those without next of kin to consent were excluded from the study. Initial assessment included haemodynamic status, type and severity of bleeding. In cases of mild bleed and stable patient history details were noted alongwith. In case of heavy bleed, history was taken after the bleeding was controlled. If there were signs of excessive blood loss and/or patient was in a state of shock, steps were taken to stabilize the patient simultaneously with control of epistaxis. Resuscitation was carried out according to Advanced Trauma Life Support (ATLS) principles. After resuscitation all patients underwent a detailed history taking and a through general examination, systemic examination and examination of the nose, throat and ears with special emphasis to identify the site of bleeding. The patients were subjected to investigations of hematological parameters and radiological evaluation. Blood samples were taken and sent for base line haemoglobin estimation and blood grouping and cross matching when indicated. Other relevant investigations were ordered based on clinical suspicion regarding a particular aetiology. The diagnosis of epistaxis was based on clinical history, physical findings, laboratory and radiological investigations with examination under anaesthesia of the nose, nasopharynx and biopsy. All patients were treated conservatively initially and surgical intervention was considered only when conservative means failed to control the epistaxis.

Conservative (non-surgical) treatment included cauterization of the bleeding site using electrocautery, anterior nasal packing and posterior nasal packing. Surgical treatment included resection of intranasal tumors. Arterial ligation and endovascular embolization were not performed as there were no patients with intractable epistaxis. Successful treatment was defined as no recurrent epistaxis following pack removal or no readmission with epistaxis within 24 hours of hospital discharge.

Data collection, management and Statistical analysis

The data was collected using a pre-tested, structured proforma prepared for the purpose. Data collected included: patient's demographics, cause of epistaxis, anatomical location of bleeding sites, management modalities, need for blood transfusion, length of hospital stay, complications and mortality. The data collected were entered in SPSS version 15.0 for analysis. In descriptive analysis, the mean and standard deviation of continuous variables and percentages of categorical variables were computed

Ethical consideration
Ethical approval to conduct the study was sought from the WBUCHS/BMC joint institutional ethic review committee before the commencement of the study.

Results
During the period under study, a total of 104 patients were studied. Eighty-one (77.9%) patients presented through the accident and emergency units and 23 (22.1%) presented in the otorhinolaryngology Clinic. There were 76 males (73.1%) and 28 females (26.9%) with a male to female ratio of 2.7:1. Their ages ranged between 4 and 82 years (mean 32.24 years). The modal age group was 31-40 years. The commonest cause of epistaxis was trauma (30.8%) followed by idiopathic (26.9%) and hypertension (17.3%) (Table 1). All patients with non-traumatic epistaxis had previous history of nasal bleeding ranging from one to five episodes with a mean of three episodes.

Twelve (11.5%) of the patients had more than one cause of the illness. According to the bleeding site, 92 patients (88.5%) had anterior nasal bleeding, 8 (7.7%) had posterior bleeding and the remaining four (3.8%) patients had non-identifiable bleeding sites. The right nasal cavity (62, 59.6%) was more affected than the left (28, 26.9%). Bilateral involvement was recorded in 14 (13.5%) of cases.

Non surgical measures were the main intervention methods in 98.1% of cases. Of this, observation alone without active intervention to arrest bleeding and anterior nasal packing were most common non-surgical measures accounting for 40.4% and 38.5% respectively. Surgical measures mainly tumor resection was carried

out in 1.9% of cases (Table 2). Blood transfusion was required in 18 (17.3%) of cases.

The overall success rate of treatment was 92.0%. Success rates for various treatment modalities are shown in table 3 below.

Prophylactic broad spectrum antibiotics were prescribed in all patients who had nasal packing, local cauterization and those who underwent surgical resection of intranasal tumors.

The majority of patients 64 (61.5%) were admitted in the ENT wards and the remaining 40 (38.5%) were treated as outpatients. Two (3.1%) patients among the inpatients had severe head injuries and were admitted in the ICU for ventilatory support. Most of in-patients were discharged between 1 day and 7 days after treatment. Six complications were recorded in four patients giving a complication rate of 3.8%. Of these, Hypovolemic shock and recurrent epistaxis were the most common complications accounting for 33.3% each respectively (Table 4).

The overall mean of duration of hospital stay (LOS) was 7.2 days (range 1 day to 24 days). On the average, patients who have undergone cauterization of the bleeding site required hospitalization for 5.6 days compared to those with anterior nasal packing who had a mean LOS stay of 6.8 days (P < 0.05). Those requiring posterior nasal packing were hospitalized for an average of 10.6 days (P > 0.05).

The majority of patients (90.4%) had good recovery. The details of outcome of patients are shown in table 5

In this study, five patients died giving a mortality rate of 4.8%. The causes of death were; associated severe head injuries in two patients, cardiac arrest during resuscitation, associated tension pneumothorax and nasopharyngeal carcinoma in one patient each respectively.

Discussion
In this review, epistaxis was found to be more prevalent in the young adults, which is in agreement with Eziyi et al [10] but contrary to findings by Pallin et al [8] who found a bimodal age-related frequency with peaks

Table 1 Causes of epistaxis

Causes of epistaxis	Frequency	Percentage
Trauma	32	30.8
Idiopathic	28	26.9
Hypertension	18	17.3
Inflammatory diseases (chronic rhinosinusitis)	6	5.8
Tumors (benign/malignancies)	5	4.8
Iatrogenic	5	4.8
Foreign bodies	4	3.8
Mucosal irritation	3	2.9
Blood dyscrasias	2	1.9
Congenital	1	1.0

Table 2 Treatment modalities

Treatment modality	Number of patients	Percentage
Observation alone	42	40.4
Anterior nasal packing	40	38.5
Posterior nasal packing ± Foley catheter balloon	12	11.5
Local cauterization (electrocautery)	8	7.7
Surgical excision of bleeding intranasal tumor	2	1.9
More than one procedure	16	15.4

Table 3 Success rates for various treatment modalities

Treatment modality	Number of patients	Number of patients treated successfully	Success rate (%)
Anterior nasal packing	40	37	92.5
Posterior nasal packing	12	11	91.7
Anterior + posterior nasal packing	13	12	92.3
Local cauterization (electrocautery)	8	7	87.5
Surgical resection of bleeding nasal tumor	2	2	100

among those younger than 10 years and aged 70-79 years. Varshney and Saxena [11] in India reported most of their patients to be older than 40 years which correlates with other reports which showed that epistaxis is a geriatric problem. The low age incidence in our study may be attributed to the fact that the majority of our patients had traumatic epistaxis and patients with traumatic epistaxis tended to be younger than those with atraumatic epistaxis [6-8].

In the present study, epistaxis was found to affect more males than females, with a male to female ratio of 2.7:1. This male preponderance has been documented in literature [10,12-14]. Globally there is a male preponderance in epistaxis except in the geriatric age group in some reports where no significant sex difference exists [11]. The male preponderance in this study may be attributed to high incidence of traumatic epistaxis which tends to affect young males because of their frequent involvement in high risk taking behaviour. Young males are the most active in the population and so are more vulnerable to trauma from nose picking especially among children, fights, road traffic accident with maxillofacial injuries causing epistaxis.

The present study shows that the most common cause of epistaxis was trauma followed by idiopathic and hypertension, which is consistent with other studies in developing countries [10,15,16]. This trauma varied from minor injury such as digital trauma to varying degrees of nasal injury from road traffic injury. The nose being a prominent feature on the face is highly susceptible in craniofacial injury. Most of our patients with epistaxis from trauma were actually victims of road traffic injury. Trauma being the most common cause of epistaxis can partly explain the frequency of this problem in males. This group is the adventurous group in our community. They are often on the road in search of economic well-being thereby making them prone to

such accidents. High incidence of traumatic epistaxis resulting from road traffic crashes in our study calls for urgent preventive measures targeting at reducing the occurrence of RTCs in order to reduce the incidence of epistaxis in this region.

Findings in most western literature, cites idiopathic causes as the commonest, followed by trauma [11-14]. In the present study, idiopathic epistaxis was the next most common form of epistaxis after trauma. This is in discordance with what was found in the Eastern part of Nigeria where it represented the dominant form [12].

Hypertension being the third commonest cause in this report shows epistaxis as evidence of poor blood pressure control. This is in keeping with an earlier report from Nigeria of some patients who had epistaxis when their hypertension was not controlled due to cessation of antihypertensive drug therapy [17]. Varsney and Saxena [11] in India recorded hypertension as the second commonest cause of epistaxis after idiopathic causes while Chaiyasate et al [15] in Thailand reported hypertension to be the commonest cause of epistaxis followed by idiopathic causes. The need for regular blood pressure check and compliance to antihypertensive medications must be emphasized.

The management of epistaxis is well summarized in an age-old dictum: resuscitate the patient, establish the bleeding site, stop the bleeding and treat the cause of epistaxis [18]. Dealing with a patient with active severe epistaxis can be bloody. The authors recommend universal precautions for all health care personnel involved in the care of these patients, including face mask with shields, gowns, hair coverage, and double-gloving. The key to controlling most epistaxis is to find the site of the bleeding and cauterizing with silver nitrate or bipolar diathermy [18,19]. The goal of treatment include:

Table 4 Frequency of complications (n = 6)

Complications	Frequency	Percentage
Hypovolemic shock	2	33.3
Recurrent epistaxis	2	33.3
Toxic shock syndrome	1	16.7
Facial edema	1	16.7

Table 5 Outcome of patients

Outcome of patients	Number of patients	Percentage
Good recovery	94	90.4
Discharged on request	2	1.9
Left against medical advice	2	1.9
Referred	1	1.0
Died	5	4.8
Total	104	100

hemostasis, short hospital stay, low complication and cost effectiveness of the method of therapy [5,11,18]. Controversy exists concerning the treatment that will best accomplish these goals. Treatment modalities can be separated into two groups; nonsurgical/ion-intervention/conservative and surgical/interventional approaches. Non-surgical approach has been reported to stop the bleeding in more than 80-90% of cases [19]. Anterior nasal packing with gauzed glove finger packing was the most frequent modality of treatment in this study. This form of treatment was reported as an effective treatment in some centers in Nigeria [12], although materials used for the packing vary from center to center. The few patients that had posterior nasal packing were mainly patients with hypertension. Posterior nasal packing was performed using gauze or balloon Foley catheters inserted in the nasopharynx via the nostrils and inflated with sterile water. Anterior nasal packing was used in 38.5% of patients and was successful in 92.5% of them, while posterior nasal packing was successful in 91.7% of the cases where it was tried. Urvashi et al [20] reported successful use of anterior nasal packing in 83.5% case while posterior nasal pack was successful in 95.6% of cases. Nasal packing has the advantage of easy placement and removal; there was no need for an anesthetist or theatre space for that treatment. It is also affordable to the patients. Complications of nasal packing include septal hematoma, sinusitis, syncope during insertion of nasal pack, pressure necrosis of the alae nasi, toxic shock syndrome [20]. Most of our patients did not suffered this due to adequate precautions such as technique of insertion of the pack, use of antibiotics and nasal decongestant were administered as some of the adjunct treatment to forestall this. Only one patient in our study developed toxic shock syndrome. The authors recommend use of prophylactic systemic antibiotics and nasal packing with antibiotic soaked gauze to minimize this complication.

Cautery of the bleeding site can be performed chemically, electrically or with laser [21] though we used only electrical cautery. Cauterization with laser or chemical (Silver nitrate) was not used in our study because of their high costs and lack of availability. Cauterization in the form of electrical cautery was carried out for a group of patients where the bleeding points could be identified during examination. Electrical cauterization was used successfully in 87.5% of cases. This figure was higher than that reported by Urvashi et al [20] in India. Nemer & Mottassim [22] in Jordan reported a success rate of 74.0% which is lower than that of ours. We did not encounter any post cautery complications such as septal perforation or cartilage exposure. Since cauterization of the bleeding point entails a good success rate and no complications it should therefore be the preferred modality of treatment where ever the bleeding site can be visualized. Rigid nasal endoscopy as part of the initial assessment in patients with epistaxis, with direct visualization and control of the bleeding point has been shown to be effective in the majority of patients, reducing the need for nasal packing [18].

In this study, surgical treatment was done only in 1.9% of patients who presented with bleeding intranasal tumor and it was successful in 100% of them. Similar finding was also reported in Nigeria [17]. No surgical ligation of any vessel or endovascular embolization was carried out on any patient in this study. Arterial ligation and embolization of feeding vessels are the last resort for intractable epistaxis [23]. Selection of the artery depends upon the area of the nasal cavity whether upper or lower half or angiographic findings. Choice is usually between anterior ethmoidal artery or internal maxillary artery through an external approach. However, Sphenopalatine artery, termination of internal maxillary artery, may be ligated endosmotically [24,25]. Embolization of feeding vessels may be an option in these cases, but carries high risk of complications [26]. The risks of surgical treatment include the risk of anaesthesia, blindness, oro-antral fistula, ophthalmoplegia, cosmetic deformity, infra orbital nerve dysfunction. These complications were not observed in our study.

The rate of blood transfusion for epistaxis has been reported in literature to range between 6.92 - 15.1% which is less than our blood transfusion rate in our study [11,14]. This high rate of blood transfusion is probably due to severe acute blood loss from the trauma sustained.

The use of antimicrobial prophylaxis in the presence of nasal packing for the treatment epistaxis remains controversial [18,27]. Most of literatures recommend that patients with high risk nasal packing should be started on prophylactic antibiotics, due to an increased risk for sinusitis and toxic shock syndrome. Blood soaked pack and raw mucosal surface are good media for bacterial multiplication resulting in infection including sinusitis and sometimes toxic shock syndromes [28].

The mean length of hospital stay in our stay was 7.2 days which is higher than that reported by other authors [10,22]. Patients who underwent local cauterization were found to have significant shorter LOS compared to those with anterior nasal packing. Those requiring posterior nasal packing remained in hospital for an average of 11.6 days which is higher compared to those with local cauterization or anterior nasal packing. From our observations of average hospital stay with different treatment modalities, we are able to infer that cauterization of the bleeding point reduces hospital stay as compared to anterior nasal packing. However, the difference was not significant comparing anterior nasal packing and posterior nasal packing. Availability of nasal endoscopes which offers both proper visualization and direct facility for endoscopic cauterization to the area that is not easily accessible may have been able to further reduce the hospital stay and the discomfort of postnasal packing.

Our mortality rate in the present study was found to be high than that reported in other studies [10,16,17]. The factors responsible for this finding in our study were; associated severe head injuries, cardiac arrest associated tension pneumothorax and nasopharyngeal cancer.

Conclusion

Trauma resulting from road traffic crush (RTC) remains the most common etiological factor for epistaxis in our setting. Most cases were successfully managed with conservative (non-surgical) treatment alone such as nasal packing and local cauterization. Non-surgical treatment is still useful to arrest nasal bleeding and it is safe and cost-effective, and surgical intervention should be the last resort. Reducing the incidence of trauma from RTC will reduce the incidence of emergency epistaxis in our centre.

Acknowledgements

The authors acknowledge all those who provided care to our patients and those who provided support in preparation of this manuscript.

Authors' contributions

JMG designed the study, contributed in literature search, data analysis, manuscript writing & editing. PLC participated in study design, data analysis, manuscript writing, editing and submission of the manuscript. All the authors read and approved the final manuscript.

Authors' information

JMG: Senior Consultant General/ENT surgeon, Senior Lecturer and Head, Department of Surgery, Well Bugando University Collage of Health Sciences. PLC: Consultant general surgeon and Lecturer, Department of Surgery, Well Bugando University Collage of Health Sciences

Competing interests

The authors declare that they have no competing interests.

References

1. Akinpelu OV, Amusa YB, Eziyi JA, Nwawolo CC: **A retrospective analysis of aetiology and management of epistaxis in a south-western Nigerian teaching hospital.** *West Afr J Med* 2009, **28**:165-8.
2. Pond F, Sizeland A: **Epistaxis. Strategies for management.** *Aust Fam Physician* 2000, **29**:933-8.
3. Yueng-Hsiang C, Jih-Chin L: **Unilateral Epistaxis.** *New England Journal of Medicine* 2009, **361**(9):14.
4. Ciaran SH, Owain H: **Update on management of epistaxis.** *The West London Medical Journal* 2009, **1**:33-41.
5. Walker TWM, Macfarlane TV, McGarry GW: **The epidemiology and chronobiology of epistaxis: an investigation of Scottish hospital admissions 1995-2004.** *Clin Otolaryngol* 2007, **32**:361-5.
6. Pope LER, Hobbs CGL: **Epistaxis: an update on current management.** *Postgrad Med J* 2005, **81**:309-314.
7. Nash CM, Field SMB: **Epidemiology of Epistaxis in a Canadian Emergency Department.** *Israeli Journal of Emergency Medicine* 2008, **8**:24-28.
8. Pallin DJ, Chng Y, McKay MP, Emond JA, Pelletier AJ, Camargo CA: **Epidemiology of epistaxis in US emergency departments, 1992 to 2001.** *Ann Emerg Med* 2005, **46**:77-81.
9. Bernius M, Perlin D: **Pediatric ear, nose, and throat emergencies.** *Pediatr Clin North Am* 2006, **53**:195.
10. Eziyi JAE, Akinpelu OV, Amusa YB, Eziyi AK: **Epistaxis in Nigerians: A 3-year Experience.** *East Cent Afr J Surg* 2009, **14**(2):93-98.
11. Varshney S, Saxena RK: **Epistaxis: a retrospective clinical study.** *Indian Journal of Otolaryngology, Head Neck Surgery* 2005, **57**:125-129.
12. Mgbor NC: **Epistaxis in Enugu: A 9 year Review.** *Nig J of otolaryngology* 2004, **1**(2):11-14.
13. Huang C, Shu C: **Epistaxis: A review of hospitalized patients.** *Chinese medical journal* 2002, **65**(2):74-78.
14. Kaygusuz I, Karlidag T, Keles E, Yalcin S, Alpay HC, Sakallioglu O: **Retrospective Analysis of 68 Hospitalized Patients with Epistaxis.** *Firat Tip Dergisi* 2004, **9**(3):82-85.
15. Chaiyasate S, Roongrotwattanasiri K, Fooanan S, Sumitsawan Y: **Epistaxis in Chiang Mai University.** *J Med Assoc Thai* 2005, **88**:1282-1286.
16. Ijaduola GTA, Okeowo PA: **Pattern of epistaxis in the tropics.** *Cent Afr J Med* 1983, **29**:77-80.
17. Iseh KR, Muhammad Z: **Pattern of epistaxis in Sokoto, Nigeria: A review of 72 cases.** *Ann Afr Med* 2008, **7**:107-11.
18. Daudia A, Jaiswal V, Jones NS: **Guidelines for the management of idiopathic epistaxis in adults: how we do it.** *Clinical Otolaryngology* 2008, **33**:607-628.
19. Rodney JS: **Epistaxis: A clinical experience.** *New England Journal of Medicine* 2009, **360**:784-9.
20. Urvashi R, Raizada RM, Chaturvedi VN: **Efficacy of conservative treatment modalities used in epistaxis.** *Indian Journal of Otolaryngology and Head and Neck Surgery* 2004, **56**(1):21-23.
21. Wurman LH, Sack GJ, Flannery JV, Lipsman RA: **The management of epistaxis.** *American Journal of Otolaryngology* 1992, **13**(4):193-209.
22. Nemer AK, Motassim AR: **Evaluation of conservative measures in the treatment of epistaxis.** *Khartoum Medical Journal* 2008, **1**(1):15-17.
23. Awan MS, Ali MM, Hussain T, Mian MY: **Management of pediatrics Epistaxis; A prospective study of 100 cases.** *Professional Med J* 2001, **8**(2):226-65.
24. Feusi B, Holzmann D, Steurer J: **Posterior epistaxis: systematic review on the effectiveness of surgical therapies.** *Rhinology* 2005, **43**(4):300-4.
25. Umapathy N, Quadri A, Skinner DW: **Persistent epistaxis: what is the best practice?** *Rhinology* 2005, **43**(4):305-8.
26. Andersen PJ, Kjeldsen AD, Nepper-Rasmussen J: **Selective embolization in the treatment of intractable epistaxis.** *Acta Otolaryngol* 2005, **125**(3):293-7.
27. Biswas D, Wilson H, Mal R: **Use of systemic prophylactic antibiotics with anterior nasal packing in England, UK.** *Clin Otolaryngol* 2006, **31**:566-567.
28. Abhay-Gupta , Agrawal SR, Sivarajan K, Vineeta Gupta: **A Microbiological study of anterior nasal packs in epistaxis.** *Indian Journal of Otolaryngology and Head and neck Surgery* 1999, **15**(1):42-46.

An observational cohort study of the effects of septoplasty with or without inferior turbinate reduction in patients with obstructive sleep apnea

Mads Henrik Strand Moxness[1] and Ståle Nordgård[2,3,4*]

Abstract

Background: The objective of this observational study was to evaluate the outcomes of intranasal surgery in patients with obstructive sleep apnea (OSA) in a single institution in Norway.

Methods: Fifty-nine patients with OSA and clinically significant nasal obstruction underwent either septoplasty alone or septoplasty with concomitant volume reduction of the turbinates from August 2008 until the end of December 2010. Subjects were scheduled for sleep polygraphy before and 3 months after treatment.
In this observational single-centre cohort study we evaluated and compared the effect of these two specific surgical procedures on sleep related parameters.

Results: There was a significant reduction in the apnea-hypopnea index (AHI) only in the group that had septoplasty with turbinate reduction (17.4, (SD 14.4) – 11.7, (SD 8.2), p <0.01), and this effect was significantly better than in the group treated with septoplasty alone. Other objective parameters remained unchanged. Subjective assessments obtained with a postoperative questionnaire showed an equally positive effect on diurnal sleepiness and nasal obstruction in both groups, and a better effect on sleep quality in the combined treatment group.

Conclusion: The effect of nasal surgery on obstructive sleep apnea seemed to be greater when there were indications for combined surgery of the inferior turbinates and the nasal septum, compared to when there were indications for septoplasty alone.

Keywords: Apnea, Nose, Surgery, Septum, Concha, Turbinate

Background

There is growing interest in the field of sleep-related disorders (SRD) and in obstructive sleep apnea (OSA) particularly. This is due to the impact of SRD on global health, and a result of more profound insight into the effects of sleep deprivation, and the biomechanical and physiological changes that occur during the development of upper airway collapse during sleep [1]. The traditional way of understanding the collapsing airway includes both theories of neuromuscular regulation [2] and theories of fluid structure interaction [3]. Surgical treatments for OSA have been performed in several forms over the last 3 decades [4]. To date, tracheotomy is the only surgical procedure with definite and lasting success, but it is regarded as a method with unwanted side effects. Multiple level surgery has gained support, as well as maxillomandibular surgery, but these are also major procedures and the same concerns regarding morbidity apply for these. The effect of limited and less extensive surgery of the upper airways still needs evaluation regarding selection of procedure and results. Nasal surgery has been performed extensively in these patients, often with good effect on quality of life (QOL) measures [5,6]. Still, there is no conclusive evidence of clinical effect, and the different nasal procedures performed are often quite randomly chosen. To our

* Correspondence: stale.nordgard@ntnu.no
[2]The department of Otorhinolaryngology, Head and Neck Surgery, St Olav University Hospital, Trondheim, Norway
[3]The Institute of Neuroscience, The Norwegian University of Science and Technology (NTNU), Trondheim, Norway
Full list of author information is available at the end of the article

knowledge, there are no other clinical studies that compare the results of different nasal procedures for nasal obstruction in patients with OSA. We have evaluated and compared the results of two specific surgical procedures in the nasal cavity, septoplasty alone and septoplasty with simultaneous turbinate volume reduction.

Methods

This study was an observational single-centre cohort study. It was approved by the national regional ethics committee and was registered in Clincaltrials.gov. (NCT01282125). Between August 2008 and December 2010, 78 patients with OSA were treated surgically for nasal obstruction in Aleris Hospital in Trondheim, Norway. Fifty-nine of these had been treated with septoplasty alone or septoplasty combined with volume reductive surgery of the turbinates. Group 1 (n = 33) consisted of patients who had undergone septoplasty alone, and group 2 (n = 26) of patients treated with combined septoplasty and volume reductive surgery. The remaining patients underwent rhinoseptoplasties (n = 8), functional endoscopic sinus surgery (n = 4) and turbinate resection (n = 7) as single procedures, but the groups were too small to be subanalyzed. All patients in the two analyzed groups underwent traditional cartilage preserving septoplasty under general anesthesia. The volume reductive surgery comprised radiofrequency tissue ablation (n = 10) (BM 780-II, Sutter Medizintechnik Gmbh), lateral fracture of the lower turbinate (n = 15), and surgical reduction of concha bullosa (n = 1).

The patients were referred to the sleep clinic for suspected OSA from either primary care physicians or ENT specialists within a specific geographical area. All patients underwent a nocturnal sleep evaluation with an Embletta™ Portable Diagnostic System (ResMed, San Diego, California, USA) or a Reggie polygraph (Camtech, Oslo, Norway) and a clinical examination. There were no prior history of nasal surgery or prolonged use of nasal steroids. None of the patients were diagnosed with chronic rhinosinusitis or enlarged adenoids. Patients with confirmed OSA and clinically significant nasal obstruction due to a septal deviation with or without hypertrophy of turbinates were offered intranasal surgery as a first line of treatment. The decision to supplement septoplasty with volume reductive surgery in selected patients was based on the clinical evaluation, and not supported by objective measurements. If there were a coherence between the patients complaints of nasal blockage on both sides, and there was obvious swelling of the inferior turbinates that was relieved after decongestion with tetracain/adrenalin over 5-10 minutes in the office, one would recommend that turbinate reduction should be performed at the time of the septal surgery. Only patients with apnea-hypopnea index (AHI) >5

and BMI <35 were included. All patients used saline irrigation 6-8 times a day for two weeks postoperatively. No intranasal steroids were administered. Optional pain relief was 50 mg of diclofenac sodium three times a day and 30-60 mg of codein phosphate in combination with 500 mg of paracetamol. The same surgeon (MM) treated all but one patient. The patients were informed of the possibility of crusting in the nose for a period up to three weeks after surgery, but there were no postoperative infections and no necrosis or loss of nasal function at the follow up three months later.

The effects of intranasal surgery on OSA were evaluated routinely after 3 months with a repeated polygraph. Subjective assessment of daytime sleepiness was evaluated using the Epworth Sleepiness Scale (ESS) preoperatively and 3 months postoperatively. In a dichotomous questionnaire, the patients were asked to evaluate the effects of surgery on nasal obstruction and the subjective quality of sleep. At the same time a written informed consent was obtained from all the participants. The alternatives in the questionnaire were: 1. Did you experience an effect on your nasal obstruction after surgery? Yes or No. 2. Did you experience an effect on your sleep quality after surgery? Yes or No. If patients reported a positive outcome, they were asked to supplement the answer with a visual analog scale (VAS) in which their agreement of surgical effect was graded in a continuous scale ranging from 0 = no agreement to 10 = full agreement. Scores between 0-3 were defined as "mild", scores >3-7 were defined as "moderate", and scores >7-10 were considered "good" [7]. The primary outcome was alterations in the AHI, oxygen desaturation index (ODI), body mass index (BMI) and Epworth Sleepiness Scale (ESS) in the two groups. The secondary outcome was to evaluate the effect of surgery on sleep quality and nasal obstruction reported in the questionnaire. SPSS 19.0 was used for the statistical evaluations. Preoperative and postoperative values were evaluated using the Wilcoxon matched-pairs test in continuous variables without normal distribution (ODI, ESS). Variables with normal distribution (BMI, AHI) were evaluated using the paired t-test. The values for AHI were transformed using natural logarithm in order to create a normal distribution. An independent t-test was used to compare the changes of the objective measures and VAS after surgery between group 1 and 2. Differences with p <0.05 were considered significant.

Results

In both groups, there was a predominance of males (97% in group 1 and 85% in group 2), and the mean age was 47.5 (30 − 68) in group 1 and 45.3 (23 - 68) in group 2. The groups did not differ significantly regarding preoperative AHI, ODI, ESS, Mallampati score, age, gender or BMI. We looked at changes in the objective parameters before and after surgery in three ways: the overall changes in both groups pooled together, changes within each group, and the changes in the mean difference between the groups (Table 1). Overall, in both groups together, there was no significant reduction in mean AHI after surgery: 18.1 (±13.7) - 16.6 (±12.9), (95% CI -1.84, 4.83), p = 0.365, mean ODI: 14.2 (±12.3) – 12.4 (±10.7), (95% CI -1.16, 4.75), p = 0.229 or mean BMI: 28.1 (±3.2) – 28.3 (±3.0), (95% CI – 0.673, 0.285), p = 0.422. The reduction in mean ESS, however, was highly statistically significant: 10.7 (±3.7) – 8.9 (±3.8), (CI 1.00, 2.61), p <0.001. In comparison, when we looked at each group separately, we found a significant reduction in group 2 in mean AHI: 17.4 (±14.4) – 11.7 (±8.2), (95% CI 0.004, 0.006), p = 0.007 and mean ESS: 9.7 (±3.4) – 7.6 (±2.2), (95% CI 0.004, 0.006), p = 0.006. In group 1 there was no significant reduction in mean AHI, ODI or BMI after surgery, but there was a significant reduction in the mean ESS score: 11.5 (±3.7) – 10.0 (±4.5), (95% CI 0.53, 2.54), p = 0.004. The changes in mean

ODI levels did not fall below the 0.05 level of significance in either category, although there were near significant values in group 2. The reduction in the difference of mean AHI after surgery was significant between the groups: 1,7 (±8,8) – 5,7 (±16,1), (95% CI 0.8, 14.0), p = 0.029, but the effects on ESS, ODI and BMI were not significant between the two groups . Success criteria defined as a postoperative drop in AHI <20 and/or 50% reduction in AHI [8] were met by 15.2% (5/33) in group 1, and by 27% (7/26) in group 2, but the difference in surgical success was not statistically significant. There were 76% questionnaire responders in group 1 and 77% in group 2. In group 1, 96% answered that the procedure was effective with regard to nasal obstruction, and 68% that it improved their quality of sleep. In group 2 the corresponding percentages were 85% and 80%. The difference between the groups was not statistically significant. A significantly larger proportion in group 2 reported a good improvement in sleep quality: mean 0.08 (±0.27) – mean 0.35 (±0.49), (95% CI 0.037, 0.503), p = 0.024 (Figure 1).

Discussion

Intranasal surgery is currently regarded as important in order to improve compliance with treatment using nasal continuous positive airway pressure (CPAP)/bilevel positive airway pressure (BiPAP) devices in patients with OSA. The impact of intranasal surgery on objective measurements in OSA patients is unclear, but is regarded as limited, as shown by Verse et al in 2002 [9]. In a rare blinded randomized controlled study with sham surgery (septal resection +/- turbinectomies) in 2008, Koutserelakis et al [10] found responders only in the real surgery group. They concluded that nasal surgery rarely treats OSA effectively. In a meta-analysis of 13 studies that dealt with nasal surgery alone in OSA patients [11], the reviewers concluded that nasal surgery for obstruction alone does not reduce AHI significantly but ameliorates daytime sleepiness and clinical symptoms of snoring. Only one of these studies described a statistically significant reduction in AHI [12]. However, the observation period in this study was only 1 month as opposed to 3 months in ours, and the study group was mixed and underwent either septal resection alone or combined with turbinate surgery. One study by Li et al [13] described a homogenous patient group comparable to ours with septal deviation and hypertrophic inferior turbinates (n = 44). They found no significant effect of surgery on AHI, and a lower success rate of 16%. The procedure differed somewhat from ours in that only septal resections were performed under local anesthesia. It may indicate that the impact of the septal deviation on nasal obstruction preoperatively or postoperatively differs from that in our study. In surgical practice different nasal procedures are often performed simultaneously, and previous clinical

Table 1 Baseline values and postoperative values

Preoperative values	Septoplasty		Septoplasty and volume reduction		Overall results	
	Mean	SD	Mean	SD	Mean	SD
AHI	18.75	13.36	17.39	14.38	18.15	13.71
ODI	14.29	12.00	14.12	12.73	14.21	12.22
ESS	11.54	3.72	9.74	3.42	10.74	3.67
BMI	28.33	3.40	27.80	3.05	28.10	3.23
Postoperative values	Mean	SD	Mean	SD	Mean	SD
AHI	20.46	14.64	11.70	8.19	16.60	12.90
ODI	14.87	12.25	9.30	7.36	12.42	10.67
ESS	10.00	4.51	7.59	2.18	8.94	3.84
BMI	28.69	3.12	27.77	2.70	28.28	2.95
P-values of the difference						
AHI	0.273		0.007		0.365	
ODI	0.671		0.064		0.229	
ESS	0.004		0.006		<0.001	
BMI	0.202		0.716		0.422	
P-values of the difference between treatment groups						
AHI			0.029			
ODI			0.069			
ESS			0.454			
BMI			0.429			

There are no significant differences at baseline between the groups. There is a significant reduction of AHI between the two surgery groups.

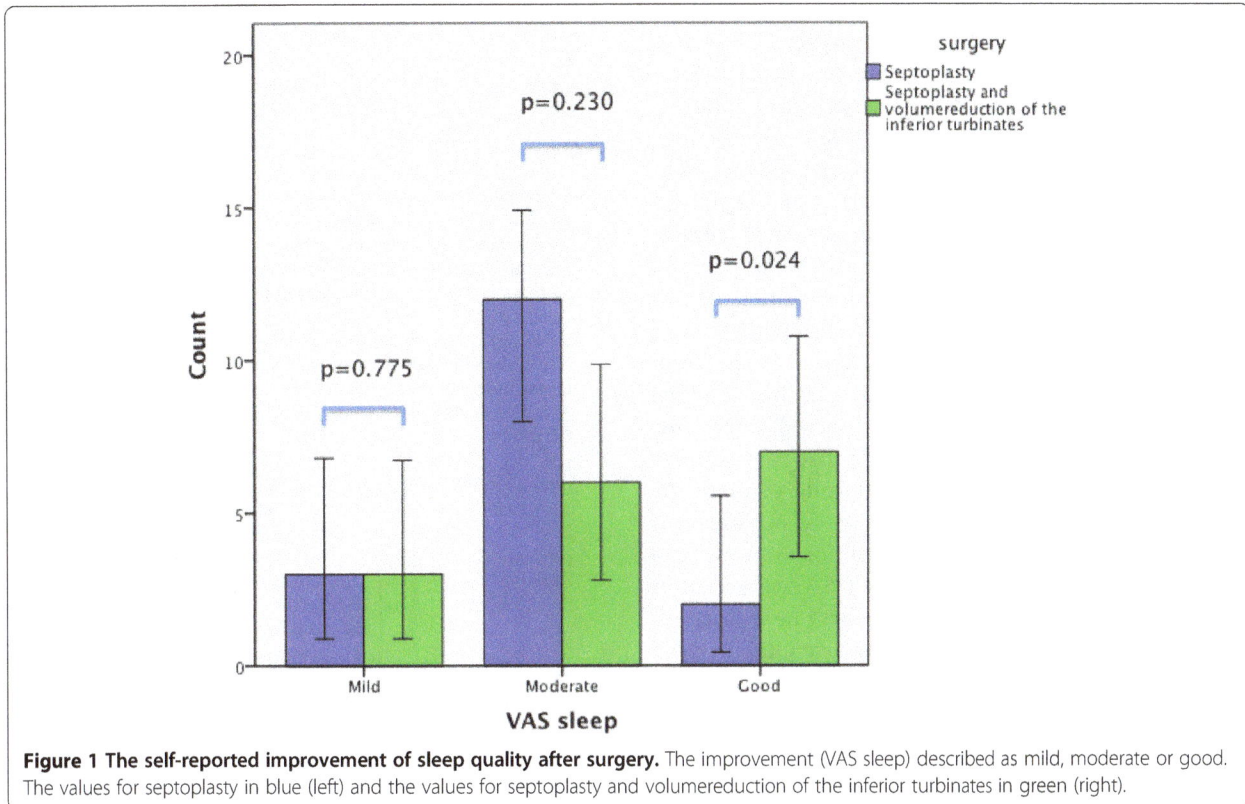

Figure 1 The self-reported improvement of sleep quality after surgery. The improvement (VAS sleep) described as mild, moderate or good. The values for septoplasty in blue (left) and the values for septoplasty and volumereduction of the inferior turbinates in green (right).

studies represent no exception [9,10,12,14,15]. If we had presented the results pooled as a single study group, without a comparison of the two different surgical approaches, we would have missed the statistically significant improvement in patients with combined surgical treatment. Assessments of the overall effect of nasal surgery on OSA predict that 16.7% will have a reduction in AHI [10] that meets the criteria by Sher [8,9]. In this observational study, we singled out two different intranasal surgical procedures for comparison and found that there were statistical differences in the outcome of AHI between septoplasty alone and septoplasty combined with volume reductive surgery in OSA patients. Using the same Sher criteria, we found a near twofold increase in treatment success in the combined surgery group compared with the septoplasty group. This difference did not reach statistical significance but it is possible that it would do so in a larger study group as the difference in AHI reduction was significant. One might anticipate that the better effect on OSA might be due to a larger effect on nasal obstruction in patients in need of combined surgery. It is also possible that the additional inferior turbinate hypertrophy affected the laminar airflow and pharyngeal walls negatively to a higher degree, and hence this group achieved a better result after surgery. Li et al [13] found that patients with a low Friedman tongue position had better results from

nasal surgery and Morinaga et al reported less effect in patients with a narrow retroglossal space and high Mallampati score. It may indicate that the increased contribution of pharyngeal structures to OSA will worsen the final results as the percentage of the nasal obstruction is diminished. On the other hand, it may also indicate that the effect of surgery was better for patients with concomitant increased volume of the turbinates and septal deviation because the total contribution of the nasal obstruction to OSA development may have been greater than in patients with septal deviation alone.

In this observational study, there are some limitations that should be taken into consideration. The number of patients in group 2 is low and could represent a statistical uncertainty. There is a higher night-to-night sleep polygraph variation regarding AHI in mild or moderate sleep apnea than in severe apnea that may influence the results on an individual basis [16]. This might suggest that a follow-up study should be performed in patients for whom there is a discrepancy between subjective and objective results. Furthermore, there is a lack of objective measuring of nasal obstruction in an outpatient setting that would otherwise help the surgeon in deciding which type of surgery to perform. Our study is an observational cohort study, and the patients were therefore not randomized to specific treatment groups. As a result, we cannot conclude that combined surgery is better than septoplasty alone in all patients with clinical indications for septal surgery. There may also be possible side effects of supplementing volume reductive surgery in all OSA patients with septal deformities, and this approach should be avoided. However, the results for OSA in our material seemed to be better when both turbinate hypertrophy and septal deviation were treated. Even though combined surgery does not imply a cure for the majority of the patients, there was a reduction of symptoms, verified by the questionnaire, which indicates that 80% perceived an improvement in their quality of sleep after the combined surgery. This study then supports the view that an effect on daytime sleepiness is observed more often than on obstructive apnea and hence that nasal surgery alone is best suited for patients with mild or moderate obstructive sleep apnea. As long as we do not have any single treatment that provides a cure for OSA and not all patients with mild and moderate OSA will accept or tolerate CPAP or oral devices, there will be a place for targeted surgical treatments that improve QOL in these patients.

Conclusion

In this observational cohort study, the effect on AHI was significantly better when indication for septoplasty combined with surgery of the inferior turbinates was present, compared to septoplasty alone. The overall effect in both groups pooled together showed no significant effect on reduction of the objective parameters but a significant reduction in the subjective ESS score. This implies that intranasal surgery has a good effect on the subjective quality of sleep in OSA patients, and that there might be an added effect on AHI in selected patients with both septal deviation and hypertrophy of the inferior turbinates. Future randomized and prospective studies that can identify responders to nasal surgery as well as what type of intranasal surgery needed.

Competing interests
The authors declare that they have no competing interests, neither financially nor non-financially.

Authors' contributions
MM performed the surgery, collected the sleep related perameters, analysed data and contributed in writing the manuscript. SN contributed to design, analysed and interpreted data, contributed in writing the manuscript, and reviewed the final version. Both authors read and approved the final manuscript.

Acknowledgements
Part of the work was funded by Unimed Innovation AS, St Olav University Hospital, Trondheim, Norway and Center for Endoscopic Nasal and Sinus surgery, Aleris Hospital Trondheim, Norway.
The authors want to thank Margaret Forbes as language editor.

Author details
[1]Center for Endoscopic Nasal and Sinus surgery, Aleris Hospital Trondheim, Trondheim, Norway. [2]The department of Otorhinolaryngology, Head and Neck Surgery, St Olav University Hospital, Trondheim, Norway. [3]The Institute of Neuroscience, The Norwegian University of Science and Technology (NTNU), Trondheim, Norway. [4]Post: Department of Neuroscience, NTNU, The Medical Faculty, N-7489 Trondheim, Norway.

References

1. Mullington JM, Haack M, Toth M, Serrador J, Meier-Ewert H: **Cardiovascular, inflammatory and metabolic consequences of sleep deprivation.** *Prog Cardiovasc Dis* 2009, **51**(4):294–302.
2. Longobardo GS, Evangelisti CJ, Cherniack NS: **Analysis of the interplay between neurochemical control of respiration and upper airway mechanics producing upper airway obstruction during sleep in humans.** *Exp Physiol* 2008, **93**(2):271–287.
3. Van Hirtum A, Pelorson X, Lagrée PY: **In vitro validation of some flow assumptions for the prediction of the pressure distribution during obstructive sleep apnea.** *Med Biol Eng Comput* 2005, **43**(1):162–171.
4. Powell NB: **Contemporary surgery for obstructive sleep apnea syndrome.** *Clin Exp Otorhinolaryngol* 2009, **2**(3):107–114.
5. Li H, Lin Y, Chen N, Lee L, Fang T, Wang P: **Improvement in quality of life after nasal surgery alone for patients with obstructive sleep apnea and nasal obstruction.** *Arch Otolaryngol Head and Neck Surg* 2008, **134**(4):429–433.
6. Georgolas C: **The role of the nose in snoring and obstructive sleep apnoea: an update.** *Eur Arch Otorhinolaryngol* 2011, **268**(9):1365–1373.
7. Fokkens WJ, Lund VJ, Mullol J, Bachert C, Alobid I, Baroody F, Cohen N, Cervin A, Douglas R, Gevaert P, Georgalas C, Goossens H, Harvey R, Hellings P, Hopkins C, Jones N, Joos G, Kalogjera L, Kern B, Kowalski M, Price D, Riechelmann H, Schlosser R, Senior B, Thomas M, Toskala E, Voegels R, Wang de Y, Wormald PJ: **EPOS 2012: European postion paper on rhinosinusitis and nasal polyps 2012. A summary for otorhinolaryngologists.** *Rhinology* 2012, **50**(1):1–12.
8. Sher AE, Schechtman KB, Piccirillo JF: **The efficacy of surgical modifications of the upper airway in adults with obstructive sleep apnea syndrome.** *Sleep* 1996, **19**(2):156–177.
9. Verse T, Maurer JT, Pirsig W: **Effect of nasal surgery on sleep-related breathing disorders.** *Laryngoscope* 2002, **112**(1):64–68.
10. Koutserelakis I, Georgoulopoulos G, Perraki E, Vagiakis E, Roussos C, Zakynthinos SG: **Randomised trial of nasal surgery for fixed nasal obstruction in obstructive sleep apnea.** *Eur Respir J* 2008, **31**(1):110–117.
11. Li HY, Wang PC, Chen YP, Lee LA, Fang TJ, Lin HC: **Critical appraisal and meta-analysis of nasal surgery for obstructive sleep apnea.** *Am J Rhinol Allergy* 2011, **25**(1):45–49.
12. Kim ST, Choi JH, Jeon HG, Cha HE, Kim DY, Chung YS: **Polysomnographic effects of nasal surgery for snoring and obstructive sleep apnea.** *Acta Otolaryngol* 2004, **124**:297–300.
13. Li HY, Lee LA, Wang PC, Fang TJ, Chen NH: **Can nasal surgery improve obstructive sleep apnea: Subjective or objective?** *Am J Rhinol Allergy* 2009, **23**:e51–e55.
14. Friedman M, Tanyeri H, Lim JW, Landsberg R, Vaidyanathan K, Caldarelli D: **Effect of improved nasal breathing on obstructive sleep apnea.** *Otolaryngol Head Neck Surg* 2000, **122**:71–74.
15. Morinaga M, Nakata S, Yasuma F, Noda A, Yagi H, Tagaya M, Suqiura M, Teranishi M, Nakashima T: **Pharyngeal morphology: A determinant of successful nasal surgery for sleep apnea.** *Laryngoscope* 2009, **119**:1011–1016.
16. Rollheim J, Tvinnereim M, Sitek J, Osnes T: **Repeatibility of sites of sleep-induced upper airway obstruction. A 2-night study based on recordings of airway pressure and flow.** *Eur Arch Otorhinolaryngol* 2001, **258**(5):259–264.

Hidden consequences of olfactory dysfunction: a patient report series

Andreas Keller[1*] and Dolores Malaspina[2,3]

Abstract

Background: The negative consequences of olfactory dysfunction for the quality of life are not widely appreciated and the condition is therefore often ignored or trivialized.

Methods: 1,000 patients with olfactory dysfunction participated in an online study by submitting accounts of their subjective experiences of how they have been affected by their condition. In addition, they were given the chance to answer 43 specific questions about the consequences of their olfactory dysfunction.

Results: Although there are less practical problems associated with impaired or distorted odor perception than with impairments in visual or auditory perception, many affected individuals report experiencing olfactory dysfunction as a debilitating condition. Smell loss-induced social isolation and smell loss-induced anhedonia can severely affect quality of life.

Conclusions: Olfactory dysfunction is a serious condition for those affected by it and it deserves more attention from doctors who treat affected patients as well as from scientist who research treatment options.

Keywords: Olfaction, Quality of life, Anosmia, Phantosmia, Parosmia, Anhedonia

Background

Two recent patient memoires describe vividly the often unanticipated consequences of changes to one's sense of smell from the patient's perspective [1,2]. Olfactory perceptual changes can be quantitative (smell loss) or qualitative (smell distortions). Smell loss can be partial, a condition called hyposmia, or total, a condition called anosmia. Patients with partial smell loss often also suffer from distorted olfactory perception. Distorted olfactory perception can be subdivided into parosmia (distorted olfactory experiences in the presence of an odor) and phantosmia (distorted olfactory experience in the absence of an odor) [for overviews, see [3,4]]. Phantosmia and parosmia often co-occur [5] and parosmia is more common than phantosmia [5-8].

Olfactory dysfunction is a very common condition with a reported prevalence between 4 and 25% [9-12]. Men are more likely to suffer from it than women [13,14] and smoking [9-11,15-17], working in a factory

environment [18], low level of education [19], and having a low household income [9] have been reported as risk factors. Olfactory dysfunction, like visual and auditory impairment, becomes more prevalent with increasing age [12,20]. Of those who suffer from smell loss, between 10 and 60% also have distorted olfactory perceptions [5,8,21,22]. Distorted perception is more common when the smell loss is less severe [22].

There are many causes of olfactory dysfunction [for an overview, see [23,24]]. The three most common causes are sinonasal disease, upper respiratory infection, and head trauma (Figure 1). Sinonasal diseases like nasal polyps or chronic inflammation of the nasal passages and/or paranasal sinuses (rhinitis, sinusitis, rhinosinusitis) are the most common cause of olfactory dysfunction (Figure 1) [for an overview see [30-32]]. Chronic inflammation in the nose and sinuses is the most common chronic medical condition in the United States of America [33-35] and more than half of the affected individuals have olfactory symptoms [36]. The cause of the olfactory problems in sinonasal diseases is in many cases nasal obstruction. The second most common cause of olfactory dysfunction are upper respiratory tract infections that result in permanent

* Correspondence: Andreas.Keller@rockefeller.edu
[1]Laboratory of Neurogenetics and Behavior, Rockefeller University, New York, NY, USA
Full list of author information is available at the end of the article

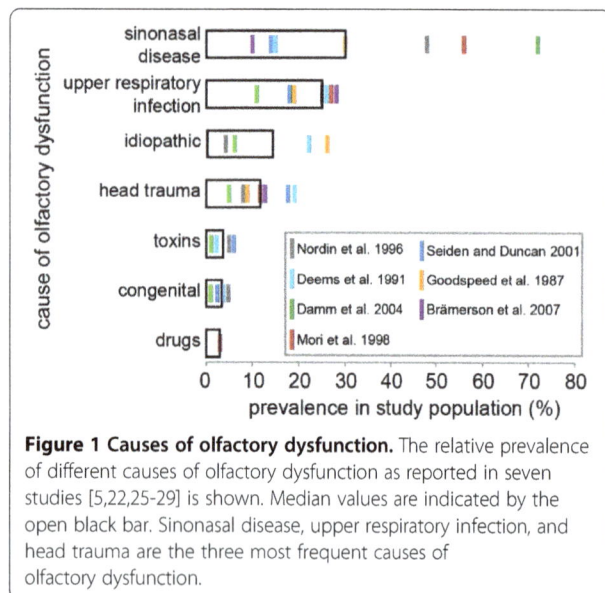

Figure 1 Causes of olfactory dysfunction. The relative prevalence of different causes of olfactory dysfunction as reported in seven studies [5,22,25-29] is shown. Median values are indicated by the open black bar. Sinonasal disease, upper respiratory infection, and head trauma are the three most frequent causes of olfactory dysfunction.

damage to the olfactory sensory system (Figure 1). As a consequence of the damage, smell loss will continue long after the infection and its other symptoms have subsided [for overviews, see [21,37,38]]. Patients with postviral olfactory loss often retain some smell capacity [22,25,39] and olfactory distortion is very common in these patients [8,21,40,41]. The third most common cause of olfactory dysfunction is head trauma (Figure 1) [for an overview, see [42-45]]. Head trauma often leads to very severe olfactory loss [41] with sudden onset. In addition to the three main causes of olfactory dysfunction, surgical procedures [46] (both sinonasal surgeries [47] and other types of surgery [48]) can affect olfactory function. Some of these cases are likely due to side-effects of the drugs used for general anesthesia [49-51]. Other drugs can also have side-effects on olfactory function [52-55]. Similarly, toxic chemicals in the environment can damage the olfactory system [56-60]. Finally, around 3% of those suffering from olfactory dysfunction have congenital anosmia: they were born without a sense of smell (Figure 1) [for an overview, see [61]]. In rare cases, olfactory perception can be disturbed due to processes in the central nervous system, as in epilepsy [62,63], migraine [64,65], Parkinson's disease [66], or schizophrenia [63,67,68].

Not all cases of olfactory dysfunction are permanent. Partial spontaneous recovery has been reported especially in younger patients [69] and in patients with postviral olfactory dysfunction [69-71]. Remarkably, spontaneous recovery can occur years after the symptoms appeared [69,71-73], but the likelihood of recovery decreases with the duration of smell loss [22,69,70]. Olfactory dysfunction caused by sinonasal disease usually fluctuates over time [25] and can be modulated, for example, by physical exercise [26] and hot showers [25]. If olfactory impairment

is a symptom of sinonasal disease, then treating the underlying disease will often improve olfactory function. Among the treatments of sinonasal disease that have been evaluated for their influence on olfactory function are antihistamines [74], nasally and systemically administered corticosteroids [25,75-79], and surgery [46,47,80-85]. For postviral and posttraumatic olfactory loss several treatments have been suggested [for an overview, see [54,86]]. Zinc [87,88], vitamin A [89], and the antibiotic minocycline [90] have been shown to be ineffective in placebo-controlled studies. α-lipoic acid [91] and the phosphodiesterase inhibitors theophylline [92,93] and pentoxifylline [94] have not been tested in placebo-controlled studies yet. Peroral caroverine, an N-methyl-D-aspartic acid (NMDA) receptor antagonist [88], as well as sodium citrate nasal spray [95] have been shown to be effective in placebo-controlled studies. In addition to drug treatments, acupuncture [96-99] and olfactory training [100,101] have also been investigated. It is likely that any successful treatment of smell loss would also improve the associated symptoms of distorted olfactory perception. However, some treatments, like the surgical excision of olfactory sensory neurons [3,102,103], bilateral olfactory nerve sections [104], and repetitive transcranial magnetic stimulation [105] have been specifically targeted at smell distortions.

None of the treatments that have been investigated are in wide use and in most cases olfactory dysfunction is untreatable. This is unfortunate because the disease burden of olfactory dysfunction is high [for an overview, see: [106-108]]. Quality of life in patients with olfactory impairments is reduced compared to matched controls [108] and patients in which the condition improves report a higher satisfaction with life than patients in which the dysfunction persists [109]. Practical problems of olfactory dysfunction include difficulties avoiding hazardous events [110] and the struggle to maintain healthy eating behaviors [70,111-113]. Without a sense of smell, natural gas leaks [109,110,114], fires [109,110,114,115], and hazardous chemical vapors [115] cannot be detected. Similarly, it is more difficult for these individuals to detect spoiled food [70,109,110,114]. In addition, food intake has been reported to be affected by olfactory dysfunction. Some patients report losing weight after losing their sense of smell, while others report gaining weight [112,113]. Weight gain is more common [112]. Both weight gain and weight loss seem to be a consequence of food being less enjoyable in the absence of olfactory input [70,112,115]. In most subjects, in addition to the change in how much food is consumed, olfactory impairment also induced a shift in food preferences. Taste and mechanosensation have to compensate for the lost olfactory input and as a consequence spicy food becomes more attractive [112,116,117].

The practical problems of not being able to sense the odorous environment are exacerbated by smell loss-induced social isolation. The social problems that the condition causes for relationships with friends, colleagues, family members, and romantic partners [27,118,119] are partially a consequence of social insecurity caused by worries about undetected body odor and partially a consequence of frustration over the perceived lack of sympathy for the patients [120]. Interactions with medical service providers can also be a source of frustration. One study showed that in Germany and Switzerland, 25% of patients felt that they had not been managed well and 6% felt that their condition had been trivialized [121].

In addition to practical and social consequences, olfactory loss also correlates with reduced ability to experience pleasure and motivation to engage in pleasurable activities: smell loss-induced anhedonia. Smell loss-induced anhedonia is the least-appreciated consequence of smell loss because affected individuals are often not aware of the connection between their olfactory dysfunction and the reduced enjoyment of formerly enjoyable activities. Although the mechanism is unknown, there is a correlation between smell loss and depressive symptoms and mood changes [22,70,115,118,120,122].

Distorted olfactory perception is even more detrimental to the quality of life than smell loss [3,4,22,123]. In one study, over half of the patients with distorted odor perception reported that their condition *severely* affected their quality of life [40]. Leopold and colleagues write about phantosmia patients that "it is usual for the patients to have thought about suicide because they had been offered no hope for resolution..." [102].

In this paper, the collected first-person accounts from 1,000 patients suffering from olfactory dysfunction confirm that severe consequences of this condition on life style and life satisfaction are common.

Methods

Between 10/16/2009 and 08/08/2012, subjects submitted their experiences with olfactory dysfunction online under the IRB-approved protocol NYU-SoM 09–0226. One thousand subjects were selected for inclusion in this paper. For edited versions of the one thousand reports, see Additional file 1. The free-form reports were not analyzed quantitatively. Excerpts of the reports are used as examples. However, in addition to submitting the free-form reports, subjects were given the chance to complete a questionnaire and the responses to this questionnaire have been quantified. A 43-point questionnaire that asked questions about specific aspects of life that are known or suspected to be affected by a change in olfactory acuity has been used. The questionnaire was adapted from the one used by Frasnelli and Hummel [123]. The complete results of the questionnaire, which was completed by 725 of the 1,000 subjects are shown in Additional file 2.

All the participants in the study gave informed consent. Due to the fact that this was an anonymous online study, they consented by responding with "I agree" in response to the question "By submitting your story you give us the right to use your story for our research and to include it in research presentations and in publications". The subjects were from 64 different countries. Because the website was in English, most reports were from English-speaking countries (Figure 2a). Sixty-two percent of the subjects who reported their gender were female and 38% male (Figure 2b). Almost three quarters self-identified as White or Caucasian (Figure 2c). The subjects range in the age at which they submitted their report from 6 to 85 with a median of 52. The median age of onset of the problems was 46, with a range from 0 to 83 (Figure 2d). Fifty-nine percent of the subjects had previously seen a doctor for their olfactory dysfunction (Additional file 2). A third to half of the subjects reported experiencing smell distortions in addition to smell loss (Figure 2e). For full methods see Additional file 3.

Results and discussion
Experiencing smell loss

Even patients with no sense of smell usually have some type of perceptual experience when they inhale high concentrations of volatile organic molecules [124]. In this study, subjects with olfactory loss report that "vapors feel differently" (subject 0002) or that smells coat their mouths (subject 0063) when there is a source of volatile chemicals nearby. Individuals with smell loss often experience their conditions as still being able to detect the presence or absence of smells, but being unable to identify smells or discriminate between different smells (subjects 0268, 0771, 0823 and 0831). Different metaphors and comparisons are employed to describe this experience. One subject (subject 0212) says that it is "like the form of a smell is there, but there really isn't a smell", another subject (subject 0248) says that her "smell is now 'black & white' and no longer 'in color'". Smelling without a sense of smell is like eating chick peas that you can feel but not taste when you eat them (subject 0818). It's like being an almost blind person who still can recognize silhouettes (subject 0723).

If the smell loss is caused by sinonasal disease it is often not due to permanent damage and the olfactory symptoms can therefore fluctuate over time [25] and can be modulated. Subjects experience improved olfactory function for example during exercise [26] (subjects 0003, 0013, 0160, 0586, 0691, 0763, and 0964). At least one subject used exercise to "switch-on" his sense of smell when desired:

> During a dinner party when a good wine was served I would excuse myself from the room and run up and down the stairs several times. This restored my sense of smell for a period. (subject 0013)

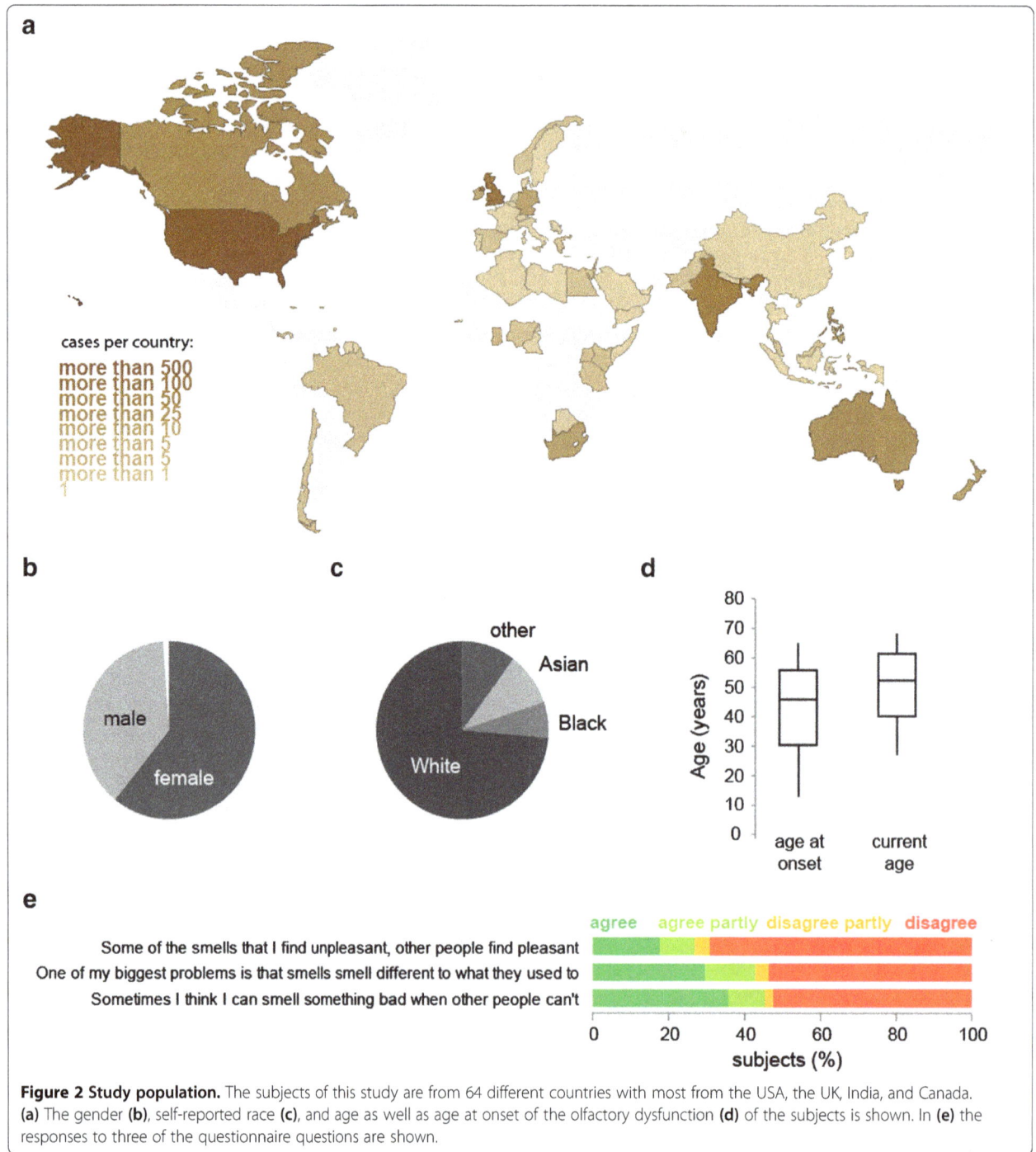

Figure 2 Study population. The subjects of this study are from 64 different countries with most from the USA, the UK, India, and Canada. (a) The gender (b), self-reported race (c), and age as well as age at onset of the olfactory dysfunction (d) of the subjects is shown. In (e) the responses to three of the questionnaire questions are shown.

Changes in altitude (and the resulting changes in air pressure) are also reported to have the effect of temporarily bringing back some olfactory perception in patients with sinonasal disease. Scuba diving (subject 0013), air travel (subject 0015), hiking in the mountains (subject 0964), or simply going to Colorado, which has a mean elevation of over 2,000 meters, (subject 0817), are all reported to improve odor detection in these patients. Hot showers have been reported to trigger this change [25] and

the subjects of this study also report that changes in the temperature of the inhaled air can temporarily improve their olfactory acuity (subjects 0140, 0160, and 0586).

Because of the large contribution of the olfactory system to flavour perception, olfactory loss also dramatically changes the experience of eating food. Subjects compare their eating experience to eating sawdust (subject 0632), cardboard (subjects 0114, 0241, 0714 and 0912), or paper with glue (subjects 0004 and 0804). Coffee and other hot beverages taste like hot water (subject 0123). Subjects cannot distinguish cola from lemonade or cream soda (subject 0712), whiskey from rum (subject 0226), or coffee from tea (subject 0160). One subject reports that she noticed that she accidentally sprinkled paprika instead of cinnamon on her oatmeal only after she had finished eating (subject 0995).

Practical problems of smell loss

The practical problems of not having a sense of smell can be grouped into three groups: problems with hazard avoidance, food-related problems, and problems with managing odors.

Hazard avoidance

72% of the subjects of this study are scared of getting exposed to dangers because of their olfactory dysfunction (Additional file 2). The main concern is the inability to detect a gas leak or a fire. Several subjects report that they have actually failed to detect a gas leak (subjects 0009, 0028, 0413, 0826, and 0985). Similarly, the inability to detect fires has resulted in dangerous situations for some subjects (subjects 0009, 0140, 0530, and 0531). For fire-fighters, olfactory loss and the resulting inability to locate fires through smell is a particular challenge (subjects 0139 and 0334). One subject (subject 0531) reports that, while cleaning the bathroom with a strong solvent that was odorless to him, he exposed himself to the volatile chemical until he was coughing up blood. Other subjects with reduced olfactory acuity also experienced adverse effects due to exposure to undetected volatile chemicals (subjects 0031, 0532 and 0913).

Food-related

Many of the practical problems of not having a sense of smell have to do with food. Among the subjects of this study, accidentally eating spoiled food is common (subjects 0009, 0066, 0285, and 0637) and subjects report that they have become overly careful and tend to discard food when in doubt (subjects 0061 and 0319). Those who have been cooking before their smell loss often no longer cook or do not enjoy cooking anymore after they lost their sense of smell (subjects 0049, 0059, 0226, 0504, 0548, 0798, 0913, and 0930). Thirty-nine percent report that since the change in their sense of smell their ability to prepare food has decreased (Figure 3a). For those who work as chefs (subjects 0041, 0199, and 0287) or sommeliers (subject 0299) olfactory dysfunction makes it extremely difficult to continue their careers.

Probably the most striking consequence of smell loss for those affected is that they no longer enjoy eating. Sixty-four percent of the subjects report that their enjoyment of food has decreased (Figure 3a). Different subjects respond with different behaviors to the reduced

hedonic value of food. Some lose the motivation to eat (subjects 0413 and 0981) and eat less (36%; Figure 3a). There are subjects reporting that they have to force themselves to eat (subjects 0421 and 0776) and a subject (subject 0875) who says "I now only eat to fill up and for no other reason". Other comments include: "I just let myself get so hungry before I eat that the taste does not matter. It's just for fuel". (subject 0284), "The only reason I eat now is to relieve hunger pains. I get no enjoyment from eating". (subject 0049), "I don't care anymore about eating, but I know I have to eat when I am hungry". (subject 0548), and "I am only eating because I'm hungry, I don't enjoy any food". (subject 0551)

These subjects respond to the reduced enjoyment they find in eating by eating less. However, other subjects (20%; Figure 3a) respond by eating more in an attempt to find the enjoyment that they remember:

> I ended up gaining almost twenty pounds before realizing I was consuming more of every food in an effort to taste it. (subject 0004)

> I think I've gained weight as a result of my loss of my sense of smell. I get the taste for certain foods, but my appetite isn't satisfied because I cannot fully enjoy the foods I eat because I can't smell them. (subject 0310)

> I have gained a substantial amount of weight and I am wondering if it is because I am never fully satisfied as a person with normal smell and taste is. (subject 0327)

> Instead of becoming disinterested in food, I find myself eating very spicy things, or sweet or sour, all in the interest of just having a sensation. But nothing much gets through except texture. I keep searching, and have even experienced weight gain since I'm ever looking for something... (subject 0560)

Some subjects will eat less and others will eat more after losing their sense of smell. As a consequence, some (19%; Figure 3a) report weight loss (subjects 0024, 0035, 0046, 0048, 0061, 0084, and 0086) while others (24%; Figure 3a) report gaining weight (subjects 0004, 0310, 0327, and 0560). This pattern has been observed before [112,113], but the factors that determine if an individual responds to food being less enjoyable by eating more or less are unexplored.

Losing their sense of smell not only influences how much affected individuals eat, but also what they eat. For 72% the taste of food changed as a consequence of the olfactory dysfunction and 19% report an increased dislike towards specific foods (Figure 3a). Many subjects of this study report that the role of texture became more important in deciding what to eat after they lost their sense of smell (subjects 0002, 0028, 0048, 0156, 0186, 0312, 0376, 0560,

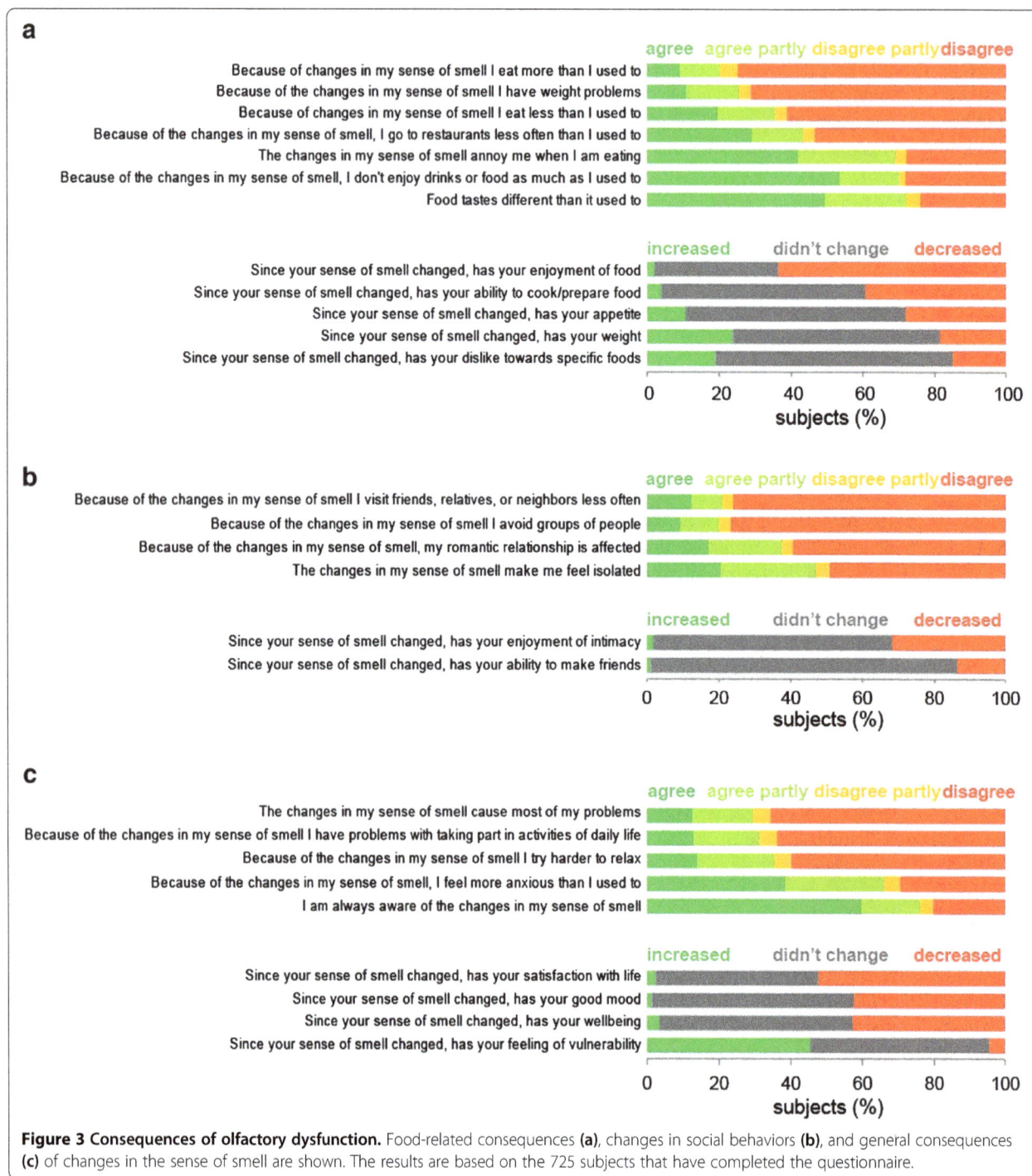

Figure 3 Consequences of olfactory dysfunction. Food-related consequences **(a)**, changes in social behaviors **(b)**, and general consequences **(c)** of changes in the sense of smell are shown. The results are based on the 725 subjects that have completed the questionnaire.

0712, and 0723). Examples of textures that are sought out by these subjects are crunchy and crispy (subjects 0312 and 0723) and smooth and creamy (subjects 0004 and 0723). Irritants also can contribute to the flavour of food through non-olfactory pathways. Pungent irritants like horseradish (subjects 0028 and 0061), chili peppers (subjects 0028, 0061), and pepper (0606) are popular. Taste is the most obvious contributor to flavour in the absence of olfactory

perception. The subjects in this study report that their loss of smell resulted in a preference for salty (subjects 0004, 0010, 0358, 0502, 0526, and 0723), sweet (subjects 0004, 0022, 0502, and 0723), and sour (subjects 0560 and 0723).

Odor management
For those who lost their sense of smell, odor management is also difficult. Without a sense of smell it is

impossible to verify that one's body, children, or home do smell acceptable:

> However, I do get paranoid about personal hygiene, how my house smells — i.e. something gone rotten in the fridge, musty smells — this has resulted in me being absolutely fanatical about both personal hygiene and household cleaning — to the point where people close to me have asked if I suffer from obsessive-compulsive disorder. (subject 0532)

> My poor kids sat in dirty diapers longer than they should have because I couldn't smell the soiled diaper. [...] I've put on way too much perfume many, many, many times. I shower every day because I'm nervous I might have body odor. (subject 0354)

The most important odor to manage is one's body odor. There are severe social consequences of failing to maintain the culturally expected body odor and many individuals who suffer from smell loss therefore are worried about their olfactory appearance. A large proportion of individuals with a diminished sense of smell complain about the difficulties of perceiving their own body odor and the resulting challenges for personal hygiene [70,115]. Of the subjects in this study, 72% report a change in the perception of their own body odor (Additional file 2). Managing their own body odor without being able to perceive it is challenging (subjects 0004, 0014, 0025, 0087, 0186, 0310, 0335, 0531, 0550, 0589, 0627, 0823, 0829, 0925). The obvious strategy is a rigid personal hygiene regime and to have others help with the assessment of one's body odors (subjects 0965 and 0984).

Another challenge for those with smell loss, especially for elderly people who live by themselves, is to manage the odor of their homes (subjects 0087, 0310, and 0756):

> I lost my sense of smell for no apparent reason five years ago at age 72. I never noticed it until my daughter said my house had a terrible odor and we then discovered a dead rodent that caused the odor. (subject 0449)

Other subjects also report that they could not perceive the foul smell of decay filling their house after an animal died underneath furniture (subjects 0637 and 0874). Living in a house filled with a foul smell can be very embarrassing and the fear of this embarrassment can lead to social isolation when the affected person refuses to let people in their house (subject 0756).

Keeping pets also poses problems for those without a sense of smell:

> [As a child] I was told I could have a pet cat as long as I took care of it and one of those responsibilities

was to change the cat box as soon as I smelled it. Needless to say I was in constant trouble and was thought to be irresponsible and lazy. Eventually I was able to convince others that I just couldn't smell. (subject 0014)

> ... just recently one of our cats urinated on a piece of carpet, and it apparently reeked, and the smell was making my boyfriend nuts, and I couldn't smell it at all. His reaction to me was complete disbelief, as if I was faking that I couldn't smell something horrid. (subject 0666)

Other subjects report having not noticed that a dog relieved itself on the floor (subjects 0087 and 0539).

Young children also need olfactory attention. Diapers need to be changed when they are "stinky" (subjects 0004, 0285, 0332, and 0747). Child care is a sensitive subject and parenting without an olfactory system can be anxiety inducing:

> Another embarrassing thing I've run into was when my last two children were babies — I wouldn't notice that they had a dirty diaper, of course. [...] I remember two different mothers who treated me with great disgust, as if I didn't care about my child or hygiene, almost as if I were abusive. I had another horrible experience when I apparently left a load of laundry in the washing machine for too long. The head of the day camp where I was sending my daughter took me aside on the third day of the week and asked why I was sending my daughter to camp in clothing that smelled of mildew [...] It's a source of enormous anxiety for me. (subject 0004)

People whose jobs involve odor management like nurses (subjects 0705 and 0782) or building managers (subject 0012) face problems in their professional lives after losing their sense of smell.

In summary, there are several practical challenges of having an olfactory impairment. Problem-focused coping strategies are available for affected individuals [115,118,119]. Fire detectors can ease anxiety about undetected fires. There are recipes designed specifically to be enjoyable for those with a reduced sense of smell [125]. Perhaps most importantly, affected individuals can learn to rely on others noses and trust their judgment. However, this social dimension of olfactory impairments causes its own set of problems, which will be discussed in the next section.

Smell loss-induced social isolation

The subjects of this study report that many of the problems that are associated with living with an olfactory dysfunction have to do with the responses by friends and family-members to the condition. It seems to be common to doubt the existence of olfactory dysfunction or to trivialize the condition. This often leads to embarrassment, alienation, anger, and withdrawal on the side of the patient. Half of the subjects report that their condition makes them feel angry (Additional file 2) and 47% report that it makes them feel isolated (Figure 3b).

Affected individuals have to continuously explain their condition and defend themselves against explicit or implicit suggestions that they are lying about their inability to smell (subjects 0008, 0272, 0666, and 0928). For those with congenital olfactory impairment the challenge starts with convincing their parents and other adults that they cannot smell (subjects 0009 and 0071). Children with congenital smell loss are usually unaware of the dysfunction and only "discover" their condition as teenagers [70,126]. One subject reports her experience when she was six years old and came home from school where cinnamon rolls were baked, wondering what this "smell" everybody else got so excited about was:

> My mother got surprised, because she had absolutely no clue about this condition before that. We went to the hospital to check it out, but with little result. I was asked to smell several different things while being blindfolded, and I couldn't smell anything. The result was however that I was a stubborn child who lied, so not much more was done. (subject 0071)

For those who lose their sense of smell as adults it is equally challenging to convince people of their condition:

> I get the feeling that people think I am lying about my sense of smell a lot; especially once they see me enjoy food. That's pretty aggravating. (subject 0020)

By many, including the patients themselves, olfactory impairment is considered to be "strange" (subjects 0078 and 0172), not "normal" (subjects 0048 and 0686), and "weird" (subjects 0005, 0078, 0729, and 0982), Those affected are labeled "freaks" (subjects 0008 and 0580) or "crazy" (subjects 0078, 0094, 0172, 0340, 0359, 0447, 0470, and 0729).

Once affected individuals have convinced others of the existence of their condition, they often face a lack of sympathy. Olfactory impairment is not considered to be a serious disability (subjects 0063 and 0072) and sometimes affected individuals are even told that they should be happy about their inability to smell unpleasant odors (subjects 0025 and 0048):

> It's a weird affliction. People don't really get it. They think it's not as big a deal as it is. After all, they figure anosmics aren't disabled. We don't need seeing-eye

dogs or sign language to interact with our environment. And they are right — partly. We can function without drawing attention to our plight. We can do virtually everything we could before we lost our sense of smell, except enjoy the immensely important aspects of human life that most people take for granted. (subject 0005)

> I have written at some length here because there seems to be a total lack of interest in the very distressing condition of anosmia — most people dismiss it as a joke: "aren't you lucky you can change babies' nappies without noticing", whereas if I had gone blind or become deaf everyone would be sympathetic. I have learned not to mention it anymore and work my way around it without letting anyone know. (subject 0025)

A symptom of the lack of sympathy for affected individuals is that others regularly keep forgetting about the condition (subjects 0008, 0029, 0063, 0292, 0589, and 0925) and are unforgiving about problems caused by it (subjects 0014, 0539, 0666, and 0897):

> Life can be hell sometimes but no one seems to take it seriously. It is a disablement that is invisible. People are always saying "smell that", "taste this". It is very annoying; you wouldn't tell a blind man to look at the lovely scenery. (subject 0029)

> If you're blind, people forgive you if you are wearing mismatched socks, but they can't see if you have anosmia and therefore a reason why you may have undetected body odor. (subject 0014)

> ...one day someone aggressively accused me of ignoring the burning meal on the stove on purpose. (subject 0897)

> I was watching TV, and my dog pooped right behind my chair, and I didn't notice until my mother came down and yelled at me for not picking it up. (subject 0539)

It is especially aggravating for the patients when members of the medical profession to which they turn for help trivialize their condition:

> My doctor did not know such a symptom existed. He was stunned that this could happen and stuck a couple things like coffee under my nose to test me. [...] When he found out it had a name, anosmia, he looked up possible causes in their computer and decided to send me to get an MRI and a CT scan. He refused to send me to an ear nose throat specialist

because "I cannot send you unless I first diagnose a condition they can treat, like sinusitis". (subject 0012)

I don't care as much ultimately about what the public awareness of this condition is; I'm resigned to anosmia being a joke for those who don't have it. I do wish that doctors took it more seriously. I have talked to too many doctors who did not believe that I cannot smell. [...] One especially ignorant fellow just didn't believe that I'm unable to smell anything at all and treated me as if I were some hysterical female, telling me it was entirely psychosomatic. This needs to change, and this is why I've just spent the last 45 minutes pouring all this out for you. (subject 0004)

My doctor first said "You're lucky! You won't have to smell the diapers!" When that upset me, he replied that loss of the sense of smell was "no big deal" and I would "probably get it back in a few weeks". That was more than a month ago and there has been no improvement. It is more terrible than I could have imagined... (subject 0079)

Other subjects also report disappointing interactions with their doctors (subjects 0030, 0035, 0054, 0073, 0080, 0121, 0133, 0196, 0238, 0267, 0271, 0395, 0402, 0428, 0571, 0897, and 0942). Doctors told them that olfactory dysfunction is "a good thing to have" (subject 0423), that it "is not a sickness" (subject 0001), "just a psychological feeling" (subject 0043), or they treated the patient's complaint as "a trivial matter" (subject 0019). These doctors are a small minority and most doctors handle complaints of olfactory impairments professionally and show compassion towards their patients. Much of the patients' frustration is caused by the lack of treatment options. However, the fact that there are some doctors who never heard of a chronic condition that affects a large percentage of the population is indicative of a problem.

The affected individuals' response to the perception that their condition is "weird" and a trivial matter is that they lie about their condition to avoid having to discuss it. Children who do not have a sense of smell often just mimic others' reactions to smell without actually perceiving any smells (subjects 0009, 0031, 0064, 0304, 0308, 0319, 0532, 0611, and 0686):

Smelling seemed to me like religion, you just had to have enough faith to make it true. (subject 0002)

When I was little I used to pretend that I was able to because I thought I had to be able to "learn" how and I just wasn't good enough at it yet. (subject 0067)

I had always figured a sense of smell was something that developed as you got older. (subject 0077)

Adults often continue to pretend having a sense of smell to avoid having to discuss their impairment with often skeptical and unsympathetic people (subjects 0002, 0186, 0292, 0666, 0883, and 0925) or because they are embarrassed about it and fear to be labeled (subjects 0021, 0064, 0074, 0172, and 0319).

It was bad when I would eat with other people. They always ask about my food or my family would ask me to taste something and I would have to explain again that I still can't taste... It seemed that in some cases my loss of taste and smell took away their pleasures, so I just started lying if someone asked me how my dinner was. (subject 0292)

... people keep asking me how I like their new perfume. Sometimes I just lie because telling my story makes me feel even worse and I don't want pity, I don't want to respond to the same questions over and over again, and I don't want the questioning looks in people's eyes starring in disbelief. (subject 0925)

The subjects of this study often comment that most people do not understand how it feels to live without a sense of smell (subjects 0005, 0008, 0023, 0027, 0137, 0530, and 0666). This perceived lack of understanding by others leads to social isolation of the affected individuals. They feel alone (subject 0102), left out (subject 0071), apart from the rest of us (subject 0030), or like outsiders (subject 0925). They are less interested in social situations (subjects 0014, 0125 and 0431), have reduced libido (subjects 0061, 0199, 0275, and 0655), and wonder if their problems with forming emotional attachments and establishing long-term romantic relationships may be due to their condition (subjects 0317 and 0912). Not being able to smell other people's odors can make it more difficult to feel close to them (subjects 0025 and 0544). Twenty and twenty-one percent of the subjects, respectively, report that since their change in olfactory perception they avoid groups of people and visit friends or relatives less frequently (Figure 3b). Thirty-eight percent report that it has affected their romantic relationship and 32% report a decreased enjoyment of intimacy (Figure 3b).

In this social isolation, affected individuals are often relieved when they find out that there are others with the same problems (subjects 0040, 0149, 0293, 0471, and 0592):

I looked it up online and found several stories about people smelling smoke just like me. [...] it was nice to know that I'm not alone. (subject 0470)

I eventually met a number of other people who lost their smell after a head injury. It didn't make us friends but it helps knowing they're out there. (subject 0020)

I have not found anyone else who has this problem and have not been able to talk about it with others. It's good to write this at least. Thanks for the opportunity. (subject 0010)

The social problems that are associated with olfactory dysfunction would be in large parts avoidable if the condition and its consequences would be more widely known:

My greatest wish (obviously right after being able to smell) is that society will know more about anosmia and that they are aware of us and that there is a broader support for affected people. (subject 0925)

Smell loss-induced anhedonia

In addition to the practical problems associated with olfactory impairment and the social consequences, not having a sense of smell can also result in anhedonia, the inability to experience pleasure from activities usually found enjoyable:

I have a two year old daughter and I've never been able to smell her. I miss the smell of pickles, early September mornings, the ocean, gasoline, matches and garlic... (subject 0008)

The sad thing, I find, is not being able to appreciate the everyday smells which we take for granted: perfume, freshly mown grass, freshly baked bread, scent of bluebells/roses/flowers in general. Living by the sea, I used to love the smell of the seaweed around the tide pools. The list is endless. (subject 0028)

My life is far less rich and my enjoyment of things (food, going to the seaside, pretty much anything) is often greatly reduced. (subject 0100)

It's made me quite sad at times as I can't get excited about a new restaurant, the smell of summer, or any other smell that brings out an emotive response. (subject 0147)

Over 40% of the affected individuals report decreased wellbeing, mood, and satisfaction with life (Figure 3c). Sixty-six percent of the subjects in this study feel more anxious than before the change in their sense of smell and 46% feel more vulnerable (Figure 3c).

One important function of smell is contributing to the experience of places. Although we are often not aware of the smells of different locations, those smells greatly contribute to our experience and enjoyment of them:

It was extremely depressing to have no sense of smell at all. You realize that rooms have smells, water has a taste, etc. (subject 0036)

It improved slightly and I forgot about it until yesterday when realized I really missed the subtle spring scents, like bluebells, grass. (subject 0701). I went to the seaside two years ago, but was unable to smell the sea and I felt quite sad about this. Also, on rainy days, I am unable to smell the damp earth or freshly cut grass... (subject 0510)

Many subjects of this study report that they miss characteristic nature smells, like the smells of flowers (subjects 0028, 0051, 0063, 0087, 0097, 0137, 0421, 0450, 0456, 0572, 0651, 0671, 0695, 0743, 0757, and 0984), grass (subjects 0058, 0587, 0701, 0705, and 0889), the forest (subject 0005), or the ocean (subjects 0008, 0028, 0058, 0100, 0441, 0510, and 0651).

Certain times or events also have characteristic smells. The subjects of this study complain about no longer being able to smell the smell of early morning (subject 0058), rain (subject 0450), an approaching snow storm (subject 0049), spring (subject 0701), summer (subject 0147), and fall (subject 0049). Similarly, holiday seasons have distinctive smells and subjects report missing the smells of Thanksgiving (subjects 0005 and 0888) and Christmas (subjects 0243, 0441, 0888, 0950, and 0998). The strong emotional effect that the characteristic smell of summer or Christmas has is partially mediated by memory. Smells are powerful elicitors of vivid personal memories [127-129] and those without a sense of smell miss these memories (subjects 0005, 0175, 0913, 0998, and 0999).

In addition to places, times, and events, people also have characteristic smells. Many subjects in this study note that they cannot smell their babies or children (subjects 0004, 0008, 0035, 0041, 0063, 0097, 0119, 0131, 0327, 0355, 0538, 0651, 0695, 0889, and 0925). Others complain about not being able to smell their romantic partner (subjects 0035, 0041, 0087, 0137, and 0912) and wonder if their olfactory impairment influences their romantic relationships (subject 0912):

I have become afraid: does my lack of sense of smell keep me from finding someone I'd like to spend the rest of my life with? (subject 0317)

Anhedonia can be subdivided into consummatory anhedonia, the inability to enjoy an activity, and motivational anhedonia, the lack of the desire to engage in enjoyable activities [130]. Motivational anhedonia can have a large negative impact on the lives of individuals suffering from smell loss. The smell of food does not only make eating food more enjoyable, it also motivates us to eat, to cook, and to go to restaurants. The smell of a romantic partner is not only a pleasant sensory experience, more importantly it motivates us to engage with him or her. An effect of smell-loss on motivation could explain the unexpectedly large life-changes experienced by patients with smell loss. The way some subjects in this study describe their experience of having no sense of smell is consistent with motivational anhedonia. They describe not having a sense of smell as dampening the colors of the world (subject 0175). The world without smells is described as "artificial" (subject 0019) and empty, like "living in a box and looking out at the world" (subject 0082). The world becomes less rich (subjects 0082 and 0100) and "smaller, darker, and sad" (subject 0925). Life becomes strange and depressing (subject 0930):

At first I felt very out of touch with myself — like I was out of step or like I had constantly forgotten something important. (subject 0606)

It is very difficult for me now to make plans, feel desire, feel good and happy. I live in a permanent present, I have lost the sensations linked to memories, I have no particular desire for the future.... (subject 0999)

Experiencing smell distortions

Between 10 and 60% of individuals with partial or complete smell loss also experience distorted smells [5,8,21,22]. The experiences of these subjects and the problems that they face are different from those of individuals with smell loss.

Quality of distorted smells

The distorted smells experienced by those with parosmia or phantosmia have been described as "burned", "foul", "rotten", "fecal", "chemical" [6]; "burned", "foul", "unpleasant", "spoiled", "rotten" [3]; "off", "rotten", "burnt" [5]; and "burned", "foul", "rotten", "sewage", "chemically" [102]. Some patients do not have any associations with the distorted smell, describing it as an unpleasant unknown odor [6]. Not all distorted odor perception is unpleasant, though [131]. It is useful to follow Leopold [3] and differentiate between two types of smell distortion. In the more common type every distorted perception is the same (for example the perception of cigarette smoke), regardless of the trigger. In the second type different triggers cause different perceptions.

Describing odors and identifying them out of their usual context is notoriously difficult [132] and this is also true for distorted smells. Regardless, many subjects attempt to describe their distorted odor perceptions:

It's not good or bad, sweet or bitter, it's not chemical or organic, it's just there. (subject 0888)

... a constant odor — not sweet, not sharp, not foul. I had never smelled it before. (subject 0017)

I cannot identify the smell; I try to associate it with something but I come up empty. (subject 0026)

Many subjects in this study label the distorted odor they perceive as "strange" (subjects 0028, 0097, 0221, 0225, 0416, 0448, 0465, 0500, 0535, 0605, 0630, 0687, 0694, 0767, 0773, 0791, 0887, and 0962) or "weird" (subjects 0028, 0060, 0097, 0164, 0427, 0470, 0752, 0785, 0916, and 0963). Based on these reports, it is tempting to speculate that the distorted smell is the consequence of random firing of neurons, similar to the smell of complex mixtures of odors with the same intensity that has been named "olfactory white" [133]. This would be analogous to white noise or the hissing sound perceived by those suffering from tinnitus [134,135]. However, many subjects who experience distorted smells describe them as readily identifiable specific odors (see below).

The distorted perception is rarely pleasant and frequently described as "unpleasant" (subjects 0011, 0018, 0025, 0040, 0041, 0100, 0164, 0169, 0172, 0182, 0260, 0381, 0383, 0509, 0544, 0606, 0694, 0814, 0825, and 0933), "foul" (subjects 0136, 0216, 0475, 0511, 0670, 0674, 0745, and 0968), or simply "bad" (subjects 0027, 0052, 0068, 0084, 0097, 0114, 0132, 0164, 0210, 0235, 0295, 0339, 0351, 0439, 0441, 0451, 0525, 0651, 0730, 0774, 0803, 0815, 0840, 0854, 0860, 0872, 0887, 0895, 0900, and 0952).

Rarely, the olfactory distortion inverts the olfactory pleasantness spectrum; pleasant smells become unpleasant and unpleasant smells become more pleasant:

Smells that I did not like before suddenly seemed pleasant to me, and some of my favorite smells from before were generally less appealing to me. (subject 0085)

The perfumes I used to use, which smelled very pleasant to me prior to anosmia, now don't smell so pleasant. Some foods don't taste as good as they used to (for example I can't stand bananas now), and other foods taste much better than they used to. Cigarette smoke smells almost minty to me, and not nearly as unpleasant as it used to. (subject 0869)

Among those who attempt to describe or identify the odor, in almost half of the cases, the odor is associated with fire. "Cigarette smoke" is the most common description used by the subjects in this study. "Car exhaust" is also a common association and some subjects are reminded of burning rubber or electrical fire. One subject describes the experience as being "stuck behind a school bus" (subject 0306). Other subject describe the distorted perception as "burnt vegetables in a fetid swamp" (subject 0832), or as "like chili that has burnt to the bottom of the pan or a coffee pot that's been on the burner all day" (subject 0592). There are also other odor categories that are commonly used to describe the distorted smell (Figure 4). Many subjects are reminded of the smell of solvents or fumes from volatile chemicals by their olfactory distortions. Diesel fumes, paint smell, and plastic smells are often mentioned in this category. The next largest category is food smells, in which a variety of different and diverse experiences from "part cooking oil, part garlic, part fish oil" (subject 0235) to "oranges and cloves mixed with mulled wine" (subject 0066) are grouped.

Other common experiences are the odors of decay, like rotten meat (subjects 0126 and 0619) or "rotten peanuts soaked in vinegar" (subject 0674) and the smell of urine/ammonia (subjects 0036, 0197, 0278, 0340, 0359, 0396, and 0998), the smell (or taste) of metal (subjects 0062, 0098, 0177, 0448, 0500, 0525, 0713, 0773, 0787, and 0906), and sweet smell (subjects 0034, 0055, 0152, 0225, 0274, 0483, 0534, 0563, and 0721). There are also idiosyncratic olfactory experiences that are only mentioned by one subject each, for example blood smell (subject 0603) and lavender (subject 0934).

For most subjects, the distorted experience is always the same. However, as has been reported previously [3],

for some subjects the distorted experiences can have different perceptual qualities:

I started to get phantom smells which ranged from the smell of the tumble dryer to oil and petrol. [...] Many other smells like peppers, celery, and perfumes also smell different than they used to smell. Eggs and certain other foods smell like urine. (subject 0895)

The odors range from floral/perfume, wood or paper smoke, petroleum or solvent based (petrol, WD-40, butane) to cooked foods. (subject 0781)

At times it is like the room is filled with cigarette smoke so full it burns the back of my throat. [...] Other odor variations are cherry pipe tobacco, the smell of brick being cut with a brick saw, jasmine, a smell so sweet it makes me sick. All body washes and shampoos make me sick; they smell like poop. (subject 0007)

Interestingly, several subjects of this study report that the distorted smell is similar to the last actual smell that they experienced; they are "stuck" with the last smell they smelled before losing their sense of smell (subjects 0078, 0116, 0150, 0173, 0225, 0234, and 0379). One subject lost her sense of smell in a car accident and now experiences an odor reminiscent of "the odor of the gray smoky powder that filled the car when the airbags deployed" (subject 0060). Other subjects report to continuously experience the lavender smell encountered on vacation (subject 0934) or the smell of caramelized sugar experienced at a friend's house while they were making fudge (subject 0065). For one subject the distorted smell alternated between two of the last smells she experienced, a sandwich served on a plane and the smell of guano from visiting a penguin colony (subject 0112).

Many subjects of this study report that their distorted experiences are not purely olfactory. The distorted "smells" are often accompanied by burning eyes (subjects 0047, 0106, 0172, 0203, 0263, 0391, 0397, 0451, 0545, and 0734), an irritated throat (subjects 0007, 0047, 0194, 0203, 0358, 0391, 0397, 0408, 0451, 0545, 0694, and 0739), and pain or burning sensation in the nose (subjects 0097, 0243, 0372, and 0860). These are experiences that cannot be mediated by the olfactory sensory system, but instead are likely to be a consequence of trigeminal nerve activity [136,137]. Furthermore, the "smells" elicit responses that are typical for trigeminal activation like sneezing (subjects 0127 and 0397) and nose rubbing (subject 0696). Subjects also report being woken up by the sensation (subjects 0178, 0412, and 0678), although actual olfactory sensations do not have the potential to wake subjects [138], and they locate the

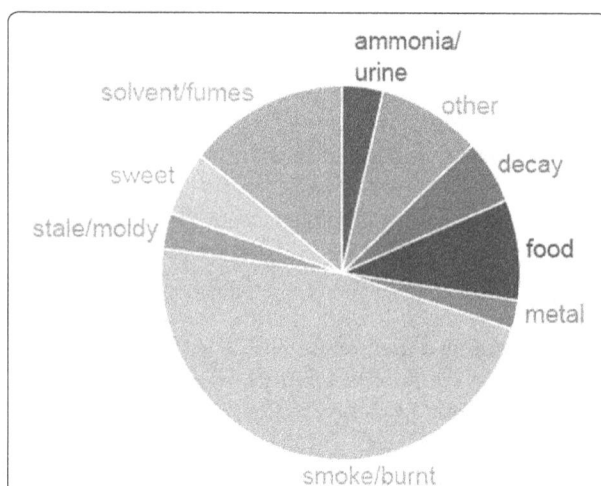

Figure 4 Perceived quality of distorted smells. Of the 161 subjects that reported quality of distorted smells, the largest group experienced a burnt or smoky smell. The second largest group reported that they experience the distorted smells as smelling like solvent or fumes.

"smell" only in one nostril, which is also possible only for trigeminal stimuli but not for olfactory stimuli [139].

Triggers of distorted smells

In most cases of distorted smell perception a trigger for the experience can be identified. Distorted perceptions can be triggered by mechanical stimuli like sneezing [3] or changes in nasal airflow [102]:

> The episodes are triggered by coughing, shouting, and sneezing. [...] Introduction of water into the nasal passages/sinus cavity (underwater swimming, saline nasal rinse, etc.) can also trigger an episode. (subject 0302)

Hot or cold air can also trigger distorted olfactory experiences. Sensations can be triggered by furnaces (subjects 0083, 0118, 0136, and 0503), the hot air inside a car that sat in the sun (subject 0766), hot weather (subject 0555), heat from a blow dryer (subject 0084) or the interior of fridges and freezers (subjects 0084 and 0321).

By far the most frequently mentioned trigger of distorted olfactory experiences among the subjects of this study are volatile chemicals (like perfumes and scented beauty products) (subjects 0007, 0040, 0097, 0136, 0164, 0199, 0249, 0274, 0322, 0326, 0370, 0388, 0397, 0441, 0465, 0468, 0475, 0576, 0605, 0774, 0825, 0869, 0916, 0936, and 0941) and food or beverages, multisensory stimuli that include volatile chemicals (subjects 0007, 0011, 0062, 0249, 0284, 0322, 0326, 0441, 0451, 0465, 0468, 0475, 0501, 0513, 0605, 0774, 0825, 0837, 0840, 0847, 0855, 0858, 0869, 0911, and 0951). It has been shown that different stimuli have different potential to trigger distorted perception. In a survey of 46 patients, the most common stimuli eliciting distorted olfaction were gasoline (30%), tobacco (28%), coffee (28%), perfume (22%), fruits (15%, mainly citrus fruits and melon), and chocolate (13%) [40]. The subjects of this study also report differences in the effectiveness of potential triggers of distorted olfactory perception:

> Within a few weeks the weird taste got stronger and started to affect more foods, including chocolate, yogurt, cottage cheese, fried foods, onions, green peppers, pancake syrup, beer, wine, grape fruit juice, and most snack foods such as chips (potato, corn, tortilla), crackers, pretzels, plus cakes and candies of all kinds. I could not even eat my birthday cake. Fruits of all kinds are at least a little bit weird with the taste becoming worse when the fruits become overripe. Water, skim milk, eggs, honey, and some cheeses taste normal. (subject 0164)

> I could not tolerate certain smells that are usually pleasant, for example coffee, cut grass, celery

(absolutely the worst), butter (especially buttered popcorn), apples, peaches, cucumbers, melons, perfumes, shampoos, soap, grilled meats, and poultry. I also discovered that I could no longer stomach certain related tastes, such as vegetable juice, carbonated beverages — especially colas, orange juice, red wines, anything melony. (subject 0027)

Some of the distorted sensations triggered by food are almost certainly triggered by heat activating the trigeminal nerve:

> Especially when food was hot it smelled so very bad. (subject 0295)

> I can smell the steam from ramen. (subject 0766)

Coffee, which is usually consumed hot, also appears to be an efficient trigger (subjects 0027, 0129, 0210, 0329, 0343, 0381, 0416, 0484, 0598, 0606, 0632, 0887, 0888, 0895, and 0911). Coffee is often mentioned together with chocolate (subjects 0164, 0445, 0632, 0855, and 0888):

> Coffee and chocolate taste horrible!! (subject 0343)

> I woke up one morning and immediately I could not stand the following smells and tastes: coffee, chocolates, all meat except processed meats like salami, peaches, watermelons, etc. (subject 0911)

> ... coffee and chocolate smelling just awful... (subject 0329)

> I started to smell coffee but not like I used to smell it. Within weeks I was getting the same smell for cigarette smoke. I still get these smells — also for chocolate. (subject 0895)

> I have never been able to smell or eat chocolate and coffee while I have the smell/taste because they are just too bad to handle. (subject 0129)

Citrus fruits like lemons (subject 0900), orange juice (subjects 0027, and 0210), citrus odors (subject 0095 and 0636), and orange peel (subject 0210) are also mentioned here as potent triggers. Melons are also often mentioned (subject 0027, 0312, 0349, 0381, and 0911), whereas other fruits appear to be less potent triggers of distorted smells (pineapple, kiwi fruit, and pears are never mentioned; strawberry and banana are mentioned by one subject each and apples by two subjects). Other foods that are indicated to be triggers by several subjects are peanuts or peanut butter (subjects 0036, 0381, 0416, and 0468), fried food (0226, 0588, and 0951), and onions (subjects 0226, 0349, 0416, 0568, and 0840).

Problems of smell distortions

Individuals with a distorted smell perception face most of the problems that those with smell loss face. It is difficult to manage odors or to avoid hazards based on odors when the perception of odors is not veridical. However, olfactory distortions have a much stronger effect on the patients' quality of life than loss of smell [40,123]. There are multiple reasons for the severity of the effect of olfactory distortions. One problem seems to be that the distorted olfactory experiences provide a constant reminder of the condition for the affected individual, thereby drawing attention to the problem. However, the three main problems that are associated with experiencing smell distortions are the (usual) unpleasantness of the experience, maladaptive responses to the condition, and the stigma that comes with experiencing things that do not exist.

Unpleasantness of distorted smells

Regularly smelling an unpleasant smell for long periods of time can have a severe impact on the affected individual's mood. Their experience is unlike any experience people with an intact sense of smell ever have because they do not adapt to the phantom smells:

It's not like perfume, where you smell it for a while and then it fades. (subject 0383)

The unpleasant distorted smell can also be triggered by all types of stimuli and can thereby complicate activities of daily living like taking public transportation:

... commuting by subway was especially difficult for some reason. (0035)

... This was particularly disturbing when I was riding on public transportation, where I was bombarded with dirty hair smell, underarm and genital body odors, strong colognes and especially bad breath and garlic odors emanating from my fellow passengers. (subject 0423)

Smell distortions can also be triggered by romantic partners, which can result in relationship problems:

My relationship with my wife has degenerated since I cringe when she comes within smelling distance. (subject 0011)

My condition is killing my sex life because when I ask "can you smell that" my partner thinks I am referring to her. (subject 0047)

I have not told my partner because I did not want him to think he smells bad to me and he has never mentioned that I have a different smell either. (subject 0052)

The most common trigger of distorted olfactory perception is food. When food elicits unpleasant olfactory experiences, it is not possible to enjoy food and it can even become difficult to eat (subjects 0043, 0045, 0046, 0284, 0429, and 0483).

A month after the accident I started having horrible phantom smells. They were so awful that I couldn't eat and was feeling horribly nauseous most of the day [...]. In a few months I had lost 30 lbs. because I wasn't eating. (subject 0035)

For the last six months I am smelling only a smell like burning vegetable oil. The smell is so strong that I use a mask, but it is of no help. [...] I am so hungry because I can't eat any food, even without oil. Everything smells the same. My life is hell. (subject 0096)

Maladaptive responses to experienced odors

Another big problem of distorted olfactory experiences is that it is an often difficult and long process for the affected individuals to determine that their perception is non-veridical. During this process the affected individuals behave as if there is a source of the unpleasant odor and these odor management behaviors can create practical and social problems:

About three years ago I started smelling diesel fumes which nobody else around me seemed to notice. This went on for about two years and I started to think that I was just oversensitive to fumes so I tried to live with it. Then, three months ago, I stayed for a few weeks in a home with a fryer that was giving off an awful chip fat smell (at least that was how I perceived it) and since then I have this smell with me everywhere I go. Until a few days ago I thought I was smelling of chip fat. I thought it was in my hair and on my clothes. I kept putting my clothes in the wash even before I wore them, kept washing my hair, really scrubbing it, and when I still smelled it, I sprayed my hair with deodorizing body spray. Whenever anyone came close to me I would pull away, conscious that they may be smelling "chip fat" on me. I then realized that there are times when I didn't notice the smell so I asked a family member to smell my hair. She said all she could smell was shampoo, which surprised me. I described what was happening to me and she assured me that there wasn't even the slightest whiff of chip fat. (subject 0116)

About a year ago I started smelling a strong unusual smell that I had never smelled before. At first I thought it was my urine. Then I thought it was my cat that had an abscess. I started smelling it more and more. I thought it was from the cat sleeping on the couch or my bed. I bought a rug shampooer and shampooed my carpets, upholstery, and washed all the linen in the house, but the smell continued. Then I started smelling it at work and on the bus; so I figured it was me. Recently, I had the nerve to start asking people if they could smell it on me. No one could. I started researching olfactory hallucinations. (subject 0070)

These two examples illustrate common phases through which people with distorted olfactory perception go as they come to realize that their perception is not caused by odor molecules. Often, they first suspect that there is an odor source in their environment. When they notice the odor in many different environments, they suspect that their body or their hair or their clothes are the source of the odor. When others assure them that they do not smell, they sometimes conclude that the source of the odor is in their nose or they start to suspect that their experience is not coinciding with reality.

If affected individuals suspect the odor source in their environment they often engage in excessive odor management efforts. Subjects in this study with distorted smell perception report cleaning their home thoroughly and repeatedly in an attempt to remove the odor source (subjects 0039, 0070, and 0278). These attempts can cause problems with those they live with (subject 0511). One subject reports that she is "gagging my family with air deodorizers" (subject 0216). Others have people come to check out their oven (subject 0392) or the drains (subject 0084). However, sometimes more drastic steps like giving away clothes and furniture (subject 0042) or changing windows to insulate them against smells entering from the outside (subject 0047) are taken. One subject started wearing a mask (subject 0096).

From the experiences reported by the subjects of this study, it seems as if subjects are more likely to have distorted olfactory experiences when resting. Consequently, distorted odor experiences are more frequent at night (subjects 0047, 0068, 0094, 0105, 0106, 0169, 0223, 0337, and 0575), and during passive activities like watching TV (subjects 0050, 0060, 0083, and 0118) and using a computer (subjects 0050, 0118, 0422, 0654, and 0887). Often the affected individuals notice

these patterns and, for a period of time, believe the smells to be associated with their TV or computer.

If affected individuals suspect that they themselves are the source of the odor, they focus on their personal hygiene (subjects 0033, 0089, and 0116). More detrimentally, they often become socially reclusive out of fear of embarrassing themselves with their unpleasant body odor (subjects 0033, 0089, 0116, and 0341):

My sense of smell within a few months' time turned to always smelling a bad distasteful smell. I first noticed it in my bedroom and then began to associate the smell with my partner first and then with myself. I have washed everything and cleaned, changed soaps, done everything I can think of but the smell seems to now follow me around and I hate it! Even when I use perfume I can still smell it. My partner and I have a good relationship. I have this nagging feeling that I am sick and that is the reason I have this bad smell around me, but I have no basis for it. (subject 0052)

Some individuals with distorted olfactory perception also suspect the source of the odor they experience in their nasal cavity, which would explain why nobody else can smell it:

The problem is that there seems to be a smell from my nose or mouth. The ear nose throat doctor says it's phantosmia, but can you have that if there is a smell? (subject 0827)

These individuals often try do manage the odor with sinus rinses and similar procedures (subjects 0150 and 0777).

Most of the ways in which affected individuals respond to odor distortion as if it were a real odor are harmless. They do however contribute to the patient's frustration because they do not result in a change in the symptoms and contribute to the feeling of not being in control. Some responses can also lead to conflict with others who have a veridical perception of the olfactory environment. One reason why affected individuals are willing to accept implausible explanations for their odor experiences, like that the smell of a sandwich got stuck in their nose for several months, is that there is a widespread unjustified stigma associated with having non-veridical sensory experiences [140].

Stigma

Phantosmia is the olfactory equivalent of phantom pain in pain perception [141,142] and tinnitus in auditory perception [134,135]. There are striking parallels between these conditions. In each case the phantom perception usually occurs with the loss of veridical perception. Phantom pain, which refers to pain in a body part that has been amputated or deafferented, is believed to be a consequence of plastic changes in the brain due to the changed sensory input [141]. Maladaptive plasticity has also been suggested to be the cause of tinnitus [135] and it has been speculated to play a role in distorted olfactory perception [4]. Phantom pain and tinnitus are both associated with a stigma and phantom pain has often been viewed as a type of mental disorder before the underlying neurological mechanisms were understood [141].

Patients with phantosmia seem to face a greater stigma than those suffering from phantom pains and tinnitus. That phantosmia is likely to be stigmatized is also clear to those that suffer from the problem and many therefore chose to not tell others (subjects 0052 and 0470). Others are worried that their phantosmia is not merely the consequence of neuronal plasticity after smell loss but a sign of a serious psychiatric problem (subject 0745). Others told their family or coworkers about their condition and have been labeled as "crazy" (subjects 0359 and 0729).

General discussion
The patient reports evaluated here show that olfactory dysfunction has a severe impact on affected individuals. This is in contrast to the low importance usually assigned to olfaction. In a survey amongst Canadian college students, for example, smell was ranked as the least important sense [143] (page 106). In the "Guides to the Evaluation of Permanent Impairment", published by the American Medical Association [144] a person's impairment due to several conditions is quantified. A complete loss of the sense of smell is suggested to be a 1% to 5% impairment. Deafness is a 35% impairment and blindness an 85% impairment. Smell loss is considered much less severe than the loss of the other modalities because: "Only rarely does complete loss of the closely related senses of olfaction and taste seriously affect an individual's performance of the usual ADLs [activities of daily living]. For this reason, a value of 1% to 5% impairment of the whole person is suggested..." (page 270). "Activities of daily living" include bathing, feeding, eating, personal hygiene, and sexual activity, activities that are shown here to be seriously affected by olfactory loss. Distorted olfactory perception is not discussed at all in the "Guides to the Evaluation of Permanent Impairment", although tinnitus, the perception of sound in the absence of an external stimulus, is considered to be a 5% impairment because it interferes with "sleep, reading (and other tasks requiring concentration), enjoyment of quiet recreation, and emotional well-being" (page 248). The reports in this paper show that in some cases a constant unpleasant smell also interferes with these activities.

It has to be noted that collecting patient reports online has two major limitations. First, it is likely that the reports collected here are not representative. The more severe the consequences of the olfactory dysfunction are experienced, the more likely is the affected individual to participate in a study about the condition. Because the subjects of this study are self-selecting and not necessarily representative, it is not possible to derive statements about the percentage of the total population of patients with olfactory dysfunction who experience any of the discussed consequences. This, however, is also true for studies of the consequences of olfactory dysfunction that enroll those patients that seek medical help for their condition (for example [27,108-110,115,123]). In fact, the barrier for participation in an online study like the one presented here is presumably lower than the barrier for participation in studies at smell clinics. Many affected individuals will be motivated enough by their condition to fill out an online survey, but not motivated enough to schedule an appointment and visit a smell clinic during office hours. An additional advantage of an online study is that there are fewer geographical and economic barriers to participation than to a study based at a smell clinic.

The major disadvantage of an online study compared to a study at a smell clinic is that the patient reports in an online study cannot be verified. This is the second major limitation of this study. Self-report of olfactory function in healthy individuals is notoriously unreliable [145,146] and although individuals with functional anosmia are generally aware of their impairment [147], the actual extend of olfactory loss in the subjects of this study is unclear. Similarly, the accuracy of all other information provided by the subjects anonymously cannot be independently verified. Confabulations by the subjects are also possible in studies in smell clinics, but olfactory function can be assessed objectively in these studies and the accuracy of basic facts about the subject such as age and gender are also more reliable. Furthermore, the higher entry barrier of smell clinic-based studies results presumably in more reliable data. It is easier to imagine that somebody mischievously submits wrong information to an online survey than that somebody takes a day off and drives to a smell clinic to lie about their condition there. Regardless of these limitations, the current study illustrates vividly the diversity and severity of the consequences of olfactory dysfunction.

Conclusion
Olfactory dysfunction, although it is often ignored or trivialized, can have severe consequences for those affected by it. While the practical problems of olfactory

dysfunction are dwarfed by those of visual impairments, smell loss-induced social isolation and smell loss-induced motivational anhedonia have outsized detrimental effects on the quality of life of these patients.

Better educating the patients, the public, and medical professionals about disorders of olfaction would improve the quality of life for those affected by reducing the practical and social problems they often face. However, a comprehensive solution can only be provided by research into an effective treatment.

Competing interests

The authors declare that they have no competing interests.

Authors' contributions

AK conceived of the study and collected and edited the patient reports and evaluated the questionnaire. AK and DM together designed the study and wrote the manuscript. All authors read and approved the final manuscript.

Acknowledgments

We would like to thank all the subjects who took the time to share their stories as part of this study. We are grateful to Conor McMeniman, Leslie Vosshall, and Jessica Keiser for comments on earlier versions of the manuscript. AK was supported by a Branco Weiss Fellowship from the Society in Science Foundation and by a NARSAD Young Investigator Grant. DM was supported by the National Institute of Mental Health (R01MH066428).

Author details

[1]Laboratory of Neurogenetics and Behavior, Rockefeller University, New York, NY, USA. [2]Department of Psychiatry, New York University School of Medicine, New York, NY, USA. [3]Creedmoor Psychiatric Center, New York State Office of Mental Health, New York, NY, USA.

References

1. Blodgett B: *Remembering Smell: A Memoir of Losing - and Discovering - the Primal Sense.* New York: Houghton Mifflin Harcourt; 2010.
2. Birnbaum M: *Season to Taste - How I Lost my Sense of Smell and Found my Way.* New York: Ecco; 2011.
3. Leopold D: **Distortion of olfactory perception: diagnosis and treatment.** *Chem Senses* 2002, 27:611–615.
4. Hong SC, Holbrook EH, Leopold DA, Hummel T: **Distorted olfactory perception: a systematic review.** *Acta Otolaryngol* 2012, 132:S27–S31.
5. Nordin S, Murphy C, Davidson TM, Quiñonez C, Jalowayski AA, Ellison DW: **Prevalence and assessment of qualitative olfactory dysfunction in different age groups.** *Laryngoscope* 1996, 106:739–744.
6. Frasnelli J, Landis BN, Heilmann S, Hauswald B, Hüttenbrink KB, Lacroix JS, Leopold DA, Hummel T: **Clinical presentation of qualitative olfactory dysfunction.** *Eur Arch Otorhinolaryngol* 2004, 261:411–415.
7. Majumdar S, Jones NS, McKerrow WS, Scadding G: **The management of idiopathic olfactory hallucinations: a study of two patients.** *Laryngoscope* 2003, 113:879–881.
8. Reden J, Maroldt H, Fritz A, Zahnert T, Hummel T: **A study on the prognostic significance of qualitative olfactory dysfunction.** *Eur Arch Otorhinolaryngol* 2007, 264:139–144.
9. Schubert CR, Cruickshanks KJ, Fischer ME, Huang GH, Klein BEK, Klein R, Pankow JS, Nondahl DM: **Olfactory impairment in an adult population: the beaver dam offspring study.** *Chem Senses* 2012, 37:325–334.
10. Brämerson A, Johansson L, Ek L, Nordin S, Bende M: **Prevalence of olfactory dysfunction: the Skövde population-based study.** *Laryngoscope* 2004, 114:733–737.
11. Vennemann MM, Hummel T, Berger K: **The association between smoking and smell and taste impairment in the general population.** *J Neurol* 2008, 255:1121–1126.
12. Murphy C, Schubert CR, Cruickshanks KJ, Klein BEK, Klein R, Nondahl DM: **Prevalence of olfactory impairment in older adults.** *J Am Med Assoc* 2002, 288:2307–2312.
13. Doty RL: **Studies of human olfaction from the university of Pennsylvania smell and taste center.** *Chem Senses* 1997, 22:565–586.
14. Wysocki CJ, Gilbert AN: **National geographic smell survey: effects of age are heterogenous.** *Ann N Y Acad Sci* 1989, 561:12–28.
15. Frye RE, Schwartz BS, Doty RL: **Dose-related effects of cigarette smoking on olfactory function.** *J Am Med Assoc* 1990, 263:1233–1236.
16. Katotomichelakis M, Balatsouras D, Tripsianis G, Davris S, Maroudias N, Danielides V, Simopouios C: **The effect of smoking on the olfactory function.** *Rhinology* 2007, 45:273–280.
17. Gilbert AN: *What the Nose Knows.* New York: Crown Publishers; 2008.
18. Corwin J, Loury M, Gilbert AN: **Workplace, age, and sex as mediators of olfactory function: data from the national geographic smell survey.** *J Gerontol Ser B-Psychol Sci Soc Sci* 1995, 50:179–186.
19. Boesveldt S, Lindau ST, McClintock MK, Hummel T, Lundstrom JN: **Gustatory and olfactory dysfunction in older adults: a national probability study.** *Rhinology* 2011, 49:324–330.
20. Doty RL, Shaman P, Applebaum SL, Giberson R, Siksorski L, Rosenberg L: **Smell identification ability: changes with age.** *Science* 1984, 226:1441–1443.
21. Seiden AM: **Postviral olfactory loss.** *Otolaryngol Clin North Am* 2004, 37:1159–1166.
22. Deems DA, Doty RL, Settle RG, Moore-Gillon V, Shaman P, Mester AF, Kimmelman CP, Brightman VJ, Snow JB Jr: **Smell and taste disorders, a study of 750 patients from the university of Pennsylvania smell and taste center.** *Arch Otolaryngol Head Neck Surg* 1991, 117:519–528.
23. Murphy C, Doty RL, Duncan HJ: **Clinical disorders of olfaction.** In *Handbook of Olfaction and Gustation.* 2nd edition. Edited by Doty RL. New York: Marcel Dekker; 2003.
24. Doty RL, Bartoshuk LM, Snow JB Jr: **Causes of olfactory and gustatory disorders.** In *Smell and Taste in Health and Disease.* Edited by Getchell TV, Doty RL, Bartoshuk LM, Snow JBJ. New York: Raven Press; 1991:449–462.
25. Seiden AM, Duncan HJ: **The diagnosis of a conductive olfactory loss.** *Laryngoscope* 2001, 111:9–14.
26. Goodspeed RB, Gent JF, Catalanotto FA: **Chemosensory dysfunction: clinical evaluation results from a taste and smell clinic.** *Postgrad Med* 1987, 81:251–257. 260.
27. Brämerson A, Nordin S, Bende M: **Clinical experience with patients with olfactory complaints, and their quality of life.** *Acta Otolaryngol* 2007, 127:167–174.
28. Damm M, Temmel A, Welge-Lüssen A, Eckel HE, Kreft MP, Klussmann JP, Gudziol H, Hüttenbrink KB, Hummel T: **Olfactory dysfunction: epidemiological data and treatment strategies in Germany, Austria, and Switzerland.** *HNO* 2004, 52:112–120.
29. Mori J, Aiba T, Sugiura M, Matsumoto K, Tomiyama K, Okuda F, Okigaki S, Nakai Y: **Clinical study of olfactory disturbance.** *Acta Otolaryngol* 1998, 118(Suppl 538):197–201.
30. Dalton P: **Olfaction and anosmia in rhinosinusitis.** *Curr Allergy Asthma Rep* 2004, 4:230–236.
31. Doty RL, Mishra A: **Olfaction and its alteration by nasal obstruction, rhinitis, and rhinosinusitis.** *Laryngoscope* 2001, 111:409–423.
32. Hummel T, Hüttenbrink KB: **Olfactory dysfunction due to sinonasal disease. causes, consequences, epidemiology, and therapy.** *HNO* 2005, 53:S26–S32.

33. Blackwell D, Collins J, Coles R: **Summary health statistics for U.S. adults. national health interview survey, 1997. National center for health statistics.** *Vital Health Statistics* 2002, **10:**15–16.

34. Benninger MS, Ferguson BJ, Hadley JA, Hamilos DL, Jacobs M, Kennedy DW, Lanza DC, Marple BF, Osguthorpe JD, Stankiewicz JA, Anon J, Denneny J, Emanuel I, Levine H: **Adult chronic rhinosinusitis: definitions, diagnosis, epidemiology, and pathophysiology.** *Otolaryngol Head Neck Surg* 2003, **129:**S1–S32.

35. Wallace DV, Dykewicz MS, Bernstein DI, Bernstein IL, Blessing-Moore J, Cox L, Khan DA, Lang DM, Nicklas RA, Oppenheimer J, Portnoy JM, Randolph CC, Schuller D, Spector SL, Tilles SA, May KR, Miller TA, Druce HM, Baroody FM, Bernstein JA, Craig TJ, Georgitis JW, Pawankar R, Rachelefsky GS, Settipane RA, Skoner DP, Stoloff SW: **The diagnosis and management of rhinitis: an updated practice parameter.** *J Allergy Clin Immunol* 2008, **122:**S1–S84.

36. Litvack JR, Fong K, Mace J, James KE, Smith TL: **Predictors of olfactory dysfunction in patients with chronic rhinosinusitis.** *Laryngoscope* 2008, **118:**2225–2230.

37. Duncan HJ: **Postviral olfactory loss.** In *Taste and Smell Disorders.* Edited by Seiden AM. New York: Thieme; 1997:72–78.

38. Jafek BW, Hartman D, Eller PM, Johnson EW, Strahan RC, Moran DT: **Postviral olfactory dysfunction.** *Am J Rhinol* 1990, **4:**91–100.

39. Cain WS, Goodspeed RB, Gent JF, Leonard G: **Evaluation of olfactory dysfunction in the connecticut chemosensory clinical research center.** *Laryngoscope* 1988, **98:**83–88.

40. Bonfils P, Avan P, Faulcon P, Malinvaud D: **Distorted odorant perception: analysis of a series of 56 patients with parosmia.** *Arch Otolaryngol Head Neck Surg* 2005, **131:**107–112.

41. Harris R, Davidson TM, Murphy C, Gilbert PE, Chen M: **Clinical evaluation and symptoms of chemosensory impairment: one thousand consecutive cases from the nasal dysfunction clinic in San Diego.** *Am J Rhinol* 2006, **20:**101–108.

42. Doty RL, Yousem DM, Pham LT, Kreshak AA, Geckle R, Lee WW: **Olfactory dysfunction in patients with head trauma.** *Arch Neurol* 1997, **54:**1131–1140.

43. Costanzo RM, DiNardo LJ, Reiter ER: **Head injury and olfaction.** In *Handbook of Olfaction and Gustation.* 2nd edition. Edited by Doty RL. New York: Marcel Dekker; 2003:629–638.

44. Collet S, Grulois V, Bertrand B, Rombaux P: **Post-traumatic olfactory dysfunction: a cohort study and update.** *B-ENT* 2009, **5:**97–107.

45. Costanzo RM, Zasler ND: **Head trauma.** In *Smell and Taste in Health and Disease.* Edited by Getchell TV, Doty RL, Bartoshuk LM, Snow JB Jr. New York: Raven Press; 1991:711–730.

46. Bonfils P, Malinvaud D, Soudry Y, Devars Du Maine M, Laccourreye O: **Surgical therapy and olfactory function.** *B-ENT* 2009, **5:**77–87.

47. Pade J, Hummel T: **Olfactory function following nasal surgery.** *Laryngoscope* 2008, **118:**1260–1264.

48. Harris AM, Griffin SM: **Postoperative taste and smell deficit after upper gastrointestinal cancer surgery: an unreported complication.** *J Surg Oncol* 2003, **82:**147–150.

49. Dhanani NM, Jiang D: **Anosmia and hypogeusia as a complication of general anesthesia.** *J Clin Anesth* 2012, **24:**231–233.

50. Henkin RI: **Altered taste and smell after anesthesia: cause and effect - reply.** *Anesthesiology* 1995, **83:**648–649.

51. Konstantinidis I, Tsakiropoulou E, Iakovou I, Douvantzi A, Metaxas S: **Anosmia after general anaesthesia: a case report.** *Anaesthesia* 2009, **64:**1367–1370.

52. Ackerman BH, Kasbekar N: **Disturbances of taste and smell induced by drugs.** *Pharmacotherapy* 1997, **17:**482–496.

53. Doty RL, Bromley SM: **Effects of drugs on olfaction and taste.** *Otolaryngol Clin North Am* 2004, **37:**1229–1254.

54. Lötsch J, Geisslinger G, Hummel T: **Sniffing out pharmacology: interactions of drugs with human olfaction.** *Trends Pharmacol Sci* 2012, **33:**193–199.

55. Henkin RI: **Drug-induced taste and smell disorders: incidence, mechanisms and management related primarily to treatment of sensory receptor dysfunction.** *Drug Saf* 1994, **11:**318–377.

56. Schiffman SS, Nagle HT: **Effect of environmental pollutants on taste and smell.** *Otolaryngol Head Neck Surg* 1992, **106:**693–700.

57. Hastings L, Miller ML: **Influence of environmental toxicants on olfactory function.** In *Handbook of Olfaction and Gustation.* 2nd edition. Edited by Doty RL. New York: Marcel Dekker; 2003:575–592.

58. Doty RL, Hastings L: **Neurotoxic exposure and olfactory impairment.** *Clin Occup Environ Med* 2001, **1:**547–575.

59. Shusterman DJ, Sheedy JE: **Occupational and environmental disorders of the special senses.** *Occup Med* 1992, **7:**515–542.

60. Upadhyay UD, Holbrook EH: **Olfactory loss as a result of toxic exposure.** *Otolaryngol Clin North Am* 2004, **37:**1185–1207.

61. Karstensen HG, Tommerup N: **Isolated and syndromic forms of congenital anosmia.** *Clin Genet* 2012, **81:**210–215.

62. Acharya V, Acharya J, Lüders H: **Olfactory epileptic auras.** *Neurology* 1998, **51:**56–61.

63. Velakoulis D: **Olfactory hallucinations.** In *Olfaction and the Brain.* Edited by Brewer WJ, Castle D, Pantelis C. Cambridge: Cambridge University Press; 2006:322–333.

64. Fuller GN, Guiloff RJ: **Migrainous olfactory hallucinations.** *J Neurol Neurosurg Psychiatry* 1987, **50:**1688–1690.

65. Schreiber AO, Calvert PC: **Migrainous olfactory hallucinations.** *Headache* 1986, **26:**513–514.

66. Bannier S, Berdagué JL, Rieu I, de Chazeron I, Marques A, Derost P, Ulla M, Llorca PM, Durif F: **Prevalence and phenomenology of olfactory hallucinations in parkinson's disease.** *J Neurol Neurosurg Psychiatry* 2012, **83:**1019–1021.

67. Arguedas D, Langdon R, Stevenson R: **Neuropsychological characteristics associated with olfactory hallucinations in schizophrenia.** *J Int Neuropsychol Soc* 2012, **18:**799–808.

68. Kopala LC, Good KP, Honer WG: **Olfactory hallucinations and olfactory identification ability in patients with schizophrenia and other psychiatric disorders.** *Schizophr Res* 1994, **12:**205–211.

69. Reden J, Mueller A, Mueller C, Konstantinidis I, Frasnelli J, Landis BN, Hummel T: **Recovery of olfactory function following closed head injury or infections of the upper respiratory tract.** *Arch Otolaryngol Head Neck Surg* 2006, **132:**265–269.

70. Temmel AFP, Quint C, Schickinger-Fischer B, Klimek L, Stoller E, Hummel T: **Characteristics of olfactory disorders in relation to major causes of olfactory loss.** *Arch Otolaryngol Head Neck Surg* 2002, **128:**635–641.

71. Duncan HJ, Seiden AM: **Long-term follow-up of olfactory loss secondary to head trauma and upper respiratory tract infection.** *Arch Otolaryngol Head Neck Surg* 1995, **121:**1183–1187.

72. Welge-Lüssen A, Hilgenfeld A, Meusel T, Hummel T: **Long-term follow-up of posttraumatic olfactory disorders.** *Rhinology* 2012, **50:**67–72.

73. Mueller CA, Hummel T: **Recovery of olfactory function after nine years of post-traumatic anosmia: a case report.** *J Med Case Reports* 2009, **3:**9283.

74. Guilemany JM, Garcia-Piñero A, Alobid I, Centellas S, Mariño FS, Valero A, Bernal-Sprekelsen M, Picado C, Mullol J: **The loss of smell in persistent allergic rhinitis is improved by levocetirizine due to reduction of nasal inflammation but not nasal nongestion (the CIRANO study).** *Int Arch Allergy Immunol* 2012, **158:**184–190.

75. Meltzer EO, Jalowayski AA, Orgel HA, Harris AG: **Subjective and objective assessments in patients with seasonal allergic rhinitis: effects of therapy with mometasone furoate nasal spray.** *J Allergy Clin Immunol* 1998, **102:**39–49.

76. Heilmann S, Huettenbrink KB, Hummel T: **Local and systemic administration of corticosteroids in the treatment of olfactory loss.** *Am J Rhinol* 2004, **18:**29–33.

77. Mott AE, Cain WS, Lafreniere D, Leonard G, Gent JF, Frank ME: **Topical corticosteroid treatment of anosmia associated with nasal and sinus disease.** *Arch Otolaryngol Head Neck Surg* 1997, **123:**367–372.

78. Golding-Wood DG, Holmstrom M, Darby Y, Scadding GK, Lund VJ: **The treatment of hyposmia with intranasal steroids.** *J Laryngol Otol* 1996, **110:**132–135.

79. Goodspeed RB, Gent JF, Catalanotto FA, Cain WS, Zagraniski RT: **Corticosteroids in olfactory dysfunction.** In *Book Corticosteroids in olfactory dysfunction.* City: Macmillan; 1986:514–518. 514–518.

80. Rudmik L, Smith TL: **Olfactory improvement after endoscopic sinus surgery.** *Curr Opin Otolaryngol Head Neck Surg* 2012, **20:**29–32.

81. Litvack JR, Mace J, Smith TL: **Does olfactory function improve after endoscopic sinus surgery?** *Otolaryngol Head Neck Surg* 2009, **140:**312–319.

82. Jiang RS, Lu FJ, Liang KL, Shiao JY, Su MC, Hsin CH, Chen WK: **Olfactory function in patients with chronic rhinosinusitis before and after functional endoscopic sinus surgery.** *Am J Rhinol* 2008, **22:**445–448.

83. Pfaar O, Hüttenbrink KB, Hummel T: **Assessment of olfactory function after septoplasty: a longitudinal study.** *Rhinology* 2004, **42:**195–199.

84. Delank KW, Stoll W: Olfactory function after functional endoscopic sinus surgery for chronic sinusitis. *Rhinology* 1998, **36**:15–19.

85. Hosemann W, Goertzen W, Wohlleben R, Wolf S, Wigand ME: Olfaction after endoscopic endonasal ethmoidectomy. *Am J Rhinol* 1993, **7**:11–15.

86. Hummel T, Stuck BA: Treatment of olfactory disorders. *HNO* 2010, **58**:656–660.

87. Henkin RI, Schecter PJ, Friedewald WT, Demets DL, Raff M: A double blind study of the effects of zinc sulfate on taste and smell dysfunction. *Am J Med Sci* 1976, **272**:285–299.

88. Quint C, Temmel AFP, Hummel T, Ehrenberger K: The quinoxaline derivative caroverine in the treatment of sensorineural smell disorders: a proof-of-concept study. *Acta Otolaryngol* 2002, **122**:877–881.

89. Reden J, Lill K, Zahnert T, Haehner A, Hummel T: Olfactory function in patients with postinfectious and posttraumatic smell disorders before and after treatment with vitamin A: a double-blind, placebo-controlled, randomized clinical trial. *Laryngoscope* 2012, **122**:1906–1909.

90. Reden J, Herting B, Lill K, Kern R, Hummel T: Treatment of postinfectious olfactory disorders with minocycline: a double-blind, placebo-controlled study. *Laryngoscope* 2011, **121**:679–682.

91. Hummel T, Heilmann S, Hüttenbriuk KB: Lipoic acid in the treatment of smell dysfunction following viral infection of the upper respiratory tract. *Laryngoscope* 2002, **112**:2076–2080.

92. Henkin RI, Velicu I, Schmidt L: Relative resistance to oral theophylline treatment in patients with hyposmia manifested by decreased secretion of nasal mucus cyclic nucleotides. *Am J Med Sci* 2011, **341**:17–22.

93. Levy LM, Henkin RI, Lin CS, Hutter A, Schellinger D: Increased brain activation in response to odors in patients with hyposmia after theophylline treatment demonstrated by fMRI. *J Comput Assist Tomogr* 1998, **22**:760–770.

94. Gudziol V, Hummel T: Effects of pentoxifylline on olfactory sensitivity: a postmarketing surveillance study. *Arch Otolaryngol Head Neck Surg* 2009, **135**:291–295.

95. Panagiotopoulos G, Naxakis S, Papavasiliou A, Filipakis K, Papatheodorou G, Goumas P: Decreasing nasal mucus Ca++ improves hyposmia. *Rhinology* 2005, **43**:130–134.

96. Vent J, Wang DW, Damm M: Effects of traditional Chinese acupuncture in post-viral olfactory dysfunction. *Otolaryngol Head Neck Surg* 2010, **142**:505–509.

97. Silas J, Doty RL: No evidence for specific benefit of acupuncture over vitamin B complex in treating persons with olfactory dysfunction. *Otolaryngol Head Neck Surg* 2010, **143**:603.

98. Damm M, Vent J: Response to: no evidence for specific benefit of acupuncture over vitamin B complex in treating persons with olfactory dysfunction, by Jonathan Silas and Richard L. Doty. *Otolaryngol Head Neck Surg* 2010, **143**:603–604.

99. Anzinger A, Albrecht J, Kopietz R, Kleemann AM, Schöpf V, Demmel M, Schreder T, Eichhorn I, Wiesmann M: Effects of laserneedle acupuncture on olfactory sensitivity of healthy human subjects: a placebo-controlled, double-blinded, randomized trial. *Rhinology* 2009, **47**:153–159.

100. Fleiner F, Lau L, Göktas O: Active olfactory training for the treatment of smelling disorders. *Ear Nose Throat J* 2012, **91**:198–203. 215.

101. Hummel T, Rissom K, Reden J, Hähner A, Weidenbecher M, Hüttenbrink KB: Effects of olfactory training in patients with olfactory loss. *Laryngoscope* 2009, **119**:496–499.

102. Leopold DA, Loehrl TA, Schwob JE: Long-term follow-up of surgically treated phantosmia. *Arch Otolaryngol Head Neck Surg* 2002, **128**:642–647.

103. Leopold DA, Schwob JE, Youngentob SL, Hornung DE, Wright HN, Mozell MM: Successful treatment of phantosmia with preservation of olfaction. *Arch Otolaryngol Head Neck Surg* 1991, **117**:1402–1406.

104. Sarangi P, Aziz TZ: Post-traumatic parosmia treated by olfactory nerve section. *Br J Neurosurg* 1990, **4**:358.

105. Henkin RI, Potolicchio SJ, Levy LM: Improvement in smell and taste dysfunction after repetitive transcranial magnetic stimulation. *Am J Otolaryngol* 2011, **32**:38–46.

106. Nordin S, Brämerson A: Complaints of olfactory disorders: epidemiology, assessment and clinical implications. *Curr Opin Allergy Clin Immunol* 2008, **8**:10–15.

107. Hummel T, Nordin S: Olfactory disorders and their consequences for quality of life. *Acta Otolaryngol* 2005, **125**:116–121.

108. Neuland C, Bitter T, Marschner H, Gudziol H, Guntinas-Lichius O: Health-related and specific olfaction-related quality of life in patients with chronic functional anosmia or severe hyposmia. *Laryngoscope* 2011, **121**:867–872.

109. Miwa T, Furukawa M, Tsukatani T, Costanzo RM, DiNardo LJ, Reiter ER: Impact of olfactory impairment on quality of life and disability. *Arch Otolaryngol Head Neck Surg* 2001, **127**:497–503.

110. Santos DV, Reiter ER, DiNardo LJ, Costanzo RM: Hazardous events associated with impaired olfactory function. *Arch Otolaryngol Head Neck Surg* 2004, **130**:317–319.

111. Ferris AM, Duffy VB: Effect of olfactory deficits on nutritional status: does age predict persons at risk? *Ann N Y Acad Sci* 1989, **561**:113–123.

112. Mattes RD, Cowart BJ, Schiavo MA, Arnold C, Garrison B, Kare MR, Lowry LD: Dietary evaluation of patients with smell and/or taste disorders. *Am J Clin Nutr* 1990, **51**:233–240.

113. Mattes RD: Nutritional implications of taste and smell disorders. In *Handbook of Olfaction and Gustation*. Edited by Doty RL. New York: Marcel Dekker; 1995:731–734.

114. Bonfils P, Faulcon P, Tavernier L, Bonfils NA, Malinvaud D: Home accidents associated with anosmia. *Presse Med* 2008, **37**:742–745.

115. Nordin S, Blomqvist EH, Olsson P, Stjärne P, Ehnhage A: Effects of smell loss on daily life and adopted coping strategies in patients with nasal polyposis with asthma. *Acta Otolaryngol* 2011, **131**:826–832.

116. Aschenbrenner K, Hummel C, Teszmer K, Krone F, Ishimaru T, Seo HS, Hummel T: The influence of olfactory loss on dietary behaviors. *Laryngoscope* 2008, **118**:135–144.

117. Van Toller S: Assessing the impact of anosmia: review of a questionnaire's findings. *Chem Senses* 1999, **24**:705–712.

118. Blomqvist EH, Brämerson A, Stjärne P, Nordin S: Consequences of olfactory loss and adopted coping strategies. *Rhinology* 2004, **42**:189–194.

119. Tennen H, Affleck G, Mendola R: Coping with smell and taste disorder. In *Smell and Taste in Health and Disease*. Edited by Getchell TV, Doty RL, Bartoshuk LM, Snow JBJ. New York: Raven Press; 1991:787–802.

120. Croy I, Negoias S, Novakova L, Landis BN, Hummel T: Learning about the functions of the olfactory system from people without a sense of smell. *PLoS One* 2012, **7**:e33365.

121. Landis BN, Stow NW, Lacroix JS, Hugentobler M, Hummel T: Olfactory disorders: the patients' view. *Rhinology* 2009, **47**:454–459.

122. Gudziol V, Wolff-Stephan S, Aschenbrenner K, Joraschky P, Hummel T: Depression resulting from olfactory dysfunction is associated with reduced sexual appetite: a cross-sectional cohort study. *J Sex Med* 2009, **6**:1924–1929.

123. Frasnelli J, Hummel T: Olfactory dysfunction and daily life. *Eur Arch Otorhinolaryngol* 2005, **262**:231–235.

124. Glaser O: Hereditary deficiencies in the sense of smell. *Science* 1918, **48**:647–648.

125. DeVere R, Calvert M: *Navigating Taste and Smell Disorders*. New York: demos health; 2011.

126. Vowles RH, Bleach NR, Rowe-Jones JM: Congenital anosmia. *Int J Pediatr Otorhinolaryngol* 1997, **41**:207–214.

127. Chu S, Downes JJ: Odour-evoked autobiographical memories: psychological investigations of Proustian phenomena. *Chem Senses* 2000, **25**:111–116.

128. Herz RS, Cupchik GC: The emotional distinctiveness of odor-evoked memories. *Chem Senses* 1995, **20**:517–528.

129. Herz RS: Are odors the best cues to memory? A cross-modal comparison of associative memory stimuli. In *Olfaction and Taste Xii: An International Symposium*, Volume 855. Edited by Murphy C. New York: New York Acad Sciences; 1998:670–674. *Annals of the New York Academy of Sciences*].

130. Treadway MT, Zald DH: Reconsidering anhedonia in depression: lessons from translational neuroscience. *Neurosci Biobehav Rev* 2011, **35**:537–555.

131. Landis BN, Frasnelli J, Hummel T: Euosmia: a rare form of parosmia. *Acta Otolaryngol* 2006, **126**:101–103.

132. Desor JA, Beauchamp GK: The human capacity to transmit olfactory information. *Percept Psychophys* 1974, **16**:551–556.

133. Weiss T, Snitz K, Yablonka A, Khan RM, Gafsou D, Schneidman E, Sobel N: Perceptual convergence of multi-component mixtures in olfaction implies an olfactory white. *Proc Natl Acad Sci* 2012, **109**:19959–19964.

134. Jastreboff PJ: Phantom auditory perception (tinnitus): mechanisms of generation and perception. *Neurosci Res* 1990, **8**:221–254.

135. Eggermont JJ, Roberts LE: The neuroscience of tinnitus. *Trends Neurosci* 2004, **27**:676–682.

136. Doty RL, Cometto-Muniz JE: Trigeminal chemosensation. In *Handbook of Olfaction and Gustation*. 2nd edition. Edited by Doty RL. New York: Marcel Dekker; 2003:981–1000.

137. Silver WL, Finger TE: The trigeminal system. In *Smell and Taste in Health and Disease*. Edited by Getchell TV, Doty RL, Bartoshuk LM, Snow JB Jr. New York: Raven Press; 1991:97–108.

138. Carskadon MA, Herz RS: **Minimal olfactory perception during sleep: why odor alarms will not work for humans.** *Sleep* 2004, **27**:402–405.

139. Radil T, Wysocki CJ: **Spatiotemporal masking in pure olfaction.** *Ann N Y Acad Sci* 1998, **855**:641–644.

140. Sacks O: *Hallucinations.* New York: Knopf; 2012.

141. Flor H, Nikolajsen L, Staehelin Jensen T: **Phantom limb pain: a case of maladaptive CNS plasticity?** *Nat Rev Neurosci* 2006, **7**:873–881.

142. Flor H, Elbert T, Knecht S, Wienbruch C, Pantev C, Birbaumer N, Larbig W, Taub E: **Phantom-limb pain as a perceptual correlate of cortical reorganization following arm amputation.** *Nature* 1995, **375**:482–484.

143. Classen C, Howes D, Synnott A: *Aroma: The Cultural History of Smell.* London: Routledge; 1994.

144. American Medical Association: *Guides to the Evaluation of Permanent Impairment.* 6th edition. Chicago: American Medical Association; 2007.

145. Landis BN, Hummel T, Hugentobler M, Giger R, Lacroix JS: **Ratings of overall olfactory function.** *Chem Senses* 2003, **28**:691–694.

146. Knaapila A, Tuorila H, Kyvik KO, Wright MJ, Keskitalo K, Hansen J, Kaprio J, Perola M, Silventoinen K: **Self-ratings of olfactory function reflect odor annoyance rather than olfactory acuity.** *Laryngoscope* 2008, **118**:2212–2217.

147. Welge-Lüssen A, Hummel T, Stojan T, Wolfensberger M: **What is the correlation between ratings and measures of olfactory function in patients with olfactory loss?** *Am J Rhinol* 2005, **19**:567–571.

9

Reappraisal of the glycerol test in patients with suspected Menière's disease

Bernd Lütkenhöner[*] and Türker Basel

Abstract

Background: Recent advances in magnetic resonance imaging make it possible to visualize the presumed pathophysiologic correlate of Menière's disease: endolymphatic hydrops. As traditional diagnostic tests can provide only indirect evidence, they are hardly competitive in this respect and need to be rethought. This is done here for the glycerol test.

Methods: The data of a previous retrospective analysis of the glycerol test in patients with suspected Menière's disease are reinterpreted using a simple model. The mean threshold reduction (MTR) in the frequency range from 125 to 1500 Hz (calculated from audiograms obtained immediately before and four hours after the glycerol intake) is used as the test statistic. The proposed model explains the frequency distribution of the observed MTR by the convolution of a Gaussian probability density function (representing measurement errors) with a template representing the frequency distribution of the true MTR. The latter is defined in terms of two adjustable parameters. After fitting the model to the data, the performance of the test is evaluated using receiver operating characteristic (ROC) analysis.

Results: The cumulative frequency distribution of the observed MTR can be explained almost perfectly by the model. According to the ROC analysis performed, the capability of the currently used audiometric procedure to detect a glycerol-induced threshold reduction corresponds to a diagnostic test of rather high accuracy (area under the ROC curve greater than 0.9). Simulations show that methodological improvements could further enhance the performance.

Conclusions: Owing to their ability to reveal functional aspects without an obvious morphological correlate, traditional test for Menière's disease could be decisive for defining the stage of the disease. A distinctive feature of the glycerol test is that it is capable of determining, with high accuracy, whether the pathophysiologic condition of the inner ear is partially reversible. Prospectively, this could help to estimate the chances of specific therapies.

Background

In 1861, Prosper Menière reported on patients who suddenly suffered from intermittent attacks of vertigo combined with tinnitus and a gradually increasing hearing loss [1]. Although more than 150 years have passed since then, the disease, now named after him, is still not fully understood, and the criteria for establishing the diagnosis have not fundamentally changed. According to the widely accepted guidelines of the Committee on Hearing and Equilibrium of the American Academy of Otolaryngology - Head and Neck Surgery [2], the diagnosis of *definite* Menière' disease requires (1) two or more definitive spontaneous episodes of vertigo 20 minutes or longer, (2) an audiometrically documented hearing loss on at least one occasion, (3) tinnitus or aural fullness in the treated ear, and (4) the exclusion of other causes; *probable* Menière' disease is diagnosed if there is only one definite episode of vertigo. These definitions show that, as yet, the identification of Menière's disease is largely dependent on the patient's medical history. By implication this means that the numerous efforts to develop a specific diagnostic test [3,4] did not lead to a practice that gained general acceptance. Recently, however, a major breakthrough was achieved. Using magnetic resonance imaging (MRI) with gadolinium as the contrast agent, Nakashima et al. [5] succeeded to visualize the presumed pathophysiologic correlate of Menière's disease:

* Correspondence: Lutkenh@uni-muenster.de
ENT Clinic, Münster University Hospital, Münster, Germany

endolymphatic hydrops. According to the above-mentioned guidelines, the diagnosis of *definite* Menière's disease becomes *certain* by such confirmation, which hitherto could be obtained only after death. Meanwhile, this seminal work has been confirmed in many subsequent studies, in which the methodology was not only improved [6,7], but also applied to specific questions [8-11].

In an MRI study by Fiorino et al. [12], each of 26 patients diagnosed with definite Menière's disease showed evidence of endolymphatic hydrops exclusively in the affected ear. Moreover, there was no such evidence in 11 of 12 patients with other inner ear diseases. Considering the conclusiveness of these results, it can be expected that MRI will soon be the method of choice if a suspected diagnosis of Menière's disease is to be confirmed by proving the hydrops. This intriguing progress appears to eliminate the need for other diagnostic procedures. However, such a conclusion would be premature. Diagnostic tests should be appraised in terms of their ability to improve patient-important outcomes [13], and in this respect, some of the traditional methods (or a combination of them) may ultimately turn out to be competitive, especially since it is not clear how important it is to prove endolymphatic hydrops in patients that were already diagnosed with definite Menière's disease. If the above-mentioned results are representative, meaning that patients so diagnosed nearly always have endolymphatic hydrops (a supposition that would be consistent with Merchant et al. [14]), verifying the hydrops by whatever method provides hardly any new information. Thus, in future, more emphasis should probably be placed on the question as to what the various diagnostic tests can tell us about the stage and manifestation of the disease and to what extent they allow us to predict the prospects of specific therapeutic measures, e.g., treatment with betahistine [15].

As proving endolymphatic hydrops appears to become the domain of imaging techniques, the possible future roles of other diagnostic tests for Menière's disease need to be rethought. This is done here for the glycerol test devised by Klockhoff and Lindblom [16], but some basic conclusions appear to be valid for other diagnostic procedures as well. The test exploits the fact that, in patients suffering from Menière's disease, oral application of glycerol can temporarily improve the threshold of hearing, whereas no systematic effect is to be expected in patients with other hearing disorders and subjects with normal hearing. The underlying idea is that the dehydrating effect of glycerol transiently reduces the endolymphatic volume, which in turn may lead to partial recovery from hearing loss. To test for the latter, a pre-test audiogram is compared with an audiogram taken a few hours after the glycerol intake. While a significant threshold reduction can be regarded as evidence of endolymphatic hydrops, the reverse is not true: Since Menière's disease is typically fluctuating and progressive [17,18], there may be hydrops despite a negative glycerol test. It is known, for example, that the probability of a positive glycerol test depends on the phase of the disease, being minimal at times of remission [19]. Moreover, the hearing loss may be irreversible at a more advanced stage so that reducing the endolymphatic volume has no effect anymore.

Several variants of the glycerol test have been proposed since its first description, and so it seems timely to scrutinize the conceptual and methodological details of the test. In a previous article [20], we presented a retrospective study of 356 cases with suspected Menière's disease (all ears fulfilled the aforementioned criteria for definite or at least probable Menière's disease). In addition to descriptive analyses of the data, we introduced a new criterion for a positive test result. Moreover, we proposed a rule of thumb that can be used to define a subpopulation of patients for whom the probability of a positive outcome is significantly higher than for the excluded patients. The rule proved to be competitive with more advanced predictive modeling approaches [21]. However, gaining a deeper understanding of the test was impeded by the fact that there is no "gold standard" to compare with and that the determination of the auditory threshold is, like any measurement, affected by errors. In the present work, these problems are overcome by fitting a simple model to the data. The model gives an idea of what the results would be if the thresholds of hearing were determined exactly. Moreover, it becomes possible to assess the performance of the test by considering its receiver operating characteristic (ROC) curve and to predict what would be gained by methodological amendments.

Methods
Data
The same data as in our previous study [20], now available from a Digital Repository [22], are used. Briefly, archived audiograms from 347 patients that underwent a glycerol test to confirm a suspected Menière's disease were transcribed into a computer-readable form. The tests had been performed following the protocol suggested by Klockhoff [19], which means that glycerol (1.2 ml/kg body weight) was orally administered with an equal amount of isotonic saline solution. The audiograms were obtained immediately before the glycerol intake (pre-test audiogram) and at hourly intervals thereafter (the last one obtained after four hours). Since *both* ears were investigated in a few patients, 356 cases are available altogether. But to restrict the data range to be plotted, two cases are excluded here as outliers (apart from that, the exclusion has no relevant impact on the results).

The effect of the administered glycerol is assessed by comparing the pre-test audiogram with the audiogram that was obtained after four hours. In the previous study [20], the aggregate threshold reduction (ATR) in a contiguous frequency range was used as a summary measure. But this quantity is inconvenient for modeling, because its calculation requires to integrate over a variable frequency range (the bounds of integration depend on the true hearing losses at the different frequencies as well as measurement errors), which makes it difficult (if not impossible) to apply standard statistical techniques. Therefore an alternative summary measure is used here: the mean threshold reduction (MTR) at the five lowest audiometric frequencies (125, 250, 500, 1000, and 1500 Hz), which represent the frequency range where the effect of glycerol is typically most pronounced. A convenient side-benefit of focusing on these frequencies is that the MTR is always an integer number (five thresholds are averaged, each of which was determined in steps of 5 dB).

Figure 1 shows that MTR (abscissa) and ATR (ordinate) are highly correlated ($R = 0.924$). In principle, each of the 354 cases considered in this study is represented by a single point, but the points partially coincide. Thus, instead of single points, circles with an area proportional to the number of points sharing the respective location are plotted. If the criterion for a positive glycerol test is that the ATR is at least 30 dB (dotted horizontal line), the false-positive rate may be expected to be about 5% [20]. Consistent decisions would be made by requiring the MTR to be at least 5 dB (dotted vertical line), apart from the few cases represented by the filled circles: In 16 cases (red circles) the test would be positive only according to the ATR-based criterion, and in 9 cases (blue circles) it would be positive only according to the MTR-based criterion.

Convolution model

Audiograms measured at different times typically show discrepancies even when there is no reason to assume that the true threshold of hearing has changed. This intrinsic uncertainty of the threshold estimation may be considered as a measurement error, which, of course, propagates to every audiogram-based measure. As a consequence, the distribution of the observed MTR values reflects, to a considerable extent, the measurement error rather than the glycerol-induced threshold reduction. If the measurement error is assumed to be additive to the glycerol

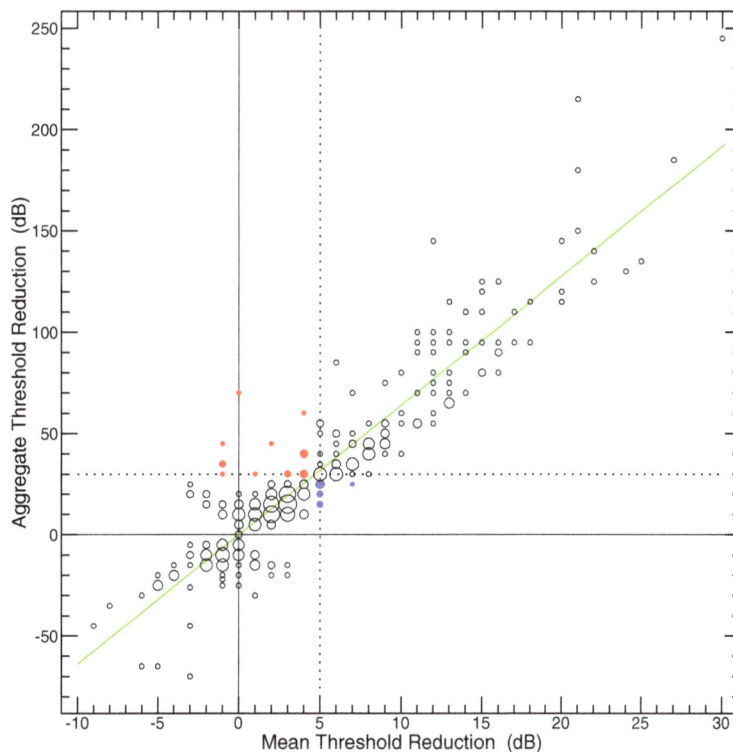

Figure 1 Correlation between mean threshold reduction (MTR) and aggregate threshold reduction (ATR). Both the MTR and the ATR can assume only a limited number of values. As a consequence, there are generally multiple occurrences for each combination of these measures so that a standard scatter plot would be problematic. The problem was solved by plotting a circle for each MTR-ATR combination and adjusting the radius so that the area of the circle is proportional to the number of occurrences. The two dotted lines (one horizontal, the other vertical) represent criteria that generally lead to consistent decisions as to the presence of a glycerol induced effect. The few exceptions are marked by filled circles: Blue indicates that the MTR is equal to or greater than the associated criterion value while the ATR falls short of the corresponding threshold. Red indicates that the situation is just the other way round.

effect, the problem can be described by a convolution formula,

$$f(x) = \int\limits_{-\infty}^{\infty} g(u)\ h(x-u)\ du, \tag{1}$$

where $f(x), g(x),$ and $h(x)$ are probability density functions. The first one, $f(x),$ characterizes the distribution of the MTR values actually observed, whereas the second one, $g(x),$ characterizes the distribution that would be observed under ideal conditions, i.e., in the absence of measurement errors. The third function, finally, is the probability density function of the measurement error. In what follows, the measurement error will be assumed to be normally distributed, with a standard deviation estimated from the data. Given $h(x),$ the unknown $g(x)$ could be calculated by deconvolving the observed $f(x),$ at least in theory. However, to be able to use this approach for the problem at hand, the number of cases would have to be increased by at least an order of magnitude [23,24]. Thus, Eq. (1) will be used here in a different way. The idea is to "guess" a suitable function $g(x)$ and to determine the parameters of this function so that the right-hand side of the equation optimally explains the observed $f(x).$

As will be shown, the data can be explained reasonably well by means of an empirical function $g(x)$ depending on only two parameters. The basic idea is outlined in Figure 2a. Conceptually, the patients are divided into two groups. Patients belonging to the first group, represented by the arrow in the figure, are assumed to show no glycerol-induced effect at all. Their proportion is denoted as p_0 (in Figure 2 having a value of 0.3). Patients belonging to the second group are assumed to have a threshold reduction that is distributed according to a gamma distribution with a shape parameter of 2 (the choice of this well-known distribution was a pragmatic decision; other distributions with similar properties could be assumed as well). The corresponding probability density function is, for $x \geq 0,$

$$g_2(x) = \theta^{-2}x\exp\left(-\theta^{-1}x\right), \tag{2}$$

where θ is called the scale parameter. Figure 2a shows this function for $\theta = 3.$ For reasons that will be explicated in the Discussion (in essence, the goal is to avoid eye-catching details that cannot be validated against the data), this initial concept of function $g(x)$ is modified as follows. In a first step, function $g_2(x)$ is replaced by a function that is constant between $x = 0$ and the maximum at $x = \theta$ (indicated by the dashed line in Figure 2a). Renormalization (to get a probability density function again) yields:

$$\tilde{g}_2(x) = \frac{1}{3\theta}\begin{cases} 1 & for\ 0 \leq x \leq \theta \\ \theta^{-1}x\exp\left(1-\theta^{-1}x\right) & for\ x > \theta \end{cases} \tag{3}$$

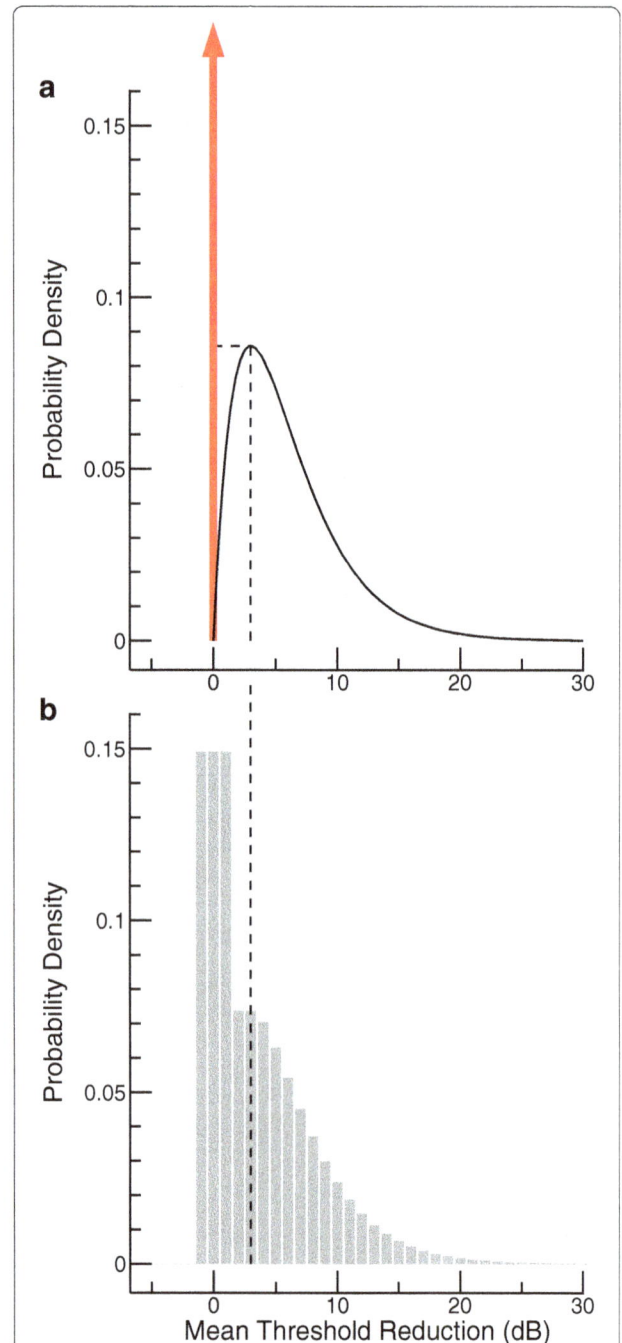

Figure 2 Model for the distribution of the "true" MTR (i.e., the MTR that would be obtained if thresholds were estimated without errors). **(a)** Basic idea. A first model parameter corresponds to the proportion of patients *without* a glycerol-induced threshold reduction (represented by the arrow), whereas a second one scales the MTR distribution of the patients showing an effect. **(b)** Discretized and smoothed version of the upper model.

In the next step, the distribution is discretized, taking into account that the MTR is an integer. Cases with an MTR not greater than 1 dB are finally combined with those showing no effect, and the resulting no-effect group is distributed equally over the MTR values $-1, 0$, and 1 dB (Figure 2b). The last step has no other purpose than to facilitate the visualization of the model parameter p_0 (which otherwise would be represented by a rather high peak).

Modeling investigator bias

A deviation of the observed error distribution from a normal distribution will be interpreted as possible evidence of a partially biased practice on the part of the investigator. To corroborate the hypothesis, some modifications are applied to the above model. For a start, we confine ourselves to considering the threshold estimation for a single frequency. To mimic the common practice in clinical audiometry, the real-valued measurement error (normally distributed) is rounded to the nearest integer divisible by 5. Bias is introduced by assuming that an investigator sometimes reuses a previously estimated threshold instead of taking the time to carefully measure a small threshold change. To mimic this behavior in the model, a threshold difference of 5 dB between previous and current audiogram is ignored with a certain probability. Correspondingly, the model provides for the possibility that an investigator occasionally determines a threshold difference of 5 dB when a more careful procedure would have resulted in a threshold difference of 10 dB. It should be emphasized that the investigator is assumed to be unprejudiced as to the sign of the threshold change.

To simulate the estimation of MTRs, it was assumed that threshold estimations at different times (and possibly for different frequencies) have statistically independent measurement errors with identical standard deviations, σ. The difference between two threshold estimations for the same frequency (test-retest reliability), then, has the standard deviation $2^{1/2}\sigma$, and averaging 5 such differences (as required for obtaining the MTR) yields a measure with the standard deviation $(2/5)^{1/2}\sigma$. The test-retest reliability of auditory threshold estimations has been investigated in many studies [25-29], and unlike in our model, the measurement error was found to be frequency-dependent. But this does not seriously compromise the validity of the model, because σ^2 can be understood as the *mean* variance for the frequencies considered.

Numerical calculations

All calculations were done with custom scripts using Matlab Version 7.14 (The MathWorks, Inc., Natick, MA, USA). The model parameters were optimized by least-squares fitting using the function FMINSEARCH (considering the cumulative distribution functions). ROC curves were calculated using the function PERF-CURVE, which readily provides also the area under the curve (AUC).

The Monte Carlo simulations for the ROC analysis were done as follows. First, "true" MTR values were assigned to each of 100,000 cases so that the resulting cumulative distribution function was in accordance with that of the assumed model. Adding normally distributed random numbers to these values then yielded the "experimentally observed" MTR values.

Results
Measurement error

Before attempts can be made to correct the distribution of observed threshold reductions for the measurement error, the latter has to be characterized. Our previous investigation (see Figure Four in [20]) suggested that the effect of glycerol barely intensifies after the third hour. Thus, the MTR distribution derived from the audiograms taken three and four hours after the glycerol intake (histogram on the left of Figure 3) is basically a fingerprint of the measurement error. Mean and standard deviation were calculated to be 0.26 dB and 2.45 dB, respectively (the curve superimposed on the histogram shows a normal distribution with a standard deviation corresponding to the calculated one, but with mean zero). The estimated mean confirms the previous observation that the threshold after 4 hours is only marginally lower than after 3 hours. The difference reached statistical significance, though (two-sided t-test yielded $P = 0.045$).

A remarkable feature of the estimated distribution is the pronounced peak at an MTR of zero, which is not fully compatible with the idea of a normally distributed measurement error. Although the reasons could be manifold, a Monte Carlo simulation using the model described in the Methods corroborates the hypothesis that this peculiarity reflects a methodological shortcoming: Knowledge of a previous audiogram biases the decision-making on part of the investigator. To obtain the histogram on the right of Figure 3, 100,000 partially biased investigations were simulated. A comparison with the histogram on the left shows that, by carefully adjusting the parameters, an excellent agreement between model and data could be achieved: It was assumed that single threshold estimations have a standard deviation of $\sigma = 4.43$ dB, that a threshold difference of 5 dB between previous and current audiogram is ignored in 80% of the cases, and that a threshold difference of 10 dB is reduced to 5 dB in 30% of the cases. Again, the solid curve represents a zero-mean normal distribution with a standard deviation corresponding to that estimated from the data (the simulated ones in this case). The dotted curve, by contrast, represents the distribution that, according to the model, would be obtained in the case of an unbiased estimation (as described in the Methods section, the standard deviation assumed for single threshold estimations, σ, was converted into the standard deviation of the MTR, yielding 2.80 dB).

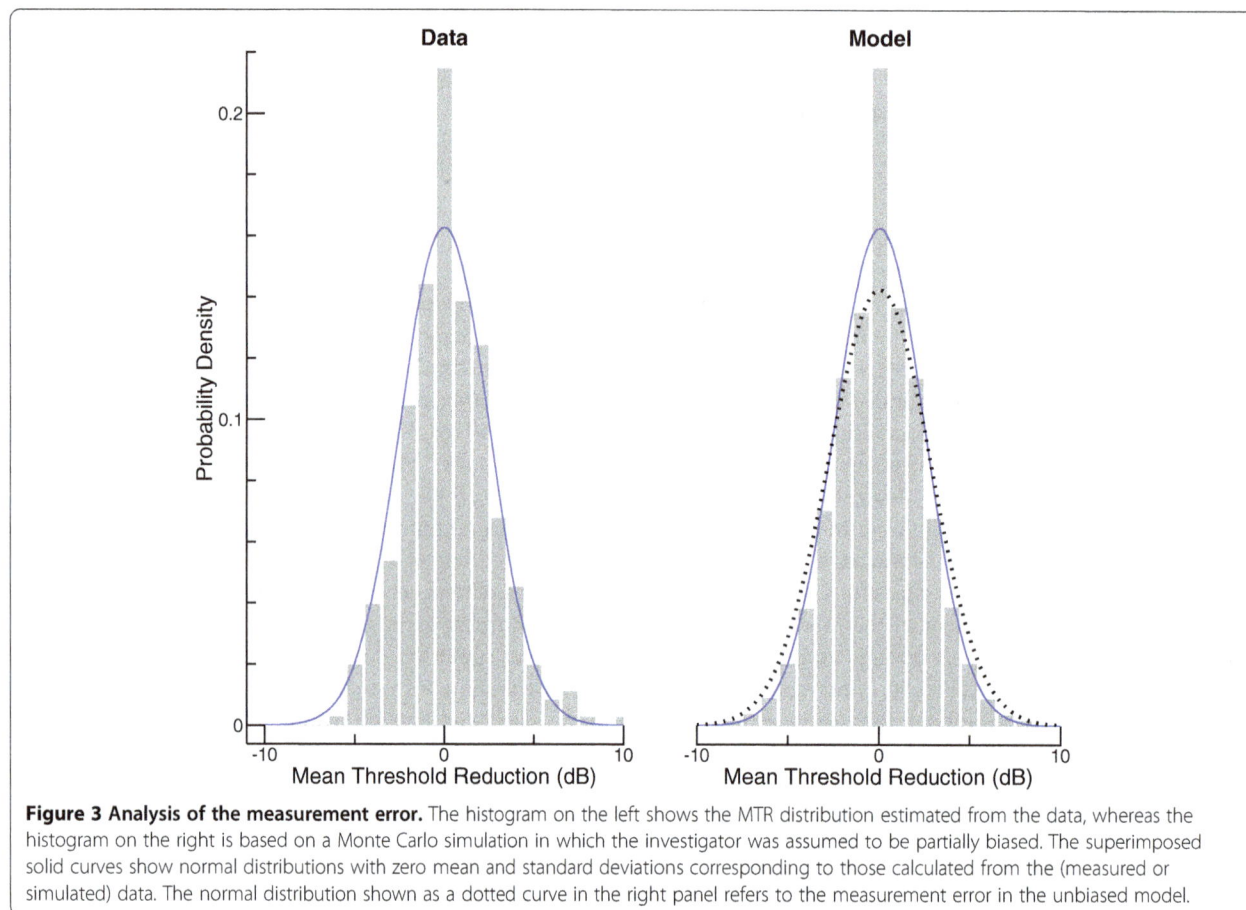

Figure 3 Analysis of the measurement error. The histogram on the left shows the MTR distribution estimated from the data, whereas the histogram on the right is based on a Monte Carlo simulation in which the investigator was assumed to be partially biased. The superimposed solid curves show normal distributions with zero mean and standard deviations corresponding to those calculated from the (measured or simulated) data. The normal distribution shown as a dotted curve in the right panel refers to the measurement error in the unbiased model.

A comparison between dotted curve and histogram illustrates that greater threshold changes are slightly underrepresented in the latter.

Frequency distribution of the mean threshold reduction

For clinical testing, the audiogram obtained 4 hours after the glycerol intake is compared with the pre-test audiogram rather than the audiogram obtained after three hours (as in the error analysis above). The frequency distribution of the MTR calculated from these two audiograms is shown in the middle of Figure 4 (histogram). The three rows represent different groups of patients. In the upper row (a), all patients are considered, whereas the other two rows represent subsets of patients who either do (c) or do not (b) fulfill the rule of thumb proposed in our previous article [20]. According to this rule, the probability of a positive outcome of the glycerol test is increased if the mean low-frequency hearing loss in the pretest audiogram is within the range 30 to 70 dB and not smaller than the mean high-frequency hearing loss. Patients for whom the rule is satisfied will be referred to as the good candidates; the others will be referred to as the poor candidates, for the sake of convenience. Consistent with this idea, large MTR values (>15 dB) are found

only for the good candidates (row c). But apart from that, the interpretation of the estimated distributions is complicated by the substantial blurring caused by the measurement error.

The goal of modeling is to eliminate the influence of the measurement error, i.e., to recover the distribution that would be obtained if hearing thresholds were determined with arbitrary accuracy. The result, represented by the histograms in the left column of Figure 4, will be referred to as the frequency distribution of the *true* MTR (the model parameters are provided in Table 1; the curves represent the function defined in Eq. (3)). A convolution of the theoretical distributions with the probability density function of the measurement error (curve on the left of Figure 3) yields the curves in the middle column, which agree reasonably well with the histograms derived from the data. If cumulative frequency distributions (right column) are considered instead of frequency distributions, the agreement between model and data appears to be almost perfect.

Comparing the three groups of patients is facilitated when the differences in the number of cases are eliminated by normalization. The cumulative distribution functions in Figure 5 (obtained by rescaling the corresponding

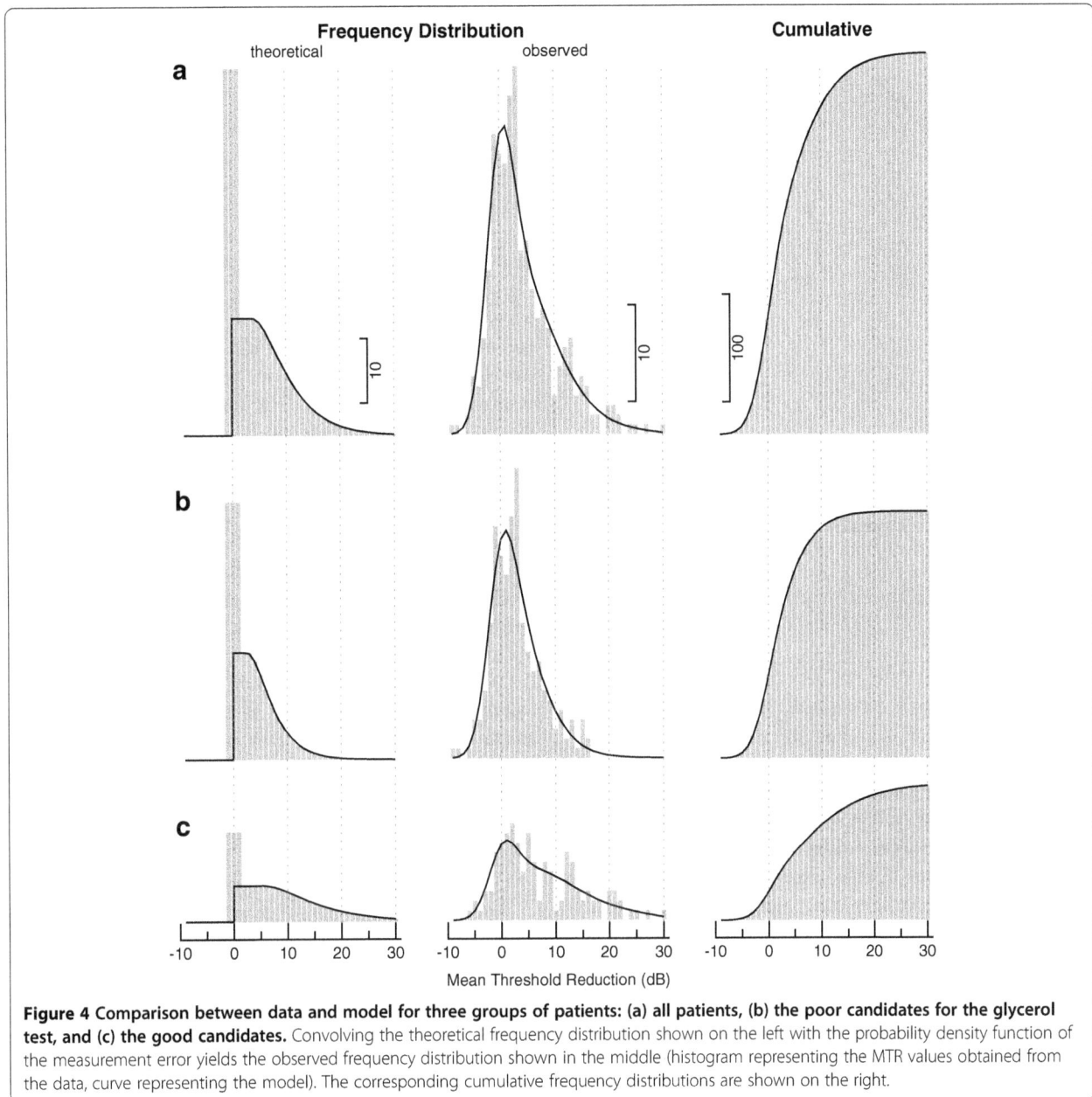

Figure 4 Comparison between data and model for three groups of patients: (a) all patients, (b) the poor candidates for the glycerol test, and (c) the good candidates. Convolving the theoretical frequency distribution shown on the left with the probability density function of the measurement error yields the observed frequency distribution shown in the middle (histogram representing the MTR values obtained from the data, curve representing the model). The corresponding cumulative frequency distributions are shown on the right.

Table 1 Model parameters and area under the ROC curve

		Model parameters		Area under the ROC curve	
	N	p_0	θ (dB)	assuming $\sigma = 2.45$ dB	assuming $\sigma = 1.2$ dB
All patients	354	0.378	3.89	0.922	0.976
Poor candidates	229	0.377	2.71	0.889	0.963
Good candidates	125	0.244	5.67	0.949	0.983

Three groups of patients are considered (N is the number of group members). In the middle, the values of the two model parameters, p_0 and θ, are provided. On the right, the area under the ROC curve is given for two assumptions about the standard deviation of the measurement error.

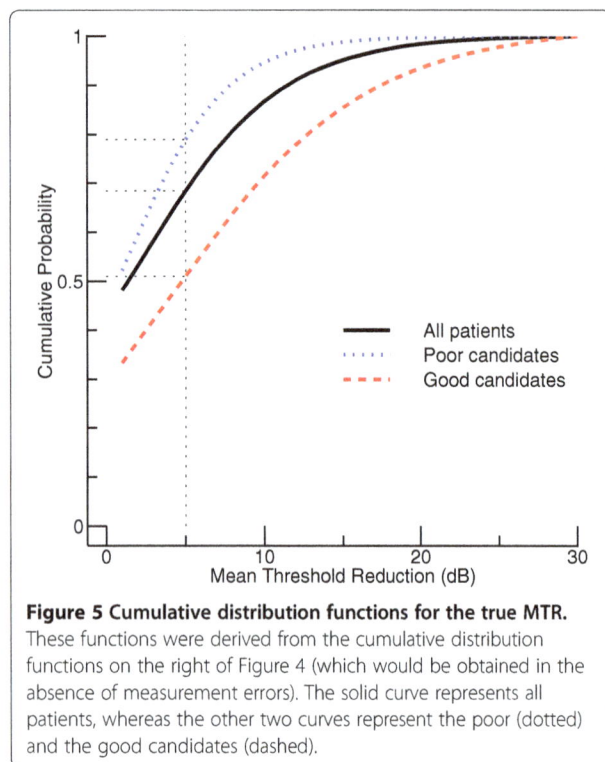

Figure 5 Cumulative distribution functions for the true MTR.
These functions were derived from the cumulative distribution
functions on the right of Figure 4 (which would be obtained in the
absence of measurement errors). The solid curve represents all
patients, whereas the other two curves represent the poor (dotted)
and the good candidates (dashed).

functions on the right of Figure 4) give the probability that
the true MTR (which would be observed in the absence of
measurement errors) does not exceed a specified value. If
all patients are considered (solid curve), no or almost no
effect (MTR ≤1 dB) is found in nearly every other case,
while this applies to only every third of the good candidates (dashed curve). For the latter group, the cumulative
distribution function increases relatively slowly, which
contrasts with the steeper increase obtained for the poor
candidates (dotted curve). As a consequence of these
differences, the probability of finding an MTR of at most
5 dB (dotted vertical line) considerably varies for the three
groups.

ROC curves

The performance of a diagnostic test is commonly characterized in terms of its specificity and sensitivity. If alternative versions of a method (or different methods) are to be
compared, these performance measures are conveniently
visualized in the so-called ROC space, where the horizontal axis represents the false-positive rate (1 – specificity)
and the vertical axis represents the true-positive rate (synonymous with sensitivity). The analysis evidently requires
that the test results can be checked against the actual facts
or the results of a superior method serving as the "gold
standard". But this turns out to be problematic in the context of Menière's disease. A Monte Carlo simulation based
on the above modeling results offers at least a partial
workaround.

To keep the simulation realistic, a "gold-standard"
method is assumed to signal a positive glycerol effect if
the true MTR exceeds a specified threshold (2 dB in
our simulations, unless stated otherwise). The assumption
of a threshold accounts for the fact that a distinction
between "no effect" and "almost no effect" is not only difficult to accomplish in reality, but may also be irrelevant
with respect to possible clinical consequences. After having defined a "gold standard", a ROC curve [30-32] is
easily derived from simulated data. The thick curve in
Figure 6 was obtained using the model parameters that
were determined on the basis of all patients, whereas the
curves above and below were obtained using the parameters determined for the good and the poor candidates,
respectively (see Table 1). The measurement error had a
standard deviation of 2.45 dB, as estimated from our real
data.

A convenient summary measure for the performance
of a test is the area under the ROC curve (AUC). An
intuitive interpretation of the AUC is as follows: If a randomly selected diseased individual is compared with a
randomly selected non-diseased individual, the AUC
corresponds to the probability that the test quantity (in
our case the MTR) is higher for the diseased individual
[33,34]. Random guessing would result in a ROC curve
corresponding to the diagonal line in Figure 6, which
has an AUC of 0.5. By contrast, an AUC greater than 0.9

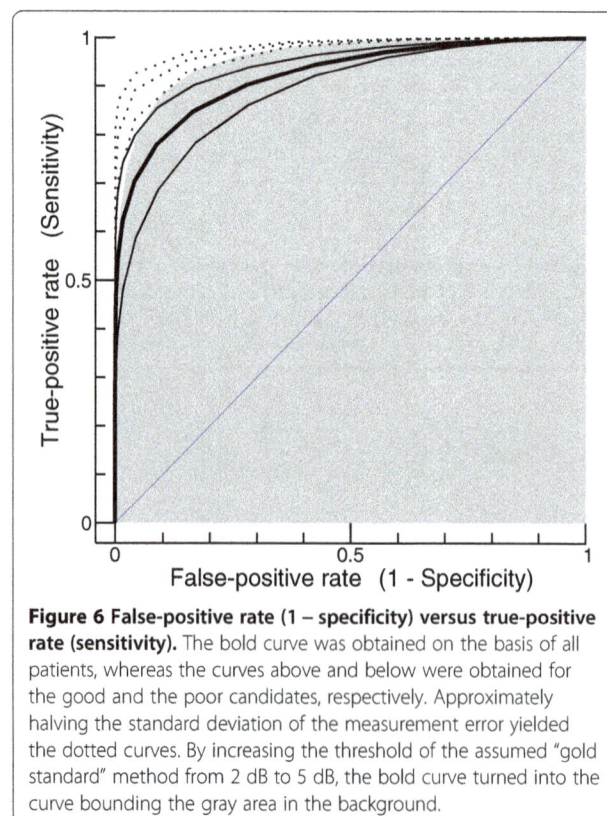

**Figure 6 False-positive rate (1 – specificity) versus true-positive
rate (sensitivity).** The bold curve was obtained on the basis of all
patients, whereas the curves above and below were obtained for
the good and the poor candidates, respectively. Approximately
halving the standard deviation of the measurement error yielded
the dotted curves. By increasing the threshold of the assumed "gold
standard" method from 2 dB to 5 dB, the bold curve turned into the
curve bounding the gray area in the background.

indicates a test of "rather high accuracy" [33]. The latter criterion is clearly fulfilled for the glycerol test, all the more if only the good candidates are considered (AUC values provided in Table 1). If methodological improvements allowed us to approximately halve the standard deviation of the measurement error (from 2.45 to 1.2 dB), the three dotted curves would be obtained instead of the three solid ones, and the AUC for the investigation of all patients would increase from 0.922 to 0.976.

The threshold of the "gold-standard" method in the above simulations (2 dB) corresponds to the lowest MTR value that, according to the model presented in Figure 2b, unequivocally represents a positive glycerol effect. But with respect to future applications it is conceivable that only patients showing stronger effects are considered good candidates for a certain clinical measure. This would require adjusting the criterion for a positive test result, which in our model is achieved by increasing the threshold of the "gold-standard" method. The curve bounding the gray area in the background of Figure 6 corresponds to the thick black curve (consideration of all patients), but the threshold was 5 dB rather than 2 dB. The differences between the two curves (the AUC increased from 0.922 to 0.960) have an obvious explanation: testing is the more accurate the greater is the effect to be detected.

Discussion

Modeling the glycerol test data

Central to this study was the attempt to explain our retrospective collection of glycerol test data [20] with a simple model that distinguishes between true effect and measurement error. The attempt turned out to be successful in that a model was found by which the cumulative frequency distribution of the observed MTR could be reproduced almost perfectly. Nevertheless, as subsequent considerations were based on the model rather than the data, a critical reflection on the model appears to be appropriate. The model builds on three main assumptions. *First*, the true MTR and the measurement error are assumed to be additive and statistically independent. Since the measurement error essentially reflects methodological imperfection and the patient's uncertainty about the threshold, this point is not considered to be critical. *Second*, the measurement error is assumed to be normally distributed. Despite the minor problem revealed in Figure 3, this assumption is considered acceptable as well. A standard deviation of 2.45 dB for the mean of five threshold reductions suggests that the standard deviation of a single threshold reduction is $2.45 \cdot 5^{1/2} = 5.48$ dB. This value is consistent with the test-retest variability of audiometric thresholds reported by others [35-37]. *Third*, the probability density function of the true MTR is postulated to correspond to the template shown in Figure 2b. While the good agreement between

model and data proves the suitability of this educated guess, a more meticulous examination is indispensable.

When trying to deduce the probability density function of the true MTR, it must be borne in mind that it is not about finding the unique solution to a well-posed problem. According to Eq. (1), the function sought, $g(x)$, is convolved with the probability density function of the measurement error, $h(x)$. The consequence is that finer details of $g(x)$ are smoothed out, making a faithful reconstruction from the data impossible. This is why we chose a parameterized model. The law of parsimony, also known as Occam's razor [38], mandates to make a model as simple as possible, and with only two adjustable parameters our model complies with this requirement. But still the problem remains that many different two-parameter models could explain the data equally well, for example the two models in Figure 2. A disadvantage of the first one (Figure 2a) is that the initial increase, from zero to the maximum, is an example of a fine structure that is inevitably smoothed out by the convolution with $h(x)$. Moreover, the model suggests that patients without a glycerol-induced threshold reduction can be unequivocally distinguished from patients showing a rather small effect, which is, of course, unrealistic. As such aspects may lead to misunderstandings we switched to the model in Figure 2b. It is in the nature of the problem that there are alternatives to this second model, too. For example, one might consider smoothing the sharp transition that occurs around 2 dB. Questions of this kind become secondary, however, if the focus is on the *cumulative* distribution of the true MTR, because seemingly discrepant probability density functions may be associated with nearly identical cumulative distribution functions. Thus, given the fact that the model explains the data so well, the curves in Figure 5 can be assumed to provide a fairly realistic view of the cumulative distribution of the true MTR, even though details of the underlying probability density function are debatable.

Performance of the glycerol test and future prospects

After having found a model that accurately reproduces the data, hitherto intractable questions could be addressed. In particular, defining a virtual "gold standard" allowed us to evaluate the performance of the glycerol test using ROC analysis. Even in its present form, the test turned out to have a "rather high accuracy" according to Swets' [33] classification of diagnostic techniques. Reducing the standard deviation of the measurement error would further enhance the performance, although it is difficult to say how much improvement is realistically possible in a clinical setting. At least there can be no doubt that the current practice of determining thresholds of hearing in steps of 5 dB sets a lower limit for the size of effects that can be proven. Moreover, Figure 3 suggested that the investigator tends to be partially biased. Thus, innovative threshold estimation techniques such as the recently proposed single-interval adaptive procedure [39] could help to significantly amend the test.

It shall be emphasized that the performance measures examined in this study do not characterize the ability of the glycerol test to fulfill what Klockhoff [19] considered to be its genuine purpose: indicating endolymphatic hydrops. Instead, they refer to the capability of the audiometric procedure to detect a glycerol-induced threshold reduction. Admittedly, the original reason for configuring the analysis this way was a lack of reliable information about the presence or absence of hydrops, which necessitated finding a workaround. However, closer inspection suggests that our solution is not at all a substitute for a superior, albeit impracticable approach. This realization is linked to the key question as to what the actual purpose of the glycerol test is. Notwithstanding the above-mentioned later view, Klockhoff and Lindblom [40] took a positive glycerol test as evidence that hydrodynamic damping of the organ of Corti is reversible and that treatment with diuretic drugs may be of value. Treatment with diuretics is commonplace now, but strong evidence to support their use in Menière patients is limited [41]. Nevertheless, if not taken too literally, the initial idea of Klockhoff and Lindblom may also guide *future* clinical practice. What distinguishes the glycerol test from other approaches is that it does not simply measure the consequence of a pathophysiologic process, but probes to what extent the patient's current medical condition responds to drug treatment, at least temporarily. Thus, the test could help to estimate the chances of success of pharmacological therapy [42,43]. Progress as to that may, consequently, increase the interest in the glycerol test.

Diagnostic testing for Menière's disease from a more general perspective

Several other approaches have been proposed for diagnosing Menière's disease. Probably the most popular technique at present is electrocochleography: Endolymphatic hydrops causes the summating potential (SP) to be enhanced compared to the compound action potential (AP) of the auditory nerve, yielding an increased SP/AP ratio [44]. However, opinions about the method are divided: A recent survey among American otologists and neurotologists showed that nearly half of the respondents had stopped ordering electrocochleography due to variability in results and lack of correlation with patients' symptoms [45].

An abnormal endolymphatic pressure is supposed to affect also the impedance of the middle ear transmission system. However, testing for this effect by means of multifrequency tympanometry has only moderate diagnostic accuracy [46]. Another option for diagnostic testing seems

to be the posture-induced phase shift of distortion-product otoacoustic emissions monitored around 1 kHz [47]. Auditory brainstem responses (ABR) have been studied as well. High-pass noise masking appears to be less efficient in patients with Menière's disease [48]. Thus, these patients show ABR with abnormal latencies if the masking level is adjusted to suit normal hearing subjects [49]. The result of a traveling-wave-velocity test was reported to be correlated with the outcome of transtympanic electrocochleography [50].

The vestibular component of Menière's disease can be tested by recording the vestibular evoked myogenic potential (VEMP), which, in the case of a unilateral manifestation of the disease, is of significantly lower amplitude on the affected side [51]. VEMP abnormalities may enable separation of Menière's disease from other peripheral vestibulopathies [52,53], although views differ as to whether Menière's disease can be distinguished from vestibular migraine [54,55].

This glimpse on recent studies shows that various possibilities are available to find objective correlates of Menière's disease. Even though most of these techniques may not be suitable yet to provide reliable diagnostic information for individual patients, revealing statistical differences between groups of patients and working out the relationships between the different tests will help to better understand the disease.

Fukuoka et al. [56] recently compared MRI, electrocochleography, and the glycerol test in 20 patients diagnosed with definite Menière's disease. While the latter two techniques yielded a positive result in only 11 and 12 patients, respectively, MRI gave evidence of hydrops in 19 patients. The authors therefore concluded that MRI is more useful for detecting hydrops than the two functional tests. Even taken together, the two functional tests were not competitive (only 15 patients showed a positive result in at least one test). This does not surprise considering that claims about the superiority of a combination of electrocochleography and glycerol test compared to the single tests [57,58] are not well founded (false positives are left unconsidered).

Paradoxically, the seeming inferiority of the functional tests could eventually prove to be an opportunity. Diagnostic testing is most useful when the presence of disease is neither very likely nor very unlikely [59], and from this point of view, MRI is less informative than the functional tests: If finding endolymphatic hydrops in a patient diagnosed with definite Menière's is rather likely, actually testing for the hydrops is wasteful unless there are compelling arguments to do so. Matters may be different if hydrops is considered in a more nuanced way, but attempts to derive a clinical benefit from this perception failed as yet: MRI neither predicted the outcome of intratympanic treatment with gentamicin [60,61] nor demonstrated a reduction of hydrops after treatment with betahistine [62]. While it is questionable at this point whether any other presently available method would have been more successful in this respect, the examples illustrate that there are clinically important questions which imaging techniques may not be able to answer: A natural limit is reached when functional aspects without an obvious morphological correlate are concerned.

Although the upsurge of imaging methodology could eventually revolutionize the study of Menière's disease, the above consideration shows that there is no reason to lose interest in functional methods. On the contrary, increased efforts should be made to improve them. As for the glycerol-induced change of state, it might be worthwhile to consider not only the threshold of hearing (classical glycerol test), but also other test quantities. And indeed, this idea has already been pursued regarding otoacoustic emissions [63], electrocochleography [64], and VEMP [65]. The ability to make useful predictions with respect to clinically important questions will ultimately decide which method (or what combination of methods) prevails. As to electrocochleography, it has been suggested, for example, that a high SP/AP ratio at the patient's initial visit may be used as a predictor of poor hearing outcomes [66]. Admittedly, even more useful would be predictions about the chances of therapies being considered. But, at present, that would perhaps be asking too much, given that management of Menière's disease is a topic which itself requires more research.

Conclusions

The three key questions for decisions about using a diagnostic test are how accurate the test is, how it adds to the information provided by the history, examination and other (cheaper or more readily available) tests, and how it improves patient outcomes [13]. With regard to the various approaches that have been proposed for diagnosing Menière's disease, these questions do not have simple, uncontroversial answers. Since different methods may target aspects of the disease that are not straightforwardly linked, premature conclusions about the relative merits of the various methods are to be avoided. This implies that defining a particular method as the "gold standard" is problematic unless the goal of diagnostic testing is clearly specified and the elected method is understood well enough to assess its suitability for that purpose.

While in the past the main focus was on getting indirect evidence of endolymphatic hydrops, MRI now provides a direct approach. However, if patients diagnosed with definite Menière's disease almost always have endolymphatic hydrops, diagnostic testing with the goal to actually prove the hydrops may not be generally justified. Instead, more attention should probably be paid to the question as to what predictions can be made about the chances of specific therapies. The glycerol test (like similar tests using other diuretics such as furosemide [67] or urea [68,69]) has the extraordinary property that it does not simply measure the consequence of a pathophysiologic condition in the inner ear, but investigates whether this condition is partially reversible. Even in its present, suboptimal form it fulfills Swets' [33] criterion for tests of "rather high accuracy". As a positive outcome proves the hearing loss to be partially reversible, the test could, prospectively, help to predict whether a patient is a suitable candidate for a certain type of therapy.

Abbreviations

ABR: Auditory brainstem response; AP: Compound action potential; ATR: Aggregate threshold reduction; AUC: Area under the ROC curve; MRI: Magnetic resonance imaging; MRT: Mean threshold reduction; ROC: Receiver operating characteristic; SP: Summating potential; VEMP: Vestibular evoked myogenic potential.

Competing interests

The authors declare that they have no competing interests.

Authors' contributions

BL built the model, analyzed the data and drafted the manuscript. TB provided the data and contributed to the interpretation of the results. Both authors read and approved the final manuscript.

Acknowledgements

The authors acknowledge support by Deutsche Forschungsgemeinschaft and the Open Access Publication Fund of the University of Munster. The funders had no role in study design, data collection and analysis, decision to publish, or preparation of the manuscript.

References

1. Atkinson M: Menière's original papers; reprinted with an English translation together with commentaries and biographical sketch. *Acta Otolaryngo (Stockh)* 1961, **Suppl. 162**:1–78.
2. Committee on Hearing and Equilibrium: Guidelines for the diagnosis and evaluation of therapy in Meniere's disease. *Otolaryngol Head Neck Surg* 1995, **113**(3):181–185.
3. Arts HA, Kileny PR, Telian SA: **Diagnostic testing for endolymphatic hydrops.** *Otolaryngol Clin North Am* 1997, **30**(6):987–1005.
4. Adams ME, Heidenreich KD, Kileny PR: **Audiovestibular testing in patients with Meniere's disease.** *Otolaryngol Clin North Am* 2010, **43**(5):995–1009.
5. Nakashima T, Naganawa S, Sugiura M, Teranishi M, Sone M, Hayashi H, Nakata S, Katayama N, Ishida IM: **Visualization of endolymphatic hydrops in patients with Meniere's disease.** *Laryngoscope* 2007, **117**(3):415–420.
6. Naganawa S, Yamazaki M, Kawai H, Bokura K, Sone M, Nakashima T: **Imaging of endolymphatic and perilymphatic fluid after intravenous administration of single-dose gadodiamide.** *Magn Reson Med Sci* 2012, **11**(2):145–150.
7. Naganawa S, Yamazaki M, Kawai H, Bokura K, Sone M, Nakashima T: **Imaging of Ménière's disease after intravenous administration of single-dose gadodiamide: Utility of multiplication of MR cisternography and HYDROPS image.** *Magn Reson Med Sci* 2013, **12**(1):63–68.
8. Colletti V, Mandala M, Carner M, Barillari M, Cerini R, Pozzi Mucelli R, Colletti L: **Evidence of gadolinium distribution from the endolymphatic sac to the endolymphatic compartments of the human inner ear.** *Audiol Neurootol* 2010, **15**(6):353–363.

9. Yamamoto M, Teranishi M, Naganawa S, Otake H, Sugiura M, Iwata T, Yoshida T, Katayama N, Nakata S, Sone M, Nakashima T: **Relationship between the degree of endolymphatic hydrops and electrocochleography.** *Audiology and Neuro-Otology* 2010, **15**(4):254–260.

10. Gürkov R, Flatz W, Louza J, Strupp M, Ertl-Wagner B, Krause E: **In vivo visualized endolymphatic hydrops and inner ear functions in patients with electrocochleographically confirmed Ménière's disease.** *Otol Neurotol* 2012, **33**(6):1040–1045.

11. Pyykkö I, Nakashima T, Yoshida T, Zou J, Naganawa S: **Ménière's disease: a reappraisal supported by a variable latency of symptoms and the MRI visualisation of endolymphatic hydrops.** *BMJ Open* 2013, **3**:e001555.

12. Fiorino F, Pizzini FB, Beltramello A, Mattellini B, Barbieri F: **Reliability of magnetic resonance imaging performed after intratympanic administration of gadolinium in the identification of endolymphatic hydrops in patients with Ménière's disease.** *Otol Neurotol* 2011, **32**(3):472–477.

13. Power M, Fell G, Wright M: **Principles for high-quality, high-value testing.** *Evid Based Med* 2013, **18**(1):5–10.

14. Merchant SN, Adams JC, Nadol JB: **Pathophysiology of Ménière's syndrome: Are symptoms caused by endolymphatic hydrops?** *Otol Neurotol* 2005, **26**(1):74–81.

15. Strupp M, Hupert D, Frenzel C, Wagner J, Hahn A, Jahn K, Zingler VC, Mansmann U, Brandt T: **Long-term prophylactic treatment of attacks of vertigo in Menière's disease - comparison of a high with a low dosage of betahistine in an open trial.** *Acta Otolaryngol* 2008, **128**(5):520–524.

16. Klockhoff I, Lindblom U: **Endolymphatic hydrops revealed by glycerol test. Preliminary report.** *Acta Otolaryngol* 1966, **61**(5):459–462.

17. Minor LB, Schessel DA, Carey JP: **Ménière's disease.** *Curr Opin Neurol* 2004, **17**(1):9–16.

18. Belinchon A, Perez-Garrigues H, Tenias JM: **Evolution of symptoms in Ménière's disease.** *Audiol Neurootol* 2012, **17**(2):126–132.

19. Klockhoff I: **Glycerol test — some remarks after 15 years experience.** In *Menière's Disease: Pathogenesis, Diagnosis and Treatment.* Edited by Vosteen KH, Schuknecht H, Pfaltz CR, Wersäll J, Kimura RS, Morgenstern C, Juhn SK. New York: Thieme-Stratton Inc; 1981:148–151.

20. Basel T, Lütkenhöner B: **Auditory threshold shifts after glycerol administration to patients with suspected Menière's disease: A retrospective analysis.** *Ear Hear* 2013, **34**(3):370–384.

21. Lütkenhöner B, Basel T: **Predictive modeling for diagnostic tests with high specificity, but low sensitivity: a study of the glycerol test in patients with suspected Meniere's disease.** *PLoS One* 2013, **8**(11):e79315.

22. Basel T, Lütkenhöner B: **Data from: Auditory threshold shifts after glycerol administration to patients with suspected Menière's disease: a retrospective analysis.** In 2013. http://datadryad.org/resource/doi:10.5061/dryad.dr78n.

23. Stefanski L, Carroll RJ: **Deconvoluting kernel density estimators.** *Statistics* 1990, **21**(2):169–184.

24. Lütkenhöner B: **A family of kernels and their associated deconvolving kernels for normally distributed measurement errors.** *J Stat Comput Simul* 2014, doi:10.1080/00949655.2014.928712.

25. Witting EG, Hughson W: **Inherent accuracy of a series of repeated clinical audiograms.** *Laryngoscope* 1940, **50**(3):259–269.

26. Gardner MB: **A pulse-tone technique for clinical audiometric threshold measurements.** *J Acoust Soc Am* 1947, **19**(4):592–599.

27. Atherley GR, Dingwall-Fordyce I: **The Reliability of Repeated Auditory Threshold Determination.** *Br J Ind Med* 1963, **20**:231–235.

28. Hickling S: **The Validity and Reliability of Pure Tone Clinical Audiometry.** *N Z Med J* 1964, **63**:379–382.

29. Chermak GD, Dengerink JE, Dengerink HA: **Test-retest reliability of auditory threshold and temporary threshold shift.** *Scand Audiol* 1983, **12**(4):237–240.

30. Brown CD, Davis HT: **Receiver operating characteristics curves and related decision measures: A tutorial.** *Chemometrics Intell Lab Syst* 2006, **80**(1):24–38.

31. Zou KH, O'Malley AJ, Mauri L: **Receiver-operating characteristic analysis for evaluating diagnostic tests and predictive models.** *Circulation* 2007, **115**(5):654–657.

32. Søreide K, Kørner H, Søreide JA: **Diagnostic accuracy and receiver-operating characteristics curve analysis in surgical research and decision making.** *Ann Surg* 2011, **253**(1):27–34.

33. Swets J: **Measuring the accuracy of diagnostic systems.** *Science* 1988, **240**(4857):1285–1293.

34. Macaskill P, Gatsonis C, Deeks JJ, Harbord RM, Takwoingi Y: **Analysing and presenting results.** In *Cochrane handbook for systematic reviews of diagnostic test accuracy.* Edited by Deeks JJ, Bossuyt PM, Gatsonis C. The Cochrane Collaboration; 2010. Available from: http://srdta.cochrane.org/sites/srdta.cochrane.org/files/uploads/Chapter%2010%20-%20Version%201.0.pdf.

35. Studebaker GA: **Intertest variability and the air-bone gap.** *J Speech Hear Disord* 1967, **32**(1):82–86.

36. Jerlvall L, Arlinger S: **A comparison of 2-dB and 5-dB step size in pure-tone audiometry.** *Scand Audiol* 1986, **15**(1):51–56.

37. Stuart A, Stenstrom R, Tompkins C, Vandenhoff S: **Test-retest variability in audiometric threshold with supraaural and insert earphones among children and adults.** *Audiology* 1991, **30**(2):82–90.

38. Wildner M: **In memory of William of Occam.** *Lancet* 1999, **354**(9196):2172.

39. Lecluyse W, Meddis R: **A simple single-interval adaptive procedure for estimating thresholds in normal and impaired listeners.** *J Acoust Soc Am* 2009, **126**(5):2570–2579.

40. Klockhoff I, Lindblom U: **Glycerol test in Ménière's disease.** *Acta Otolaryngol* 1967, **Suppl 224**:449–451.

41. Coelho DH, Roland JT Jr, Rush SA, Narayana A, St Clair E, Chung W, Golfinos JG: **Small vestibular schwannomas with no hearing: comparison of functional outcomes in stereotactic radiosurgery and microsurgery.** *Laryngoscope* 2008, **118**(11):1909–1916.

42. Pierce NE, Antonelli PJ: **Endolymphatic hydrops perspectives 2012.** *Curr Opin Otolaryngol Head Neck Surg* 2012, **20**(5):416–419.

43. Strupp M, Brandt T: **Peripheral vestibular disorders.** *Curr Opin Neurol* 2013, **26**(1):81–89.

44. Gibson WPR, Moffat DA, Ramsden RT: **Clinical electrocochleography in the diagnosis and management of Menière's disorders.** *Int J Audiol* 1977, **16**(5):389–401.

45. Nguyen LT, Harris JP, Nguyen QT: **Clinical utility of electrocochleography in the diagnosis and management of Ménière's disease: AOS and ANS membership survey data.** *Otol Neurotol* 2010, **31**(3):455–459.

46. Sugasawa K, Iwasaki S, Fujimoto C, Kinoshita M, Inoue A, Egami N, Ushio M, Chihara Y, Yamasoba T: **Diagnostic usefulness of multifrequency tympanometry for Ménière's disease.** *Audiol Neurootol* 2013, **18**(3):152–160.

47. Avan P, Giraudet F, Chauveau B, Gilain L, Mom T: **Unstable distortion-product otoacoustic emission phase in Menière's disease.** *Hear Res* 2011, **277**(1–2):88–95.

48. Don M, Kwong B, Tanaka T: **A diagnostic test for Ménière's disease and cochlear hydrops: Impaired high-pass noise masking of auditory brainstem responses.** *Otol Neurotol* 2005, **26**(4):711–722.

49. Kingma CM, Wit HP: **Cochlear Hydrops Analysis Masking Procedure results in patients with unilateral Ménière's Disease.** *Otol Neurotol* 2010, **31**(6):1004–1008.

50. Claes GM, Wyndaele M, De Valck CF, Claes J, Govaerts P, Wuyts FL, Van de Heyning PH: **Travelling wave velocity test and Ménière's disease revisited.** *Eur Arch Otorhinolaryngol* 2008, **265**(5):517–523.

51. Kingma CM, Wit HP: **Asymmetric vestibular evoked myogenic potentials in unilateral Ménière patients.** *Eur Arch Otorhinolaryngol* 2011, **268**(1):57–61.

52. Taylor RL, Wijewardene AA, Gibson WP, Black DA, Halmagyi GM, Welgampola MS: **The vestibular evoked-potential profile of Ménière's disease.** *Clin Neurophysiol* 2011, **122**(6):1256–1263.

53. Winters SM, Berg IT, Grolman W, Klis SF: **Ocular vestibular evoked myogenic potentials: frequency tuning to air-conducted acoustic stimuli in healthy subjects and Ménière's disease.** *Audiol Neurootol* 2012, **17**(1):12–19.

54. Taylor RL, Zagami AS, Gibson WP, Black DA, Watson SR, Halmagyi MG, Welgampola MS: **Vestibular evoked myogenic potentials to sound and vibration: characteristics in vestibular migraine that enable separation from Ménière's disease.** *Cephalalgia* 2012, **32**(3):213–225.

55. Zuniga MG, Janky KL, Schubert MC, Carey JP: **Can vestibular-evoked myogenic potentials help differentiate Ménière disease from vestibular migraine?** *Otolaryngol Head Neck Surg* 2012, **146**(5):788–796.

56. Fukuoka H, Takumi Y, Tsukada K, Miyagawa M, Oguchi T, Ueda H, Kadoya M, Usami S: **Comparison of the diagnostic value of 3 T MRI after intratympanic injection of GBCA, electrocochleography, and the glycerol test in patients with Meniere's disease.** *Acta Otolaryngol* 2012, **132**(2):141–145.

57. Kimura H, Aso S, Watanabe Y: **Prediction of progression from atypical to definite Ménière's disease using electrocochleography and glycerol and furosemide tests.** *Acta Otolaryngol* 2003, **123**(3):388–395.

58. Taguchi D, Kakigi A, Takeda T, Sawada S, Nakatani H: **Diagnostic value of plasma antidiuretic hormone, electrocochleography, and glycerol test in patients with endolymphatic hydrops.** *ORL* 2009, **71**(suppl 1):26–29.
59. Fletcher RH, Fletcher SW: *Clinical epidemiology: the essentials.* 4th edition. Philadelphia: Lippincott Williams & Wilkins; 2005.
60. Claes G, Van den Hauwe L, Wuyts F, Van de Heyning P: **Does intratympanic gadolinium injection predict efficacy of gentamicin partial chemolabyrinthectomy in Menière's disease patients?** *Eur Arch Otorhinolaryngol* 2012, **269**(2):413–418.
61. Fiorino F, Pizzini FB, Barbieri F, Beltramello A: **Variability in the perilymphatic diffusion of gadolinium does not predict the outcome of intratympanic gentamicin in patients with Menière's disease.** *Laryngoscope* 2012, **122**(4):907–911.
62. Gürkov R, Flatz W, Keeser D, Strupp M, Ertl-Wagner B, Krause E: **Effect of standard-dose betahistine on endolymphatic hydrops: an MRI pilot study.** *Eur Arch Otorhinolaryngol* 2013, **270**(4):1231–1235.
63. Mom T, Gilain L, Avan P: **Effects of glycerol intake and body tilt on otoacoustic emissions reflect labyrinthine pressure changes in Menière's disease.** *Hear Res* 2009, **250**(1–2):38–45.
64. Gibbin KP, Mason SM, Singh CB: **Glycerol dehydration tests in Menière's disorder using extratympanic electrocochleography.** *Clin Otolaryngol Allied Sci* 1981, **6**(6):395–400.
65. Magliulo G, Cuiuli G, Gagliardi M, Ciniglio-Appiani G, D'Amico R: **Vestibular evoked myogenic potentials and glycerol testing.** *Laryngoscope* 2004, **114**(2):338–343.
66. Moon IJ, Park GY, Choi J, Cho YS, Hong SH, Chung WH: **Predictive value of electrocochleography for determining hearing outcomes in Menière's disease.** *Otol Neurotol* 2012, **33**(2):204–210.
67. Futaki T, Kitahara M, Morimoto M: **A comparison of the furosemide and glycerol tests for Meniere's disease. With special reference to the bilateral lesion.** *Acta Otolaryngol* 1977, **83**(3–4):272–278.
68. Angelborg C, Klockhoff I, Stahle J: **Urea and hearing in patients with Meniere's disease.** *Scand Audiol* 1977, **6**(3):143–146.
69. Van de Water SM, Arenberg IK, Balkany TJ: **Auditory dehydration testing: glycerol versus urea.** *Am J Otol* 1986, **7**(3):200–203.

10

Allergic rhinitis and its associated co-morbidities at Bugando Medical Centre in Northwestern Tanzania; A prospective review of 190 cases

Said A Said[1†], Mabula D Mchembe[2†], Phillipo L Chalya[1*], Peter Rambau[3†] and Japhet M Gilyoma[1†]

Abstract

Background: Allergic rhinitis is one of the commonest atopic diseases which contribute to significant morbidity world wide while its epidemiology in Tanzania remains sparse. There was paucity of information regarding allergic rhinitis in our setting; therefore it was important to conduct this study to describe our experience on allergic rhinitis, associated co-morbidities and treatment outcome in patients attending Bugando Medical Centre.

Methods: This was descriptive cross-sectional study involving all patients with a clinical diagnosis of allergic rhinitis at Bugando Medical Centre over a three-month period between June 2011 and August 2011. Data was collected using a pre-tested coded questionnaire and analyzed using SPSS statistical computer software version 17.0.

Results: A total of 190 patients were studied giving the prevalence of allergic rhinitis 14.7%. The median age of the patients was 8.5 years. The male to female ratio was 1:1. Adenoid hypertrophy, tonsillitis, hypertrophy of inferior turbinate, nasal polyps, otitis media and sinusitis were the most common co-morbidities affecting 92.6% of cases and were the major reason for attending hospital services. Sleep disturbance was common in children with adenoids hypertrophy ($\chi^2 = 28.691$, P = 0.000). Allergic conjunctivitis was found in 51.9%. The most common identified triggers were dust, strong perfume odors and cold weather (P < 0.05). Strong perfume odors affect female than males ($\chi^2 = 4.583$, P = 0.032). In this study family history of allergic rhinitis was not a significant risk factor (P =0.423). The majority of patients (68.8%) were treated surgically for allergic rhinitis co morbidities. Post operative complication and mortality rates were 2.9% and 1.6% respectively. The overall median duration of hospital stay of in-patients was 3 days (2 – 28 days). Most patients (98.4%) had satisfactory results at discharge.

Conclusion: The study shows that allergic rhinitis is common in our settings representing 14.7% of all otorhinolaryngology and commonly affecting children and adolescent. Sufferers seek medical services due to co-morbidities of which combination of surgical and medical treatment was needed. High index of suspicions in diagnosing allergic rhinitis and early treatment is recommended.

Keywords: Allergic rhinitis, Co-morbidities, Treatment outcome, Tanzania

Background

Allergic rhinitis is recognized as one of the most common otorhinolaryngological condition which has considerable effects on quality of life and can have significant consequences if left untreated [1]. Globally allergic rhinitis constitutes a worldwide public health problem with a prevalence of 10% to 40% and the trend is increasing [2-5]. About 20 to 40 million people in the United States alone are estimated to be affected, [6] with 3.5 million lost workdays and 2 million lost schooldays annually [1]. Local population-based studies have reported a prevalence of allergic rhinitis of 44% in Singaporean school children [7]. In UK intermittent allergic rhinitis (also known as seasonal allergic rhinitis or hay fever affects up to 30% of adults and 40% of children at some time in their lives [8].

Allergic rhinitis is associated with significant co-morbidities and health care costs [9] and has been

* Correspondence: drphillipoleo@yahoo.com
†Equal contributors
[1]Department of Surgery, Catholic University of Health and Allied Sciences Bugando, Mwanza, Tanzania
Full list of author information is available at the end of the article

identified as one of the top ten reasons for visits to primary care clinics [10]. The total burden of allergic rhinitis lies on impaired physical and social functioning and also in a financial burden for treatment of its co-morbid diseases [1]. Allergic rhinitis commonly causes sleep disturbance, fatigue, listlessness irritability, and poor concentration leading to developmental delay, impaired learning ability and poor school performance in children [11-14]. Socially unacceptable behavior such as sniffing, sneezing, noisy breathing and coughing may lead to isolation and rejection at school and home. Further morbidity results from associated conditions such as sinusitis, adenoids, tonsil hypertrophy and otitis media [11].

Time trend studies of the prevalence of allergies in Africa show a consistent increase over a period of 7–10 years [15]. In South African epidemiological data are scarce but the overall prevalence of allergic rhinitis in children is at least 20% to 24% and there is evidence of increasing prevalence [11]. In Tanzania the data concerning allergic rhinitis are limited. Observation from Bugando Medical centre E.N.T clinical records reveals that allergic rhinitis and its associated co morbidities are common problem encountered with increasing trend for the past three years. Despite adverse sequalae, allergic rhinitis remains unrecognized and miss managed condition. Further more many patients do not recognize allergic rhinitis as a disease and therefore do not consult a physician [16].

The aim of this study was to describe our experience on allergic rhinitis, associated co-morbidities and treatment outcome among patient attending Bugando Medical Centre. Early identification of patient with allergic rhinitis and its co-morbidities would suggest development of guideline for early detection and proper treatment of allergic rhinitis and so reduce development of co-morbidities.

Methods
Study design and setting
This was a descriptive prospective hospital-based study of patients with clinical Allergic rhinitis carried out at Bugando Medical Centre in Northwestern Tanzania over a period of three months from July to September 2011. Bugando Medical Centre is located in Mwanza city along the shore of Lake Victoria in the northwestern part of Tanzania. It is a tertiary care and teaching hospital for the Catholic University of Health and Allied Sciences- Bugando (CUHAS-Bugando) and other paramedics and has a bed capacity of 1000. Bugando Medical Centre is one of the four largest referral hospitals in the country and serves as a referral centre for tertiary specialist care for a catchment population of approximately 13 million people from Mwanza, Mara, Kagera, Shinyanga, Tabora and Kigoma regions.

Study subjects and procedures
The study included all patients with clinical diagnosis of allergic rhinitis presented with two or more recurrent nasal symptoms of excessive sneezing, watery nasal discharge, nasal congestion and itching of nose and eyes in all age group and sex attended Bugando Medical Centre ENT clinic and ENT wards during the study period. Patients with co-morbid conditions associated with allergic rhinitis like otitis media, nasal polyps, tonsillitis, hypertrophied turbinate and sinusitis were also included in the study. Patient who refused investigations i.e. nasal scrapings and those received intranasal steroid one week prior to the enrollment into the study were excluded from the study. Recruitment of patient to participate in the study was done at ENT clinics and wards. Patients were screened for inclusion criteria and those who met the inclusion criteria were given an explanation about the study and requested to sign a written informed consent for the study before being enrolled in the study. In case of children below 18 years the Guardian/Parents were asked to consent on their behalf. Convenient sampling of patients who met the inclusion criteria was performed until the sample size was reached.

Data were collected using a pre-tested coded questionnaire and physical examination. Data administered in the questionnaire included; patients characteristics (e.g. age, sex, occupation), nasal symptoms, eye symptoms, age of onset of symptoms, triggering factors, presence or absence of family history of allergic rhinitis and asthma in the first and second degree relatives, presence of co morbidity and the effects to the quality of life (defined as interference with daily activities and sleep disturbances). Appropriate examination was done to all patients where candidate with nose complaints were examined using anterior rhinoscopy. All candidates with ear complaints were inspected using otoscope for evidence of eustachian tube dysfunction and otitis media. Children who showed features of allergic rhinitis and history of sleep noisy snoring or apnoea their posterior oropharyngeal wall were examined for adenoid hypertrophy with the aid of wooden tongue spatula. Sinusitis in atopic patient was defined by clinical presentation of facial pain, blocked nose, thicker and purulent rhinorrhoea and or anosmia. Paranasal sinus radiographs X - Ray submental vertical (water) view was taken in all suspected respondents for air/fluid level, septal deviation and thickening mucosa and was interpreted by an experienced radiologist. Extracapsular tonsillectomy and adenoidectomies were done in selected patients who had enlarged tonsils and adenoid hypertrophy which obstruct breathing, causing snoring, and sleep apnoea, difficult in feeding and recurrent bacterial infection.

In selected patients with hypertrophy of inferior turbinate with obstructive nasal symptoms electrical cauterization of submucosa of inferior turbinate under general anaesthesia was done. Patient with chronic maxillary sinusitis were treated by Caldwell-luc procedure.

The research assistant and Principle Investigator gathered relevant information regarding history and physical examination and the Scrapings of secretions and nasal mucosa cells [17] were taken from all patients and eosinophils, neutrophils and basophils count was done. Nasal Eosinophil infiltration is the cornerstone of allergic inflammation [18] and was found to be sensitive for the diagnosis of allergic rhinitis [19,20]. Nasal mucosal specimens were scraped from the surfaces of the middle thirds of inferior turbinate with specially made wooden spatula as rhinoprobes. They transferred onto plain glass slides, fixed in 95% ethyl alcohol for at least 1 minute, excess alcohol was drained. The collected slides were sent to the laboratory for staining. The slides were dipped sequentially in modified Wright- Giemsa stain, for 15 seconds, in Volu-Sol buffer for 30 seconds, and in Volu-Sol hematology rinse for 5 seconds. The slides were drained of excess fluid between the procedures. After air drying, the slides were examined under oil immersion by light microscopy [21,22]. At least 10-well spread, high power epithelium fields were examined. It was known from literature that nasal cytology assist in (1) distinguishing inflammatory from non-inflammatory rhinopathies; (2) distinguishing between allergic, nonallergic, and infectious rhinitis; (3) distinguishing between viral and bacterial infections; (4) following the course of a disease; and (5) following the response to treatment.

The quantitative score of nasal eosinophils and metachromatic cells were rated according to a scale previously described by Meltzer [23]. The grading were semiquantitative on a scale of 0 to 4 + [21]. It was shown that the presence of either nasal eosinophilic or basophilic metachromatic cell provides the best sensitivity and specificity [20,24]. Eosinophil scores and/or basophilic metachromatic cell scores of 1 was considered positive cut-off points for the diagnosis of allergic rhinitis. The diagnosis of patient with allergic rhinitis and associated co-morbidities was made clinically based on the validated questionnaire derived from international studies of allergic rhinitis i.e. Score For Allergic Rhinitis (SFAR) and International Study of Asthma and Allergies in Childhood (ISAAC) questionnaire where they had satisfactory sensitivity and specificity, in the absence of any allergic test in developing countries [3]

All patients with no co morbidities were treated conservatively with intra nasal corticosteroids (Fluticasone) and oral antihistamine citerizine and selected patients with co morbidities were operated accordingly. Patients were followed up until the day of discharge or death. After discharge patients were followed up at our ENT

clinic for one month (30 days) period. Length of hospital stay (LOS) and mortality were recorded at the end of study period.

Statistical data analysis

Data was analyzed using SPSS software version 17.0 with the guide of medical statistician. Data was summarized in the form of proportions frequency tables, bar and pie charts for categorical variables. Appropriate summary was used for continuous variables such as Mean, median, mode, standard deviation and histogram. Chi- square test was used to test for significance of association between predictors and outcome variables in the categorical variable. Odds ratio was calculated to test the strength of association between predictor and outcome variables in the continuous variables. Significance was defined as a p-value of less than 0.05. Multivariate logistic regression analysis was used to determine the predictor variables that are associated with outcome.

Ethical consideration

Ethical approval to conduct the study was obtained from the CUHAS-Bugando/BMC joint institutional ethic review committee before the commencement of the study. Informed consent was sought from each patient before being enrolled into the study.

Results

During the study period, a total of 1294 ENT patients were seen at Bugando Medical Centre. Of these, 200 patients had a clinical diagnosis of Allergic rhinitis. Ten patients were excluded from the study due to failure to meet inclusion criteria. Thus, 190 patients were studied representing 14.7% of cases. There were 95 (50.0%) males and 95 (50.0%) females with a male to female ratio of 1:1. The age of the patients raged from 5 months to 56 years with a median age of 8.5 years. The model age group was 0 −10 years accounting 55.8% of cases (Table 1).

Table 1 Distribution of patients according to age group

Age group (Years)	Frequency	Percentage
0 – 10	108	56.8
11 – 20	23	12.1
21 – 30	27	14.2
31 -40	15	7.9
41 – 50	11	5.8
51- 60	5	2.6
61+	1	0.5
Total	**190**	**100.0**

The majority of patients, 77 (40.5%) were in the pre school age group and occupation of the patients is as shown in the Table 2.

The age of onset of allergic rhinitis symptoms ranged from 2 months to 56 years with a median age of 3 years. The onset of symptoms were significantly associated with co-morbidities (χ^2 = 10.963, P = 0.001).

The majority of patients, 189 (99.5%) presented with nasal symptoms, of which blocked nose was the most common presentation affecting 75.0% of patients (Table 3). There was statistically significant association between the blocked nose and age below 12 years in the study population. (χ^2 = 9.513, P = 0.002). Ninety-eight (51.6%) patients had eye symptoms (rhinoconjunctivitis), of which watery eye discharge was the most common symptoms affecting 33.2% of cases.

Most patients 112 (58.9%) were able to identify the triggers of their allergic symptom and dust was reported to be the most common triggering factor in 39.5% of patients (Table 3). There was a significant association between the dust allergens and sneezing in patient with allergic rhinitis (χ^2 = 12.391, P = 0.002), there was also significant association between sex and strong perfume odors (χ^2 = 4.583, P = 0.032). Seventy-four (38.9%) patients reported to have family history of allergic rhinitis.

In this study, associated sleep disturbance was reported in 141 (74.2%) patients. There was a strong statistical association between sleep disturbance and presence of adenoid hypertrophy (χ^2 = 28.691, P = 0.000) but not with chronic tonsillitis (χ^2 = 2.914, P = 0.088).

One hundred and seventy-seven (93.3%) patients admitted to have interference with their daily activities.

Majority of patients 179 (92.6%) had co-morbidities associated with allergic rhinitis as shown in Table 4.

Table 2 Distribution of patients according to education and occupation

Variable	Response	Frequency	Percentage
Level of education	Pre school	77	40.5
	Primary education	44	23.3
	Secondary education	51	26.8
	Tertiary education	18	9.5
	Total	**190**	**100**
Occupation	Students	68	60.1
	Peasants	18	15.9
	Business	13	11.5
	Teachers	8	7.1
	Mining workers	2	1.8
	Industrial workers	2	1.8
	Health workers	2	1.8
	Total	**113**	**100.0**

Table 3 Distribution of patients according to nasal and eye symptoms

Symptoms	Response	Frequency	Percentage
Nasal symptoms	Blocked nose	144	75.8
	Runny nose	124	65.3
	Recurrent sneezing	111	58.4
	Nasal itching	101	53.2
Eye symptoms	Watery eyes	63	33.2
	Eye itching	62	32.6
Triggers of the symptoms	Dust	75	39.5
	Cold weather	53	27.9
	Perfume	34	17.9
	Smoke	7	3.7

Patients who had allergic rhinitis with co-morbidities had significant interference with quality of life (sleep disturbance and work) compared to allergic rhinitis patients without co-morbidities (χ^2 = 20.711, P = 0.000), and younger age at onset had significant association with development of co-morbidities (χ^2 = 76.040, P = 0.01).

X-ray was taken in 14 patients who had symptoms of sinusitis. Out of these 5 (35.7%) were found to have radiological features of chronic sinusitis. Nasal scrapings were taken in all 190 patients. Neutrophils were found in 177 (77.4%), esinophils 139 (73.2%) and there were no cells found in 18 (9.47%) slides. Eosinophils were higher in females (χ^2 = 7.746, P = 0.005) and in patient with family history of AR (χ^2 = 5.309, P = 0.021).

One hundred and four (54.7%) patients were admitted to hospital for surgical intervention resulting from co morbidities associated with allergic rhinitis (Table 5). Of these, tonsillectomy was the most frequent type of surgical procedure performed accounting for 68.3% of cases. The remaining 86 (45.3%) patients were treated by non-surgical approach (conservatively).

The overall hospital stay for the admitted patients ranged from 2 to 28 days with a mean of 4.6 ± 3.6 days. The median was 3 days.

Table 4 Distribution of patients according to their co morbidities

Co morbidities	Number of patients	Percentage
Recurrent tonsillitis	105	55.3
Adenoid hypertrophy	88	46.3
Inferior turbinate hypertrophy	77	40.5
Nasal polyps	18	9.5
Ear discharge	16	8.4
Sinusitis	10	5.3

Table 5 Distribution of patients according to the type of surgical procedure performed (N = 104)

Type of procedure	Number of patients	Percentage
Tonsillectomy	71	68.3
Adenoidectomy	55	52.9
Polypectomy	7	6.7
Caldwell luc	3	2.9
Turbinectomy	3	2.9

Postoperative complications were reported in 3 (2.8%) patients who had bleeding post-adenotonsillectomy.

Nine (4.7%) patients were discharged against medical advice. Of these 5 (55.5%) patients were due to long hospital stay before operation. Two (22%) patients were due to financial constrains, and 2 (22%) patient were due to unknown reason.

In this study 3 patients died giving mortality rate of 1.6%. All deaths were attributed to post operative and anesthetic complications. Two (1.9%) patients died from respiratory arrest post operative and one (0.9%) patient died of cardiopulmonary arrest during recovery period.

Discussion

Allergic rhinitis represents a global healthy problem with considerable prevalence especially in children [25]. The majority of patients in this study were children which is comparable with previous studies done else where [26-29]. The reason for increased number of children with allergic rhinitis to attend medical services in this study may be due to the fact that allergic rhinits is associated with severe and troublesome symptoms which are exacerbated by recurrent viral infections making parents to seek medical attention while majority of symptoms of allergic rhinitis are ignored by adult patients.

In this study, no gender predilection was observed which is in agreement with other studies [30]' but at variant with other studies which reported female [29,31,32] and male [33] predominance respectively.

The prevalence of allergic rhinitis is increasing in developing countries [34] due to the introduction of Western life style [35] and environmental factors [25] and it differs among countries and even among regions within the same country [20]. In industrial countries like USA the allergic rhinitis is one among the well documented disease and high prevalence of allergic rhinitis have been reported to be more than 40% [36]. In the present study the point prevalence of allergic rhinitis at Bugando Medical Centre was 14.7%. This prevalence is comparable to 13.7%,13% found in Kinshasa [37] Nairobi Kenya [30] respectively. Higher prevalence of allergic rhinitis have been reported in African countries such as 29.6% in Nigeria [29] and more than 30% in Cape Town South Africa [11]. Several theories for the increasing

prevalence of allergic rhinitis are climatic factors, increasing in winter and rainy seasons, dietary changes, environmental factors including industrial pollution. These factors may also influence the prevalence in our study and therefore it is recommended that future studies should be done in different periods within a year to determine the variations. The prevalence of allergic rhinitis in our study may actually be underestimate as majority of patients with this condition are treated in the peripheral hospitals and only patients with severe symptoms or associated co-morbidities present to ENT surgeon. A better picture of the magnitude of Allergic rhinitis in this region requires comprehensive data collection including both hospital and population-based study.

Clinically allergic rhinitis is defined as allergen induced inflammation of the nasal membrane and surrounding tissues that results in sneezing, rhinorrhoea, conjunctivitis, nasal congestion, and pruritis of the nose, palate, throat and ears [38]. Nasal obstruction is associated with sleep disorders, which can have a profound effect on quality of life, mental health, learning, behavior and attention [39]. Vast majority of respondents in this study had nasal symptoms of which blocked nose was found in many patients and it was found to be the most troublesome symptom. The same observation was also reported in other studies done else where [40,41]. The reason for the nasal obstruction was due to the co-existence with adenoid hypertrophy, nasal congestion, inferior turbinate hypertrophy and nasal polyps in majority of our study population. In this study blocked nose showed significant association with adenoid hypertrophy in children.

In the present study, the high proportion of patients had runny nose (rhinorrhoea) compared to other studies found in literature [42]. The reason for increased proportion of runny nose is the fact that runny nose is common in small children which is commonly associated with viral and bacteria infection especially in under five which were the majority in our study.

The rate of allergic conjunctivitis found in this study is higher as compared to other studies [26,43] and majorities of patients had watery eye discharge as compared to eye itching. Ocular symptoms were considered trivial illness by most of our patients and were not complained. The reason for the high proportion of allergic conjunctivitis could be due to dusty environment which causes symptoms in majorities of our study population. The high prevalence of rhinoconjunctivitis was also found in majorities of the centers of Africa and raises number of questions and non allergic factors are found to be responsible [44]. Further studies are needed to determine the factors responsible for rhinoconjunctivitis.

In the present study it was shown that the allergic rhinitis symptoms could begins as early as one month old child. This is earlier compared to 18 month old reported in Paris [45]. This could be due to differences in environment between the two countries. The study also shows that the early onset of symptoms of allergic rhinitis is significantly associated with the development of co-morbidities. This explains the needs for public awareness and early medical intervention.

Various environmental factors were found to increase the risk of allergic rhinitis especially in children. Pollution factors such as environmental tobacco smoke exposure, moulds, road traffic pollution and dusts seem to be important risk factors of allergic rhinitis [25]. In this study exposure to dust, weather changes, strong perfume order, and smoke were most common self reported triggers for allergic rhinitis where dust reported by majorities of patients. This observation is in agreement with other studies reported elsewhere [2,46].

The proportion of patients with self-reported allergy to dust was 39.5% which is lower than reported in Nigeria [29] and South Africa [11]. Seventy three percent of respondents noted trouble symptoms inside their houses. The reason for these findings could be due to the plenty of dust in our immediate environment and house dust which mainly consists of dust mite, moulds, insects and animal dander may be the etiological trigger in the study population. In this study dust was found to have statistical significant association with sneezing. Sneezing aims to expel mucus containing irritating allergens and cleanse the nasal cavity.

It was found in the present study that 17.9% and 27.9% of patients were affected by strong perfume and cold weather respectively. This rate is lower compared to 31.1% and 32.4% respectively reported in the literature [47]. Female patients with allergic rhinitis showed statistical significant association with strong perfume odor. This might be due to the social habits of using strong perfumes which is commonly in female compared to males.

Many patients with allergic rhinitis had their first degree relatives suffering from the disease. Similar findings were reported in other studies [11,48,49]. Unlike in other studies where family history was significant risk factor for allergic rhinitis [11,45], in the current study family history of allergic rhinitis did not reach statistical significance. The reason for poor association could be due to small sample as compared to the general population. However family history of allergic rhinitis showed statistical significant association with early onset nasal symptoms, which leads to early development of co-morbidities.

The quality of life is often impaired in patients with allergic rhinitis, due to the classic symptoms of the disease (sneezing, pruritis, rhinorrhoea and nasal obstruction). In addition, the pathophysiology of allergic rhinitis often disrupt sleep, leading to fatigue, daytime sleepiness, irritability and memory deficit [39]. Sleep disturbance was reported in most of our study population. Similar observation was also reported from other studies [50]. While 74.2% of our patient had their sleep affected, Machimu *at al* [51] reported sleep disturbance in 76.6% of the study population. Nasal obstruction and nasal congestion were responsible for the sleep disturbances. In this study nasal obstruction and congestion cause day time sleepiness in more than 70% of respondents especially those who had sleep disturbance during night time. This is in agreement with previous study [52]. The reason for the nasal obstruction was adenoid hypertrophy in one hand and hypertrophy of inferior turbinate in another hand. Adenoid hypertrophy was complained in majority of patients and it was significantly associated with sleep disturbance in children. Another cause of nasal obstruction was rhinorrhoea triggered by allergens.

Most of our patients 93.3% reported to have interference with their daily activities such as playing, working etc. and thus they have impaired social life. This is in agreement with other studies found in literature [53,54] and it is higher than that reported by Bousquet [55]. The reason for the interference with daily activities is probably due to severe symptoms of nasal blockage and rhinorrhoea which also causes embarrassment to patients.

Besides its direct effect on the quality of life, allergic rhinitis has significant co-morbid disorders such as asthma, sinusitis, otitis media, conjunctivitis and adenoid hypertrophy [25]. In the present study, more than 90% of patients had associated co-morbidities which is contrary with other studies [34]. Many other studies reported low incidence of associated co-morbidities. We could not find the reason for these differences, this call for further studies to explain these differences.

Multidisciplinary approach is needed in the treatment of allergic rhinitis and its co-morbidities involving paediatricians, allergists and the otolaryngologists [25]. Allergen avoidance require aggressive environmental control which is effective but often practically difficult [56]. Intranasal steroids are the treatment of choice and are more effective than antihistamines for relief of nasal obstruction however surgical therapy is reserved for co-morbidities refractory to medical treatment. Immunotherapy may also be used [57].

With regard to treatment patterns, majority of patients (54.7%) in this study underwent surgical treatment which is at variant with findings from other studies [11] where majority of allergic rhinitis patient were treated conservatively and surgical management was reserved for minority of cases who were refractory to medical treatment. The most common indications for surgical treatment in the present study were adenoid hypertrophy, recurrent tonsillitis, nasal obstruction due to hypertrophy of inferior turbinate, nasal polyps and sinusitis. The high rate of surgical treatment found in this study is attributed to high proportion of patients with associated co-morbidities requiring surgical interventions

In agreement with previous report [58], conservative treatment in this study was done using mono therapy with steroid nasal spray fluticasone which does not result in complete relief of symptoms and so prolongs the hospital visit and affect compliance with long term use.

Allergen exposure in atopic individual activates mast cells resulting in the release of mediators and cytokines capable of inducing inflammatory cell recruitment including eosinophils, neutrophils and basophils at the target organ level. Eosinophils in the nasal smear has shown to display the best correlation with clinical allergic rhinitis [59], and can be used not only to establishes the diagnosis of allergic rhinitis but also useful in the follow up of patients with this condition [22]. In this study oesinophils were found in 73.2% of patients and were significantly associated with female sex and family history of allergic rhinitis. The reason for this association was not known

Polymorpho-nuclear cells were found in 77.4% of our patients. Since the presence of neutrophils provides evidence substantiating the diagnosis of nasal infections, high rate of nasal neutrophils in this study indicate that nasal infections is common in these groups.

Nasal smears for oesinophils, basophils and neutrophils were negative in 9.7% of the slides. Unlike observation from other studies that nasal mucosa scrapings in allergic rhinitis patients had large numbers of basophilic metachromatic cells [60] in this studies no basophils was found. The reason could be due to the fact that basophil cells are found predominately in the nasal mucosa [23], where proper nasal curettes (rhino-probe) are required for acquisition of a large number of intact cells to interpret. In contrary neutrophils and oesinophils are present in both nasal secretion and within the nasal mucosa.

The overall average length of hospital stay for in patients was 4.6 days. However for the patient underwent adenotonsillectomy the average hospital stay was 3 days. This was in contrary with other studies done in Malaysia where adenotonsillectomy was done safely as day care surgery [46].

While gender was not found to be a risk factor, younger age group was significantly associated with increased length of hospital stay post adenotonsillectomy. Same observation was also reported in the literature [61]. This is contrary with other studies [62]. The reason for increased length of hospital stay was mostly due to delay in conduction of the procedure, where patients stayed in the ward for days awaiting surgery.

Patients who had chronic sinusitis were found to have statistical significant association with increased length of hospital stay. The reason for this is that during post operative period, most of patients had associated oedema and prolonged catheter placed for sinus drainage.

In the present study post operative bleeding was the most post surgical complication. This is consistent with other study [63]. The rate of post operative bleeding of 2.88% in the present study was in agreement to the rate of 2.4% found in other studies [64]. The low rate of post tonsillectomy bleeding was attributed to the suture tie techniques used to arrest bleeding during tonsillectomy at Bugando Medical Centre and also weekly follow up post surgery was found to be effective in early detection of delayed and episodic bleeding which can be corrected before the development of life-threatening anaemia.

Majority of patients were discharged against medical advice in the current study was caused by long hospital stay especially before surgery. This is attributed to inadequate operating days for ENT patients despite of high number of patients demanding surgical services. Further more lack of essential surgical equipments such as oxygen, gauze and surgical gowns during the study period led to delay of surgical procedures.

AR is not common to cause death but it may occur from its co-morbid conditions as 1.5% mortality rate reported in a study done in Sweden [65] or as a result of surgical complications. In the current study death rate post adenotonsillectomy was 1.6%. High mortality rate was previously reported [66] although there was no postoperative deaths reported in study done in Germany [67]. In our study death occurred within the first 24 hours post adenotonsillectomy in younger children who had severe obstructive symptoms. Aspiration and respiratory arrest may probably be the cause of death. This calls for improvement of pediatric post operative care.

There was no death caused by bleeding in this study. The reason was careful inspection of the nasopharynx before performing surgery and curettage in a piecemeal fashion under visual control which was done during each adenoidectomy in order to prevent direct injury to aberrant arteries.

The potential limitations of this study include the absence of allergy testing, short study period, presence of neutrophils in the nose and failure of estimating the measure of quality of life based on a standardized and validated (generic or disease-related) questionnaires. However, despite these limitations, the study has provided local data that can help health care workers develop guideline for early detection and proper treatment of allergic rhinitis and so reduce development of co-morbidities.

Conclusion

Allergic rhinitis is common condition which is under diagnosed in patients attending otorhinolaryngology department at Bugando Medical Centre and accounts for

14.7% of all otorhinolaryngology admissions. Allergic rhinitis causes considerable morbidities especially in children. Many of the allergic rhinitis triggers are commonly found in our environment and houses. It is therefore recommended that:

- High index of suspicion and improvement of laboratory diagnostic facilities for allergic rhinits are needed in order elevate the prevalence of this disease.
- Early detection and treatment of allergic rhinitis in children is needed to improve healthy of the sufferers
- Avoidance of allergic rhinitis trigger is the best first line of management of allergic rhinits and so all patients should be given education on avoidance of the triggering factors.
- Further study on incidence and risk factors of allergic rhinitis at Bugando Medical Centre ENT patients is highly recommended.

Competing interests
The author declares that they have no competing interest.

Authors' contributions
SAS designed the study, contributed in literature search, data collection and management of patients. JMG participated in study design, treatment of patient and performed surgery. PLC designed the study, data analysis, editing, writing and submission of the manuscript. PR participated in editing and preparation of nasal smears and microscopic interpretations. MDM participated in data analysis, supervising the study. All the authors read and approved the final manuscript.

Acknowledgements
The authors acknowledge all those who were involved in the care of our patients and those who provided support in the preparation of this manuscript.

Author details
[1]Department of Surgery, Catholic University of Health and Allied Sciences Bugando, Mwanza, Tanzania. [2]Department of Surgery, Muhimbili University of Health and Allied Sciences, Dar Es Salaam, Tanzania. [3]Department of Pathology, Catholic University of Health and Allied Sciences Bugando, Mwanza, Tanzania.

References
1. Nathan RA: The burden of allergic rhinitis. *Allergy Asthma Proc* 2007, **28**(1):3–9.
2. Rondon C, Fernandez J, Canto G, Blanca M: Local allergic rhinitis: concept, clinical manifestations, and diagnostic approach. *J Investig Allergol Clin Immunol* 2010, **20**(5):364–371.
3. Piau JP, Massot C, Moreau D, Ait-Khaled N, Bouayad Z, Mohammad Y, Khaldi F, Bah-Sow O, Camara L, Koffi NB, M'Boussa J, El Sony A, Moussa OA, Bousquet J, Annesi-Maesano I: Assessing allergic rhinitis in developing countries. *Int J Tuberc Lung Dis* 2010, **14**(4):506–512.
4. Bousquet J, Bousquet J, Khaltaev N, Cruz AA, Denburg J, Fokkens WJ, Togias A, Zuberbier T, Baena-Cagnani CE, Canonica GW, van Weel C, Agache I, Ait-Khaled N, Bachert C, Blaiss MS, Bonini S, Boulet LP: **Allergic Rhinitis and its Impact on Asthma (ARIA) 2008 update (in collaboration with the World Health Organization, GA(2)LEN and AllerGen).** *Allergy* 2008, **63**:8–160.
5. Saleem T, Khalid U, Sherwani UU, Ghaffar S: **Clinical profile, outcomes and improvement in symptoms and productivity in rhinitic patients in Karachi Pakistan.** *BMC Ear Nose Throat Disord* 2009, **9**:12.
6. Skoner DP: **Allergic rhinitis: definition, epidemiology, pathophysiology, detection, and diagnosis.** *J Allergy Clin Immunol* 2001, **108**(1):S2–S8.
7. Lim MY, Leong JL: **Allergic rhinitis: evidence-based practice.** *Singapore Med J* 2010, **51**(7):542–550.
8. Hammersley VS, Walker S, Elton R, Sheikh A: **Protocol for the adolescent hayfever trial: cluster randomized controlled trial of an educational intervention for healthcare professionals for the management of school-age children with hayfever.** *Trials* 2010, **11**:84.
9. Bunnag C, Jareoncharsri P, Tantilipikorn P, Vichyanond P, Pawankar R: **Epidemiology and current status of allergic rhinitis and asthma in Thailand – ARIA Asia-Pacific Workshop report.** *Asian Pac J Allergy Immunol* 2009, **27**(1):79–86.
10. Hayden ML: **Allergic rhinitis: a growing primary care challenge.** *J Am Acad Nurse Pract* 2001, **13**(12):545–551.
11. Mercer MJ, Van der Linde GP, Joubert G: **Rhinitis (allergic and nonallergic) in an atopic pediatric referral population in the grasslands of inland South Africa.** *Ann Allergy Asthma Immunol* 2002, **89**(5):503–512.
12. Juniper EF: **Impact of upper respiratory allergic diseases on quality of life.** *J Allergy Clin Immunol* 1998, **101**(2):S386–S391.
13. Spector S: **Pathophysiology and pharmacotherapy of allergic rhinitis.** *J Allergy Clin Immunol* 1999, **103**(3):S377.
14. Green RJ, Luyt DK: **Clinical presentation of chronic non-infectious rhinitis in children.** *S Afr Med J* 1997, **87**(8):987–991.
15. Obeng BB, Hartgers F, Boakye D, Yazdanbakhsh M: **Out of Africa: what can be learned from the studies of allergic disorders in Africa and Africans?** *Curr Opin Allergy Clin Immunol* 2008, **8**(5):391–397.
16. Sibbald B: **Epidemiology of allergic rhinitis.** *Monogr Allergy* 1993, **31**:61–79.
17. Quillen DM, Feller DB: **Diagnosing rhinitis: allergic vs. non-allergic.** *Am Fam Physician* 2006, **73**(9):1583–1590.
18. Crobach M, Hermans J, Kaptein A, Ridderikhoff J, Mulder J: **Nasal smear eosinophilia for the diagnosis of allergic rhinitis and eosinophilic non-allergic rhinitis.** *Scand J Prim Health Care* 1996, **14**(2):116–121.
19. Takwoingi Y, Akang E, Nwaorgu G, Nwawolo C: **Comparing nasal secretion eosinophil count with skin sensitivity test in allergic rhinitis in Ibadan, Nigeria.** *Acta Otolaryngol* 2003, **123**(9):1070–1074.
20. Miri S, Farid R, Akbari H, Amin R: **Prevalence of allergic rhinitis and nasal smear eosinophilia in 11- to 15 yr-old children in Shiraz.** *Pediatr Allergy Immunol* 2006, **17**(7):519–523.
21. Meltzer EO, Orgel HA, Rogenes PR, Field EA: **Nasal cytology in patients with allergic rhinitis: effects of intranasal fluticasone propionate.** *J Allergy Clin Immunol* 1994, **94**(4):708–715.
22. Jirapongsananuruk O, Vichyanond P: **Nasal cytology in the diagnosis of allergic rhinitis in children.** *Ann Allergy Asthma Immunol* 1998, **80**(2):165–170.
23. Meltzer EO: **Evaluating rhinitis: clinical, rhinomanometric, and cytologic assessments.** *J Allergy Clin Immunol* 1988, **82**(5):900–908.
24. Miller RE, Paradise JL, Friday GA, Fireman P, Voith D: **The nasal smear for eosinophils. Its value in children with seasonal allergic rhinitis.** *Am J Dis Child* 1982, **136**(11):1009–1011.
25. Hardjojo A, Shek LP, Van Bever HP, Lee BW: **Rhinitis in children less than 6 years of age: current knowledge and challenges.** *Asia Pac Allergy* 2011, **1**(3):115–122.
26. Yuksel H, Dinc G, Sakar A, Yilmaz O, Yorgancioglu A, Celik P, Ozcan C: **Prevalence and comorbidity of allergic eczema, rhinitis, and asthma in a city in western Turkey.** *J Investig Allergol Clin Immunol* 2008, **18**(1):31–35.
27. Osman M, Hansell AL, Simpson CR, Hollowell J, Helms PJ: **Gender-specific presentations for asthma, allergic rhinitis and eczema in primary care.** *Prim Care Respir J* 2007, **16**(1):28–35.
28. Masuda S, Fujisawa T, Katsumata H, Atsuta J, Iguchi K: **High prevalence and young onset of allergic rhinitis in children with bronchial asthma.** *Pediatr Allergy Immunol* 2008, **19**(6):517–522.
29. Desalu OO, Salami AK, Iseh KR, Oluboyo PO: **Prevalence of self reported allergic rhinitis and its relationship with asthma among adult Nigerians.** *J Investig Allergol Clin Immunol* 2009, **19**(6):474–480.
30. Gathiru C, Macharia I: **The prevalence of allergic rhinitis in college students at Kenya Medical Training College-Nairobi,Kenya.** *World Allergy Organization Journal* 2007, S84–S85.

31. Borges WG, Burns DA, Felizola ML, Oliveira BA, Hamu CS, Freitas VC: **Prevalence of allergic rhinitis among adolescents from Distrito Federal, Brazil: comparison between ISAAC phases I and III.** *J Pediatr (Rio J)* 2006, **82**(2):137–143.

32. Min YG, Jung HW, Kim HS, Park SK, Yoo KY: **Prevalence and risk factors for perennial allergic rhinitis in Korea: results of a nationwide survey.** *Clin Otolaryngol Allied Sci* 1997, **22**(2):139–144.

33. Alsowaidi S, Abdulle A, Bernsen R, Zuberbier T: **Allergic rhinitis and asthma: a large cross-sectional study in the United Arab Emirates.** *Int Arch Allergy Immunol* 2011, **153**(3):274–279.

34. Esamai F, Ayaya S, Nyandiko W: **Prevalence of asthma, allergic rhinitis and dermatitis in primary school children in Uasin Gishu district, Kenya.** *East Afr Med J* 2002, **79**(10):514–518.

35. Cruz AA, Popov T, Pawankar R, Annesi-Maesano I, Fokkens W, Kemp J, Ohta K, Price D, Bousquet J: **Common characteristics of upper and lower airways in rhinitis and asthma: ARIA update, in collaboration with GA(2) LEN.** *Allergy* 2007, **62**:1–41.

36. Blaiss MS: **Pediatric allergic rhinitis: physical and mental complications.** *Allergy Asthma Proc* 2008, **29**(1):1–6.

37. Nyembue TD, Jorissen M, Hellings PW, Muyunga C, Kayembe JM: **Prevalence and determinants of allergic diseases in a Congolese population.** *Int Forum Allergy Rhinol* 2012, Epub ahead of print.

38. Gelfand EW: **Pediatric allergic rhinitis: factors affecting treatment choice.** *Ear Nose Throat J* 2005, **84**(3):163–168.

39. Camelo-Nunes IC, Sole D: **Allergic rhinitis: indicators of quality of life.** *J Bras Pneumol* 2011, **36**(1):124–133.

40. Juniper EF, Guyatt GH, Dolovich J: **Assessment of quality of life in adolescents with allergic rhinoconjunctivitis: development and testing of a questionnaire for clinical trials.** *J Allergy Clin Immunol* 1994, **93**(2):413–423.

41. Shedden A: **Impact of nasal congestion on quality of life and work productivity in allergic rhinitis: findings from a large online survey.** *Treat Respir Med* 2005, **4**(6):439–446.

42. Montnemery P, Svensson C, Adelroth E, Lofdahl CG, Andersson M, Greiff L, Persson CG: **Prevalence of nasal symptoms and their relation to self-reported asthma and chronic bronchitis/emphysema.** *Eur Respir J* 2001, **17**(4):596–603.

43. Ait-Khaled N, Odhiambo J, Pearce N, Adjoh KS, Maesano IA, Benhabyles B, Bouhayad Z, Bahati E, Camara L, Catteau C, El Sony A, Esamai FO, Hypolite IE, Melaku K, Musa OA, Ng'ang'a L, Onadeko BO, Saad O, Jerray MM, Kayembe JM, Koffi NB, Khaldi F, Kuaban C, Voyi K, M'Boussa J, Sow O, Tidjani O, Zar HJ: **Prevalence of symptoms of asthma, rhinitis and eczema in 13- to 14-year-old children in Africa: the International Study of Asthma and Allergies in Childhood Phase III.** *Allergy* 2007, **62**(3):247–258.

44. Weiland SK, Bjorksten B, Brunekreef B, Cookson WO, von Mutius E, Strachan DP: **Phase II of the International Study of Asthma and Allergies in Childhood (ISAAC II): rationale and methods.** *Eur Respir J* 2004, **24**(3):406–412.

45. Herr M, Clarisse B, Nikasinovic L, Foucault C, Le Marec AM, Giordanella JP, Just J, Momas I: **Does allergic rhinitis exist in infancy? Findings from the PARIS birth cohort.** *Allergy* 2011, **66**(2):214–221.

46. Nurliza I, Norzi G, Azlina A, Hashimah I, Sabzah MH: **Daycare tonsillectomy: a safe outpatient procedure. Hospital Sultanah Bahiyah, Alor Setar Malaysia experience.** *Med J Malaysia* 2011, **66**(5):474–478.

47. Zhu LP, Wang F, Sun XQ, Chen RX, Lu MP, Yin M, Cheng L: **Comparison of risk factors between patients with non-allergic rhinitis and allergic rhinitis.** *Zhonghua Er Bi Yan Hou Tou Jing Wai Ke Za Zhi* 2011, **45**(12):993–998.

48. Alyasin S, Amin R: **The evaluation of new classification of Allergic Rhinitis in patients referred to a clinic in the city of Shiraz.** *Iran J Allergy Asthma Immunol* 2007, **6**(1):27–31.

49. Lee JT, Lam ZC, Lee WT, Kuo LC, Jayant V, Singh G, Lee J: **Familial risk of allergic rhinitis and atopic dermatitis among Chinese families in Singapore.** *Ann Acad Med Singapore* 2004, **33**(1):71–74.

50. Meltzer EO: **Stuffy is also related to Sleepy and Grumpy--the link between rhinitis and sleep-disordered breathing.** *J Allergy Clin Immunol* 2004, **114**(5):S133-S134.

51. Green RJ, Davis G, Price D: **Concerns of patients with allergic rhinitis: the Allergic Rhinitis Care Programme in South Africa.** *Prim Care Respir J* 2007, **16**(5):299–303.

52. Juniper EF, Stahl E, Doty RL, Simons FE, Allen DB, Howarth PH: **Clinical outcomes and adverse effect monitoring in allergic rhinitis.** *J Allergy Clin Immunol* 2005, **115**(3):S390–S413.

53. Engel-Yeger B, Engel A, Kessel A: **Differences in leisure activities between children with allergic rhinitis and healthy peers.** *Int J Pediatr Otorhinolaryngol* 2011, **74**(12):1415–1418.

54. Stuck A, Czajkowski J, Hagner AE, Klimek L, Verse T, Hormann K, Maurer JT: **Changes in daytime sleepiness, quality of life, and objective sleep patterns in seasonal allergic rhinitis: a controlled clinical trial.** *J Allergy Clin Immunol* 2004, **113**(4):663–668.

55. Bousquet J, Neukirch F, Bousquet PJ, Gehano P, Klossek JM, Le Gal M, Allaf B: **Severity and impairment of allergic rhinitis in patients consulting in primary care.** *J Allergy Clin Immunol* 2006, **117**(1):158–162.

56. Berger WE: **Overview of allergic rhinitis.** *Ann Allergy Asthma Immunol* 2003, **90**(6):7–12.

57. Turner PJ, Kemp AS: **Allergic rhinitis in children.** *J Paediatr Child Health* 2010, **48**(4):302–310.

58. Chauhan B, Patel M, Padhc H, Nivsarkar M: **Combination therapeutic approach for asthma and allergic rhinitis.** *Curr Clin Pharmacol* 2008, **3**(3):185–197.

59. Ciprandi G, Vizzaccaro A, Cirillo I, Tosca M, Massolo A, Passalacqua G: **Nasal eosinophils display the best correlation with symptoms, pulmonary function and inflammation in allergic rhinitis.** *Int Arch Allergy Immunol* 2005, **136**(3):266–272.

60. Okuda M, Ohtsuka HS, Kawabori S: **Basophil leukocytes and mast cells in the nose.** *Eur J Respir Dis Suppl* 1983, **128**(1):7–15.

61. Michael M, Carr GC, Dhave S: **Predictive Factors of Prolonged Hospital Stay in Tonsillectomy Patients.** *Otolaryngol Head Neck Surg* 2011, **145**(2):243.

62. Zhao YC, Berkowitz RG: **Prolonged hospitalization following tonsillectomy in healthy children.** *Int J Pediatr Otorhinolaryngol* 2006, **70**(11):1885–1889.

63. Stevenson AN, Shuler MD, Myer CM, Singer PS: **Complications and legal outcomes of tonsillectomy malpractice claims.** *Laryngoscope* 2012, **122**(1):71–74.

64. Wong BYH, Hui YN: **A 10 year Review of Tonsillectomy in a Tertiary Centre.** *HK J Paediatr* 2007, **12**:297–299.

65. Wiebert MS, Lindberg M, Hemmingsson T, Lundberg I, Nise G: **Mortality, Morbidity and occupational exposure to air way - irritating agent among men with respiratory diagnosis in adolescence.** *Occup Environ Med* 2008, **65**:120–125.

66. Windfuhr JP, Schloendorff G, Sesterhenn AM, Prescher A, Kremer BA: **Devastating outcome after adenoidectomy and tonsillectomy: ideas for improved prevention and management.** *Otolaryngol Head Neck Surg* 2009, **140**(2):191–196.

67. Stuck BA, Gotte K, Windfuhr JP, Genzwurker H, Schroten H, Tenenbaum T: **Tonsillectomy in children.** *Dtsch Arztebl Int* 2008, **105**(49):852–860.

Prevalence and psychopathological characteristics of depression in consecutive otorhinolaryngologic inpatients

Thomas Forkmann[1*], Christine Norra[2], Markus Wirtz[3], Thomas Vehren[1], Eftychia Volz-Sidiropoulou[1], Martin Westhofen[4], Siegfried Gauggel[1] and Maren Boecker[1]

Abstract

Background: High prevalence of depression has been reported in otorhinolaryngologic patients (ORL). However, studies using a semi-structured interview to determine the prevalence of depression in ORL are lacking. Therefore the present study sought to determine the depression prevalence in ORL applying a semi-structured diagnostic interview and to further characterize the pathopsychological and demographic characteristics of depression in these patients.

Methods: One-hundred inpatients of the otorhinolaryngologic department of a German university hospital participated voluntarily (age M = 38.8 years, SD = 13.9; 38.0% female). Depression was assessed using a clinical interview in which the International Diagnostic Checklist for depression (IDCL) was applied. Patients completed the Brief Symptom Inventory (BSI) which constitutes three composite scores and nine symptom scales and the Beck Depression Inventory (BDI). Multivariate analyses of variance, correlations and effect sizes were conducted.

Results: A prevalence of depression of 21.0% was determined, 38.0% of the depressed patients were female. Depressed patients showed higher scores on the BSI-scales "interpersonal sensitivity", "depression", "anxiety", "phobic anxiety" and "psychoticism" with medium effect sizes.

Conclusions: High prevalence of depression was found which is in accordance with results of prior studies. Depressed patients showed higher psychological distress as compared to non-depressed patients. The results call for carrying on in engaging in depression research and routine depression screening in ORL.

Keywords: prevalence, pathopsychology, depression, otolaryngologic inpatients, otorhinolaryngology

Background

Depressive disorders are among the most prevalent mental disorders of our times [1,2], coinciding with increased symptom burden, functional impairment, and immense socio-economical costs. Prevalence was found to be especially high in populations of patients with physical diseases [3-6]. Furthermore, depression may affect the course of comorbid physical illnesses and worsen their outcomes [5]. In general, depression reduces functional, emotional, cognitive and physical capacities needed to recover from coexisting somatic diseases.

Concerning depression in otorhinolaryngologic (ORL) diseases, prior studies mostly report high prevalences. Values range from 10% to 26% [7-11] indicating that patients with ORL are at high risk for depression. This is not surprising considering that characteristics of ORL diseases may entail severe consequences on subjective functioning and everyday quality of life [12].

However it is important to note, that in most published studies only self-report instruments were used to assess depression, e.g., the Hospital Anxiety and Depression Scale [HADS; 7,8]. Those studies that applied a higher diagnostic standard, e.g. the use of diagnostic interviews, mostly referring to head and neck cancer, reported highly divergent prevalence rates depending for example on the subsample of ORL patients [13-15]. In some studies, no

* Correspondence: tforkmann@ukaachen.de
[1]Institute of Medical Psychology and Medical Sociology, University Hospital of RWTH Aachen, Pauwelsstraße 30, 52074 Aachen, Germany
Full list of author information is available at the end of the article

standardized instrument was applied at all [9,10], or no information about how depressive diagnoses were determined were reported [11]. This is critical since validity and reliability of epidemiological studies depend largely on the quality of the instrument applied to collect diagnostic information.

The international accepted "gold standard" for diagnosing mental disorders like depression is a semi-structured diagnostic interview conducted by trained personnel. Self-report instruments are often used instead for economical reasons. However, to allow for reliable and sound conclusions in studies on the prevalence of depression, applying the diagnostic gold standard is strongly demanded. Nevertheless, studies using a semi-structured interview to determine the prevalence of depression in ORL are lacking.

Therefore, the present study had two major aims: (a) to determine the prevalence of depression in consecutive ORL inpatients applying a semi-structured diagnostic interview; (b) to compare the pathopsychological and demographic characteristics of depressed and non-depressed ORL inpatients in order to gain further insight into the characteristics of patients suffering from depressive disorders in this population.

Methods
Design
This was a cross-sectional study with consecutive inpatients of the department for otorhinolaryngology of a German university hospital. Prevalence of depressive disorders was determined. Depressive status served than as independent variable while measures of mental symptom burden (Somatisation, Obsessive-Compulsive, Interpersonal Sensitivity, Depression, Anxiety, Hostility, Phobic Anxiety, Paranoid Ideation, Psychoticism) were assessed as dependent variables.

Sample
One-hundred and two consecutive inpatients of the department for otorhinolaryngology of a German university hospital participated voluntarily. Two participants suffering from chronic diseases for more than 30 years were excluded from analyses because this time period exceeded the mean duration of disease in the sample by much more than two standard deviations. Overall mean age of the remaining 100 patients was 38.8 years (SD = 13.9) and 38.0% were female. See table 1 for sample details. Participants took part voluntarily without payment and signed an informed consent prior to testing. General inclusion criteria were German language skills and the ability to concentrate for at least 1 hour. Test administration was conducted by trained personnel. The study was approved by the local ethics committee of the

Medical Faculty of the RWTH Aachen University (EK 172/05) and performed according to the Declaration of Helsinki [16].

Procedures
Test sessions took place at admission and started with the conduction of a clinical interview in which the International Diagnostic Checklist for depression [IDCL; 17] was conducted. Afterwards, participants completed a demographic data sheet, and filled in further questionnaires.

Measures
Clinical Interview
Depression was assessed in all participants using a clinical interview in which the International Diagnostic Checklist for depression [IDCL; 17] was employed to verify the diagnosis. The IDCL is a checklist that can be used to make a careful evaluation of the symptoms and classification criteria, and thus help to arrive at precise diagnoses according to the 10th edition of the International Classification of Diseases (ICD-10) criteria for a depressive episode [18]. Persons who conducted the clinical interview were either psychologists or medical students in their last year with a major in psychiatry. All interviewers received one week training in completing this interview consisting of three steps: First, the interview guidelines were presented and the trainee observed a couple of interviews conducted by the principal author. Second, the trainee did role-play interviews with the principal author as "participant". Third, the trainee conducted interviews with real participants supervised by the principal author. If the trainee's diagnoses were in accordance with the trainer's, then the trainee was eligible as an interviewer in the present study.

Brief Symptom Inventory (BSI)
The Brief Symptom Inventory is a short form of the Symptom Checklist 90-R [SCL-90-R; 19] and contains 53 items that are Likert-scaled, referring to the previous week, with a range from 0 ("not at all") to 4 ("very much"). The instrument provides information on overall psychological distress. Furthermore, the 53 items of the inventory constitute three composite scores and nine symptom scales (Somatisation, Obsessive-Compulsive, Interpersonal Sensitivity, Depression, Anxiety, Hostility, Phobic Anxiety, Paranoid Ideation, Psychoticism) allowing the calculation of psychopathological profiles. The three composite scores reflect the complete answer pattern of the respondent: the "global severity index" (GSI) measures the overall mental symptom burden, the "positive symptom distress index" (PSDI) measures symptom intensity, and the "positive symptom total" (PST) reflects the total number of the respondent's symptoms. The raw scale and composite scores are transformed to standardized T-scores with a

Table 1 Detailed sample description according to ICD-10; multiple diagnoses possible

	N	age (SD)	% female	duration of disease[a] (SD)	duration of stay[a] (SD)	Impairment ADL[b] (SD)	Impairment QoL[c] (SD)	BDI sum
whole sample	100	38.8 (13.9)	38.0	151.8 (401.4)	8.3 (4.4)	1.9 (1.5)	1.8 (1.3)	6.7 (7.7)
diseases of external ear (H60-H62)	2	47.5 (3.5)	33.3	3.5 (0.7)	5.5 (0.7)	1.5 (2.1)	1.0 (1.4)	4.0 (1.4)
diseases of middle ear & mastoid (H65-H75)	1	30.0 (–)	75.0	4.0 (–)	4.0 (–)	0.0 (–)	0.0 (–)	5.0 (–)
diseases of inner ear (H80-H83)	2	42.0 (7.1)	57.1	12.0 (1.4)	10.5 (7.1)	2.5 (2.1)	3.0 (1.4)	7.0 (7.1)
hearing loss (H90-H91)	11	44.7 (13.2)	63.6	87.6 (241.0)	10.3 (5.3)	2.8 (1.3)	2.3 (1.3)	8.6 (7.9)
diseases of nose and paranasal sinuses (J01, J32, J34)	16	44.1 (17.8)	18.8	222.2 (626.4)	8.6 (5.1)	2.5 (1.4)	1.7 (1.3)	5.2 (4.3)
diseases of mouth, throat & pharynx (J03, J35-J38, K07, K11-K13)	37	34.0 (13.5)	40.5	131.3 (305.2)	8.1 (3.7)	1.3 (1.5)	1.7 (1.5)	7.9 (9.2)

[a] in days; [b] ADL: Activities of Daily Living; [c] QoL: Quality of Life

mean of 50 and a standard deviation (SD) of 10. T-scores > 60 reflect heightened mental burden [20].

Beck Depression Inventory (BDI)

The BDI [21] contains 21 items. Each item consists of four self-referring statements (e.g. "I am sad"). Item scores range from 0 to 3 and participants are supposed to choose one or more statements per item that represents best their mental state during the last week. A total score > 10 indicates mild to moderate depression and a total score > 18 moderate to severe depression. The BDI has not been validated in ORL inpatients so far, so that all conclusions based on the BDI in this study should be handled with care.

Further materials

All participants completed a demographic data sheet. Furthermore, the level of impairment in activities of daily living (ADL) and in quality of life (QoL) was inquired by a 5-point Likert-scale (0 = no impairment, 1 = little, 2 = moderate, 3 = strong, 4 = very strong). Clinical data were taken from medical records. Data were acquired within the scope of a comprehensive research project, so that participants filled in further questionnaires that are reported elsewhere [22].

Data analysis

The number of depressed and non-depressed ORL patients according to IDCL was determined. Mean age and standard deviations and number of male and female participants in both groups were calculated.

A mulitivariate analysis of variance (MANOVA) with "group" (depressed vs. non-depressed ORL patients) as between-subjects-factor was conducted. Prior to MANOVA, homogeneity of error variances was tested with the Mauchly test for sphericity. Homogeneity of error variances is important in order to interpret the results of MANOVA validly. Therefore, in case of significant results of the Mauchly test and thus violation of homogeneity of error variances, a Greenhouse-Geisser-correction was conducted. Effect sizes according to Hedges and Olkin [23] were calculated. Effect sizes amend significance tests reasonably since they allow for an estimation of the clinical relevance of empirical differences which is less sensitive to sample size than significance tests (e.g., t-tests). Cohen [24] recommended to interpret an effect size d of $.20 < d \leq .50$ as small, an effect size of $.50 < d \leq .80$ as medium and an effect size of $d \geq .80$ as large. Following the recommendations of Dunlap [25] in the present study effect sizes were calculated for independent variables instead of dependent variables because effect sizes for dependent variables often overestimate the actual size of effect.

Bivariate correlation analyses were performed to further characterize those patients who were assigned a depressive disorder. Classificatory (IDCL) as well as dimensional (BDI) information about the depressive status of the participants were correlated with age, gender, marital status, levels of impairment in ADL and in QoL, duration of disease, and duration of stay in hospital. All analyses were performed using SPSS 17 for Windows.

Results

Prevalence of depression

Considering the remaining sample (N = 100), the semi-structured interview based on the IDCL-checklist for depression revealed that 21 participants suffered from a depressive disorder, which corresponds to a prevalence rate of 21.0%. The mean score of BDI was 14.2 (SD = 12.2) in the depressed and 4.8 (SD = 4.2) in the non-depressed group. In fourteen patients (14%) a single depressive episode was found, 5 patients (5%) exhibited a recurrent depressive disorder. Nearly forty-eight percent (47.6%) of those patients with any depressive disorder were women (table 2). The mean age of patients with depression was 39.4 years (SD = 11.7) and the mean age of those without depression was 38.6 years (SD = 14.5; see table 2 for details).

Psychopathological and demographic characteristics of depressed vs. non-depressed ORL patients

The Mauchly test for sphericity revealed inhomogeneity of error variances (Mauchly-W = .013; p < .001). Thus, a Greenhouse-Geisser correction was performed prior to MANOVA. Depressed patients had higher scores than non-depressed patients on all scales (Somatisation, Obsessive-Compulsive, Interpersonal Sensitivity, Depression, Anxiety, Hostility, Phobic Anxiety, Paranoid Ideation, Psychoticism) and all three composite scores GSI, PSDI and PST. However, the corresponding main effect "group" was not significant (F = .85; df = 1; p = .60).

Univariate tests of between subjects effects showed significant differences between depressed and non-depressed patients on the scales "depression" (F = 4.53; df = 1; p = .04) and "anxiety" (F = 4.84; df = 1; p = .03) and for the global score PSDI (F = 4.38; df = 1; p = .04). Analyses of effect sizes showed relevant effect sizes between depressed and non-depressed patients of medium size for "interpersonal sensitivity", "depression", "anxiety", "phobic anxiety", "psychoticism" and the PSDI (see table 3). Most mean scores in both groups were within the range of normal mental symptom burden (T-value = 50 +/- 10). Only the mean score on the composite score PST in the depressed group was greater than a T-value of 60.

Bivariate correlation analyses between classificatory (IDCL) as well as dimensional (BDI) information about the depressive status of the participants, age, gender, marital status, levels of impairment in ADL and QoL, duration of disease, and duration of stay in hospital were performed. Gender correlated significantly with

Table 2 Prevalence rates according to ICD-10, divided by gender and diagnosis

	all patients		female		male	
Diagnosis	frequency	percentage	frequency	percentage	frequency	percentage
no depressive disorder	79	79.0	28	35.4	51	64.6
any depressive disorder	21	21.0	10	47.6	11	52.4
F31.3: Bipolar affective disorder, current episode mild or moderate depression	1	1.0	1	100.0	0	0.0
F31.4: Bipolar affective disorder, current episode severe depression	1	1.0	1	100.0	0	0.0
F32.0: Mild depressive episode	8	8.0	2	25.0	6	75.0
F32.1: Moderate depressive episode	4	4.0	1	25.0	3	75.0
F32.2: Severe depressive episode without psychotic symptoms	1	1.0	0	0.0	1	100.0
F32.4: depressive episode, in partial remission	1	1.0	0	0.0	1	100.0
F33.1: Recurrent depressive disorder, current episode moderate	2	2.0	2	100.0	0	0.0
F33.2: Recurrent depressive disorder, current episode severe without psychotic symptoms	3	3.0	3	100.0	0	0.0
total	100	100	38	38.0	62	62.0

dimensional information about the depression status (BDI) of participants (r = .25; p = .013) which persisted when controlling for age: depressed patients were slightly more likely to be male. No further significant correlations were found.

Discussion

The calculated overall prevalence of depression was 21.0%. Gender was significantly correlated with classificatory information about the patients' affective status. This is largely in accordance with published data on the prevalence of depression in this patient collective [7-10]. The fact that slightly more male than female patients exhibited depressive symptoms might be explainable by the higher base rate of male patients (62%) in the study sample. Generally, the present study confirms results of

Table 3 effect sizes between depressed and non-depressed patients for all BSI scores

BSI score	nondepressed			depressed			d	SE
	mean	n	SD	mean	n	SD		
somatisation	54.1	72	11.6	58.1	19	11.7	-0.34	0.26
obsessive-compulsive	47.6	73	10.9	53.2	19	15.6	-0.46	0.26
interpersonal sensitivity	47.3	74	9.6	54.6	19	15.2	-0.66	0.26
depression	48.2	74	8.6	54.9	19	13.8	-0.68	0.26
anxiety	50.1	74	10.9	58.1	18	13.9	-0.69	0.27
hostility	49.3	74	10.2	52.3	18	11.9	-0.28	0.26
phobic anxiety	49.9	74	9.3	55.5	19	9.6	-0.59	0.26
paranoid ideation	50.3	73	10.4	54.8	19	13.1	-0.40	0.26
psychoticism	49.4	72	9.7	56.5	19	13.1	-0.67	0.26
GSI	49.4	68	12.5	54.8	17	17.8	-0.39	0.27
PSDI	54.8	65	12.2	61.7	16	10.2	-0.58	0.28
PST	48.0	68	13.1	53.8	17	18.6	-0.40	0.27

Note: d = effect size, bias corrected according to Hedges & Olkin (1985); SE = standard error of effect size estimate.

previous investigations. However, a more reliable technique for determination of the diagnostic information was applied here (semi-structured interview) as compared to most other published studies on the prevalence of depression in ORL, so that we further substantiated previous findings. Above, analyses were conducted with data of an unselected sample of consecutive ORL inpatients. Therefore, the prevalence rate reported here reflects more directly the situation that clinicians encounter in their routine clinical practice than most previous studies did.

Depressed patients reported to suffer more from symptoms referring to anxiety, depression, interpersonal sensitivity, psychoticism, and phobic anxiety than nondepressed patients. Differences were moderate in terms of effect sizes. However, total symptom burden on most BSI-scales was only moderate in *both* groups. Nevertheless, all mean scores coincided with a huge standard deviation indicating that patients *within* both groups differed largely in terms of symptom burden.

The present study largely replicated the picture of depression that is known from a multiplicity of studies on this disease in other samples: It is a well known fact that depression often co-occurs with anxiety and obsessive-compulsive or phobic disorders, respectively [26-28].

The prevalence rate of depression found in the present study is largely consistent with prevalence rates of depression reported in other medical illnesses, e.g., cardiac diseases (17-27%) [29], cerebrovascular diseases (14-19%) [30], obesity (20-30%) [31], cancer (22-29%) [32] or HIV/AIDS (5-20%) [33]. Simultaneously, it is considerably higher than the prevalence found in the general population (10.3%) [2]. Evans [5] assembled studies that indicate a bi-directional relation between depression and comorbid medical illnesses: severe medical illness is an accepted risk factor for developing a depressive disorder. However, at the same time, it is under debate whether depression might be a causal factor itself in the development and course of medical illnesses, e.g., in cardiac diseases [34]. In this light, the relatively high prevalence rate of depression found in the present study might be interpreted as further evidence for a strong link between depression and medical illnesses of ORL in particular. Thus, one could assume that depression might impair treatment and outcome of otolaryngologic diseases like the data of Bhattacharyya & Wasan suggest [7]. Still, further research is needed, and especially longitudinally designed studies are required to gain further insight into the complex relation of depression and physical disease.

In general, the conduction of a full semi-structured diagnostic interview to assess mood in ORL-patients would be desirable. However, since this technique is laborious and time-consuming for both, the patient and the investigator, it is not likely that it will become routine diagnostic practice in ORL clinics. Still, given the general impact of depression in patients with various physical diseases [34,35] a routine screening for depression with more economical instruments is highly demanded. Therefore, future studies should engage in expanding our body of knowledge about the screening performance (sensitivity, specificity) of existing self-report instruments for depression (e.g., BDI) in this patient group. A new instrument that shows promising psychometric quality in both patients with physical and mental illnesses is the Rasch-based Depression Screening (DESC), which was developed on the basis of data from patients with mental, cardiologic, and otorhinolaryngologic diseases [36].

A limitation of the present study is that no detailed data on those patients who declined participation is available. Patients were approached at admission if their treating physicians considered them eligible and most (approximately > 80%) agreed to participate. Nevertheless, a potential bias of over- or underreporting of depression can not be ruled out. Overreporting would occur if those persons with more severe symptoms of depression would have been more likely to participate - e.g., because they felt that study aims were important for people in their present situation. Underreporting would have occurred if those persons with more severe depression would have been more likely to decline participation - e. g., because symptom burden was too high. Both directions of bias may be present in most studies of this kind and have to be kept in mind when interpreting the current results.

Another limitation is that although published research suggests that especially diagnoses like head and neck cancer might be related to elevated depression [14,32], limited sample size made it impossible to report reliable prevalence rates for ORL subsamples with different

diagnoses so that we decided to report prevalence data only divided by gender.

Conclusion
The results of our study call for carrying on in engaging in research about depression in ORL inpatients and further intensifying collaborative health care in a multidisciplinary setting to foster optimal outcome and treatment of both, the physical and psychic disorder.

List of abbreviations used
ADL: activities of daily living; BDI: Beck Depression Inventory; BSI: Brief Symptom Inventory; DESC: Rasch-based Depression Screening; GSI: global severity index; HADS: Hospital Anxiety and Depression Scale; ICD-10: International Classification of Diseases 10th Revision; IDCL: International Diagnostic Checklist for depression; MANOVA: analysis of variance for repeated measures; ORL: otorhinolaryngology; PSDI: positive symptom distress index; PST: positive symptom total; QoL: quality of life; SCL-90-R: Symptom Checklist 90-R; SD: standard deviation

Acknowledgements and funding
This research project was supported by the START-program of the Faculty of Medicine, RWTH Aachen and the German Research Foundation (DFG, WI3210/2-1).

Author details
[1]Institute of Medical Psychology and Medical Sociology, University Hospital of RWTH Aachen, Pauwelsstraße 30, 52074 Aachen, Germany. [2]Dept. of Psychiatry and Psychotherapy, LWL-University-Clinic, Ruhr-University Bochum, Alexandrinenstr. 1-3, 44791 Bochum, Germany. [3]Institute of Psychology, University of Education Freiburg, Kartäuserstr. 61b, 79117 Freiburg, Germany. [4]Clinic for Otorhinolaryngology, University Hospital of RWTH Aachen, Pauwelsstraße 30, 52074 Aachen, Germany.

Authors' contributions
TF contributed to conception and design of the study, conducted the statistical analysis and wrote the manuscript. CN participated in the analysis and interpretation of the data. MW participated in the design of the study and the statistical analysis. MW and TV participated in the design of the study and coordinated the data acquisition. SG has been involved in drafting and revising the manuscript, and coordinated the study and data acquisition. MB contributed to the analysis and interpretation of the data. All authors read and approved the final manuscript.

Competing interests
The authors declare that they have no competing interests.

References
1. Waraich P, Goldner EM, Somers JM, Hsu L: Prevalence and incidence studies of mood disorders: a systematic review of the literature. *Can J Psychiatry* 2004, **49**:124-138.
2. Kessler RC, McGonagle KA, Zhao S, Nelson CB, Hughes M, Eshleman S, Wittchen HU, Kendler KS: Lifetime and 12-month prevalence of DSM-III-R psychiatric disorders in the United States. Results from the National Comorbidity Survey. *Arch Gen Psychiatry* 1994, **51**:8-19.
3. Sadovnick AD, Remick RA, Allen J, Swartz E, Yee IM, Eisen K, Farquhar R, Hashimoto SA, Hooge J, Kastrukoff LF, Morrison W, Nelson J, Oger J, Paty DW: Depression and multiple sclerosis. *Neurology* 1996, **46**:628-632.
4. Verdelho A, Henon H, Lebert F, Pasquier F, Leys D: Depressive symptoms after stroke and relationship with dementia: A three-year follow-up study. *Neurology* 2004, **62**:905-911.
5. Evans DL, Charney DS, Lewis L, Golden RN, Gorman JM, Krishnan KR, Nemeroff CB, Bremner JD, Carney RM, Coyne JC, Delong MR, Frasure-Smith N, Glassman AH, Gold PW, Grant I, Gwyther L, Ironson G, Johnson RL,

Kanner AM, Katon WJ, Kaufmann PG, Keefe FJ, Ketter T, Laughren TP, Leserman J, Lyketsos CG, McDonald WM, McEwen BS, Miller AH, Musselman D, et al: Mood disorders in the medically ill: scientific review and recommendations. Biol Psychiatry 2005, 58:175-189.

6. Bankier B, Januzzi JL, Littman AB: The high prevalence of multiple psychiatric disorders in stable outpatients with coronary heart disease. Psychosom Med 2004, 66:645-650.

7. Bhattacharyya N, Wasan A: Do anxiety and depression confound symptom reporting and diagnostic accuracy in chronic rhinosinusitis? Ann Otol Rhinol Laryngol 2008, 117:18-23.

8. Wasan A, Fernandez E, Jamison RN, Bhattacharyya N: Association of anxiety and depression with reported disease severity in patients undergoing evaluation for chronic rhinosinusitis. Ann Otol Rhinol Laryngol 2007, 116:491-497.

9. Mace J, Michael YL, Carlson NE, Litvack JR, Smith TL: Effects of depression on quality of life improvement after endoscopic sinus surgery. Laryngoscope 2008, 118:528-534.

10. Brandsted R, Sindwani R: Impact of depression on disease-specific symptoms and quality of life in patients with chronic rhinosinusitis. Am J Rhinol 2007, 21:50-54.

11. Chandra RK, Epstein VA, Fishman AJ: Prevalence of depression and antidepressant use in an otolaryngology patient population. Otolaryngol Head Neck Surg 2009, 141:136-138.

12. Hellgren J, Balder B, Palmqvist M, Löwhagen O, Tunsäter A, Karlsson G, Torén K: Quality of life in non-infectious rhinitis and asthma. Rhinology 2004, 42:183-188.

13. Bronheim H, Strain JJ, Biller HF: Psychiatric aspects of head and neck surgery. Part I: New surgical techniques and psychiatric consequences. Gen Hosp Psychiatry 1991, 13:165-176.

14. Kugaya A, Akechi T, Okuyama T, Nakano T, Mikami I, Okamura H, Uchitomi Y: Prevalence, predictive factors, and screening for psychologic distress in patients with newly diagnosed head and neck cancer. Cancer 2000, 88:2817-2823.

15. Singer S, Herrmann E, Welzel C, Klemm E, Heim M, Schwarz R: Comorbid mental disorders in laryngectomees. Onkologie 2005, 28:631-636.

16. World Medical Association: Proposed revision of the Declaration of Helsinki. Bull Med Ethics 1999, 150:18-22.

17. Hiller W, Zaudiga M, Mombour W: ICD International Diagnostic Checklists for ICD-10 and DSM-IV Göttingen: Hogrefe & Huber Pub; 1999.

18. World Health Organization: The ICD-10 classification of mental and behavioral disorders: clinical descriptions and diagnostic guidelines Geneva: World Health Organization; 1992.

19. Derogatis LR: The Symptom Checklist-90-revised Minneapolis: NCS Assessments; 1992.

20. Derogatis LR: The Brief Symptom Inventory (BSI): Administration, scoring and procedures manual. 3 edition. Mineapolis: National Computer System; 1993.

21. Beck AT, Steer RA: Beck Depression Inventory San Antonio: The Psychological Corporation Inc.; 1987.

22. Forkmann T, Boecker M, Norra C, Eberle N, Kircher T, Schauerte P, Mischke K, Westhofen M, Gauggel S, Wirtz M: Development of an item bank for the assessment of depression in persons with mental illnesses and physical diseases using Rasch analysis. Rehabil Psychol 2009, 54:186-197.

23. Hedges LV, Olkin I: Statistical Methods for Meta-Analysis Orlando: Academic Press; 1985.

24. Cohen J: Statistical power for the behavioural science. 2 edition. Hillsdale: Erlbaum; 1988.

25. Dunlap WP, Cortina JM, Vaslow JB, Burke MJ: Meta-analysis of experiments with matched groups or repeated measures designs. Psychol Methods 1996, 1:170-177.

26. Wittchen HU, Jacobi F: Size and burden of mental disorders in Europe- a critical review and appraisal of 27 studies. Eur Neuropsychopharmacol 2005, 15:357-376.

27. Abramowitz JS: Treatment of obsessive-compulsive disorder in patients who have comorbid major depression. J Clin Psychol 2004, 60:1133-1141.

28. DeVane CL, Chiao E, Franklin M, Kruep EJ: Anxiety disorders in the 21st century: status, challenges, opportunities, and comorbidity with depression. Am J Manag Care 2005, 11:S344-S353.

29. Rudisch B, Nemeroff CB: Epidemiology of comorbid coronary artery disease and depression. Biol Psychiatry 2003, 54:227-240.

30. Robinson RG: Poststroke depression: prevalence, diagnosis, treatment, and disease progression. Biol Psychiatry 2003, 54:376-387.

31. Stunkard AJ, Faith MS, Allison KC: Depression and obesity. Biol Psychiatry 2003, 54:330-337.

32. Raison CL, Miller AH: Depression in cancer: new developments regarding diagnosis and treatment. Biol Psychiatry 2003, 54:283-294.

33. Cruess DG, Evans DL, Repetto MJ, Gettes D, Douglas SD, Petitto JM: Prevalence, diagnosis, and pharmacological treatment of mood disorders in HIV disease. Biol Psychiatry 2003, 54:307-316.

34. Bush DE, Ziegelstein RC, Tayback M, Richter D, Stevens S, Zahalsky H, Fauerbach JA: Even minimal symptoms of depression increase mortality risk after acute myocardial infarction. Am J Cardiol 2001, 88:337-341.

35. Norra C, Skobel EC, Arndt M, Schauerte P: High impact of depression in heart failure: early diagnosis and treatment options. Int J Cardiol 2008, 125:220-231.

36. Forkmann T, Boecker M, Wirtz M, Eberle N, Westhofen M, Schauerte P, Mischke K, Kircher T, Gauggel S, Norra C: Development and validation of the Rasch-based depression screening (DESC) using Rasch analysis and structural equation modelling. J Behav Ther Exp Psychiatry 2009, 40:468-78.

Incidental findings in MRI of the paranasal sinuses in adults: a population-based study (HUNT MRI)

Aleksander Grande Hansen[1,3]*, Anne-Sofie Helvik[1,2], Ståle Nordgård[1,3], Vegard Bugten[1,3], Lars Jacob Stovner[3], Asta K Håberg[3], Mari Gårseth[4] and Heidi Beate Eggesbø[5]

Abstract

Background: Diagnostic imaging of the head is used with increasing frequency, and often includes the paranasal sinuses, where incidental opacifications are found. To determine the clinical relevance of such findings can be challenging, and for the patient such incidental findings can give rise to concern if they are over-reported. Studies of incidental findings in the paranasal sinuses have been conducted mostly in patients referred for diagnostic imaging, hence the prevalence in the general population is not known. The purpose of this study was to determine the prevalence and size of incidental opacification in the paranasal sinuses in a non-selected adult population using magnetic resonance imaging (MRI) without medical indication, and to relate the results to sex and season.

Methods: Randomly and independent of medical history, 982 participants (518 women) with a mean age of 58.5 years (range, 50–66) underwent MRI of the head as part of a large public health survey in Norway. The MRIs included 3D T1 weighted volume data and 2D axial T2 weighted image (WI). Opacifications, indicating mucosal thickenings, polyps, retention cysts, or fluid, were recorded if measuring more than 1 mm.

Results: Opacifications were found in 66% of the participants. Mucosal thickenings were found in 49%, commonly in the maxillary sinuses (29%) where 25% had opacifications that were less than 4 mm in size. Other opacifications occurred in the anterior ethmoid (23%), posterior ethmoid (21%), frontal sinus (9%), and sphenoid (8%). Polyps and retention cysts were also found mainly in the maxillary sinuses in 32%. Fluid was observed in 6% of the MRIs. Mucosal thickening was observed more frequently in men than in women (P <0.05). No seasonal variation was found.

Conclusions: In this large non-selected sample, incidental opacification in the paranasal sinuses was seen in two out of three participants, and mucosal thickening was seen in one out of two. Fluid was rare. Knowledge of incidental opacification is important because it can affect clinical practice.

Keywords: Incidental findings, Paranasal sinuses, MRI, Opacification, Mucosal thickening, Polyps, Retention cysts, Fluid, Population-based study

Background

Diagnostic imaging of the head and neck is used with increasing frequency [1] and often includes the paranasal sinuses where incidental opacifications, such as mucosal thickening, polyps, retention cysts, and fluid, are often found [2,3], but the clinical relevance of these findings often remains uncertain for radiologists and ear, nose and throat surgeons. For the patient, such findings can

cause unnecessary concern, and for the health system, they can potentially lead to unnecessary costs [4]. Different studies have used a variety of methods, and the findings in the paranasal sinus in both adult [2,5-14] and paediatric populations [15,16] have varied. In all studies on adults, the participants have been recruited from clinical settings, where the diagnostic imaging was performed primarily for diagnostic reasons [2,5-8,12,17]. We therefore believe they cannot be considered a non-selected population. In previous studies the effect of sex and season on incidental findings has varied [3,5,12].

* Correspondence: aleksandergrandehansen@gmail.com
[1]Department of Ear, Nose and Throat, Head and Neck Surgery, St. Olavs Hospital NTNU, Trondheim, Norway
[3]Department of Neuroscience, St. Olavs hospital NTNU, Trondheim, Norway
Full list of author information is available at the end of the article

The HUNT study is a large public health survey in Nord-Trøndelag county in Norway that has been conducted in three waves between 1984 and 2009 (HUNT I, II and III). As a part of HUNT III, a random selection of persons between 50 and 65 years of age underwent an MRI of the head (the HUNT MRI study).

The purpose of this study was to estimate on MRI of a non-selected population, the prevalence and size of incidental opacifications of the paranasal sinuses, and to determine their relation to sex and seasonal variation.

Methods

The Nord-Trøndelag health study (Helseundersøkelsen i Nord-Trøndelag, HUNT) is a large-scale epidemiological study conducted in three waves: HUNT I (1984 to 1986), HUNT II (1995 to 1997), and HUNT III (2007 to 2009), as a collaboration between the Norwegian Institute of Public Health, the Faculty of Medicine at the Norwegian University of Science and Technology, and Nord-Trøndelag County Council [18]. For each wave, the entire population aged 20 years or older and living in the Norwegian county of Nord-Trøndelag was invited to participate. Detailed questionnaires about health status, biomedical measurements, and blood samples were collected [18]. HUNT I resulted in 74,977 completed surveys, HUNT II resulted in 66,140, and in HUNT III resulted in 50,839.

From those participating in all three waves and who were aged between 50 and 65 years in HUNT III (n = 14,033), 1560 participants were randomly invited for an MRI study of the head [19]. Selection was made with no regard to health status. Exclusion criteria were travelling distance greater than 45 minutes to the MRI examination centre in Levanger and general MRI contraindications such as cochlear implants, severe claustrophobia, weight greater than 150 kg, cardiac pacemaker, or clipped cerebral aneurysm. Written informed consent was obtained from 1088 invitees (69%), and 82 of these did not come to the MRI examination [20]. In the period between July 21, 2007 and December 10, 2009, 1006 participants underwent an MRI. Of these, 21 were excluded due to artefacts, or if opacifications were seen on T1WI, but not fully demonstrated in T2WI (e.g. the base of the maxillary sinuses), and three due to extensive paranasal sinus surgery. Finally, 982 participants met all inclusion criteria

(63% overall participation rate, 518 women, 464 men). Mean age was 58.5 years, age range 50–66 years (eight participants turned 66 years before the MRI had been done). The Regional Ethics Committee in Sør-Trøndelag, Norway approved the study (2011/2199-1).

For each participant, MRI was performed using a 1.5 T HDx scanner (Sigma, GE Healthcare, Waukesha, WI) equipped with an eight channel head coil and software version pre-14.0 M4. The scan protocol included axial T1 weighted images (WI), T1W magnetization prepared rapid acquisition gradient echo (MPRAGE) volume, scan axial T2WI, T2*WI and fluid attenuated inversion recovery (FLAIR) sequences, and a time of flight (TOF) 3D angio sequence. For this study we applied the axial T2WI (4 mm slices) and the T1W MPRAGE volume scan (1 mm slices). Scan parameters for the applied parameters are listed in Table 1.

Within two weeks after the MRIs were taken two experienced radiologists did a clinical evaluation of all MRIs in order to detect any pathology of the brain and the rest of the head with clinical significance for the participants. This evaluation was not particularly focused on sinus pathology. Three to four years later, in the period between April 2012 and July 2013, MRI readings and measurements of the sinuses were done independently and blinded for all participant data by an ear, nose and throat resident with 4 years' experience (A.G.H), and a head and neck radiologist specialized in paranasal sinus radiology (H.B.E). A DICOM reader and associated software (Osirix version 3.2.4, 32 bit; Osirix Foundation, Geneva, Switzerland) were employed. In 21% of the cases there was a discrepancy in measurements or interpretation, and in these cases the MRIs were re-examined and a consensus was reached.

Each sinus was examined separately (i.e., left and right maxillary, anterior ethmoid, frontal, posterior ethmoid, and sphenoid sinuses) using both 3D T1W volume data with coronal, sagittal and axial reconstruction and 2D axial T2WI. Aplasia was recorded to calculate the prevalence of outcomes related to the number of sinuses. Frontal sinus aplasia [21] was defined as a lack of pneumatisation of the frontal bone with no ethmoid cells extending above a line tangential to the supraorbital margin, and sphenoid sinus aplasia [21] as pneumatisation limited to the pre-sphenoid bone.

Table 1 MRI sequences and acquisition parameters

MRI sequences	Matrix (pixels)	NSA	TR (ms)	TE (ms)	Flip-angle	Slice thickness (mm)	Gap (mm)	Overlap (mm)	FOV (mm)
T1WI 3D GRE	192 × 192	1	10	4	10°	1.2	0	0	240
T2WI	512 × 320	2	7840	95	90°	4.0	1.0	0	230

All imaging was performed on the same 1.5 T General Electric Sigma HDx 1.5 T magnetic resonance imaging (MRI) scanner equipped with an eight channel head coil and software version pre-14.0 M4. T1WI: T1 weighted image, GRE: gradient echo, T2WI: T2 weighted image, NSA: number of signal averages, TR: repetition time, TE: Time of echo, FOV: field of view.

Opacifications were categorized and defined as follows: i) Mucosal thickening, identified by a high signal on T2WI and a low signal on T1WI following the peripheral border of the sinus. ii) Polyps and retention cysts, identified as circumscribed, homogeneous, dome-shaped areas with high signals on T2WI. Polyps and retention cysts cannot be unambiguously differentiated by MRI [21], and were therefore merged in one group. iii) Fluid, identified on T2WI by a distinct air-fluid level, and measured from the sinus border to the air-fluid level. In each paranasal sinus, all opacifications were measured in millimetres (mm). The opacifications were visually determined at their maximum thickness, using both the T1WI and the T2WI. The opacifications visible, but measuring less than 1 mm were categorized as 0 mm. The superior walls of the paranasal sinuses are challenging to evaluate on axial images, and they were therefore mainly investigated on the coronal and sagittal T1WI. When mucosal thickening, polyps and retention cysts, and/or fluid were found in one and the same sinus, all opacifications were measured separately.

The sex and month of MRI was recorded. Seasons were defined as follows: April through October was categorized as summer, and November through March was categorized as winter.

Statistical analysis

The prevalence and size of the three groups of opacifications were determined for all subjects and each sinus, and related to sex and season. The data were analysed using SPSS version 18 (released July 30, 2009). For comparison between men and women, and between seasons of MRI scan, the Mann–Whitney test was used for continuous variables (e.g. mean thickness of mucosal thickening, polyps/retention cysts, and fluid), and the Chi-squared test was used for proportions of participants with opacification (e.g. mucosal thickening yes/no, polyps/retention cysts yes/no, and fluid yes/no) for each sinus. In addition, prevalence of participants with opacifications in several sinuses was calculated. $P \leq 0.05$ was considered statistically significant.

Results

The prevalence of each group of opacification for each sinus, and for each sex is shown in Table 2. Frontal and sphenoid sinus aplasia was seen in respectively 49/982 (5%) and 1/982 (0.1%). Opacifications were observed more frequently in men (342/464, 73%) than in women (308/518, 59%), P <0.01. This was true both for mucosal thickening (men: 267/464, 57%, women: 17/518, 42%, P <0.01), and for polyps and retention cysts (men: 213/

Table 2 Opacification defined as mucosal thickening, polyps, retention cysts and fluid level ≥1 mm in the right (R) and left (L) paranasal sinuses in 982 individuals (518 men and 464 women) on MRI

Sinus	Maxillary		Anterior ethmoid		Frontal		Posterior ethmoid		Sphenoid	
	R	L	R	L	R	L	R	L	R	L
Mucosal thickening ≥1 mm in each sinus, n and (%)										
Men	154 (33.2)	147** (31.2)	125** (26.9)	125** (26.9)	47** (10.1)	57** (8.8)	115** (24.7)	129** (27.8)	49** (10.5)	37* (7.9)
Women	127 (24.5)	104 (20.0)	98 (18.9)	88 (16.9)	29 (5.5)	30 (5.7)	68 (13.1)	80 (15.4)	27 (5.2)	23 (4.4)
Mean mucosal thickening in each sinus (mm ± SD)										
Men	3.32 ± 3.61	3.52 ± 4.01	1.96 ± 1.09	2.06 ± 1.24	1.80 ± 1.32	1.54 ± 1.01	2.19 ± 1.29	2.14 ± 2.1	2.40 ± 2.70	2.20 ± 2.19
Women	2.55 ± 2.23	2.75 ± 1.78	1.96 ± 1.11	1.78 ± 1.29	2.17 ± 1.39	1.56 ± 0.86	1.95 ± 1.15	1.68 ± 0.9	2.70 ± 2.10	2.20 ± 1.52
Polyps/retention cysts ≥1 mm in each sinus, n and (%)										
Men	123** (26.5)	118** (25.4)	14 (3.0)	11 (2.3)	10 (2.1)	6 (1.2)	12 (2.5)	11 (2.3)	12 (2.5)	8 (1.7)
Women	85 (16.4)	79 (15.2)	8 (1.5)	8 (1.5)	1 (0.02)	5 (0.1)	9 (1.7)	7 (1.3)	12 (2.3)	6 (1.1)
Mean polyp/retention cyst diameter in each sinus (mm ± SD)										
Men	8.16 ± 5.17	9.14 ± 6.26	4.28 ± 2.33	3.81 ± 2.04	5.00 ± 1.88	5.83 ± 1.72	5.41 ± 2.42	3.63 ± 0.9	6.00 ± 4.19	6.87 ± 4.45
Women	8.24 ± 6.81	7.05 ± 4.44	2.12 ± 0.64	3.00 ± 0.92	-	4.00 ± 2.23	3.55 ± 1.23	6.42 ± 4.2	5.16 ± 2.08	5.33 ± 2.33
Fluid ≥1 mm in each sinus, n (%)										
Men	8 (1.7)	14 (3.0)	1 (0.2)	1 (0.2)	0	1 (0.2)	1 (0.2)	1 (0.2)	4 (0.8)	4 (0.8)
Women	12 (2.3)	16 (3.0)	1 (0.2)	0	0	0	0	0	5 (1.0)	5 (1.0cps)
Mean fluid level in each sinus (in mm)										
Men	6.6	7.5	-	-	-	-	-	-	7.3	5.3
Women	8.2	6.7	-	-	-	-	-	-	6.6	5.6

**p < 0.01, *p < 0.05 comparing men and women.
Number of sinuses is less than 982 due to aplasia in the right frontal (46/982, 6%), in the left frontal (46/982, 5%) and in the right sphenoid sinus (1/982, 0.1%).
Mean calculated if n > 1.

464, 46%, women: 166/518, 32%, P <0.01). Fluid was a rare finding, observed in one or several sinuses in 24/464 (5%) of the men and 32/518 (6%) of the women (P = 0.5). The majority occurred in the maxillary sinus.

In both men and women, the highest prevalence of mucosal thickening was in the maxillary sinus, followed by the ethmoid (anterior and posterior) sinuses. For polyps and retention cysts, the great majority was found in the maxillary sinuses, and 317 of the 982 participants (32%) had either unilateral or bilateral polyps/retention cysts in the maxillary sinuses. Of these, 88 (9%) had this bilaterally. The proportion of mucosal thickening is demonstrated in Figure 1 and to the size of polyps and retention cysts in Figure 2. The results with alternative cut-offs for the mucosa (3 and 4 mm) are presented in Table 3.

For each opacification group and each paranasal sinus, no seasonal variation was observed, except mucosal thickening in the left anterior ethmoid sinus, which was significantly more prevalent in MRIs taken during the summer (131/533 participants) than winter (82/449 participants), P = 0.01. Month-by-month comparisons revealed no significant variation.

Discussion

To our knowledge, this is the first large MRI study reporting incidental findings in the paranasal sinuses in an adult, non-selected population, recruited for study purposes only. This is in contrast to previous studies [2,5-8,12,17], where participants were examined for medical reasons. This study shows the prevalence and the range of mucosal thickening, polyps and retention cysts, and fluid in the different sinuses. Knowledge about opacifications of the paranasal sinuses in the general population is useful, because such findings are frequent, and can represent clinical challenges and give rise to costly additional investigations and unnecessary concern for the patient if interpreted wrongly.

It is a strength of the study that a detailed analysis of the participants has been published [19], showing that the HUNT MRI population was not considerably different from the general HUNT population. While the participants were non-selected in terms of health, they had somewhat higher education levels and were less likely to be overweight or have hypertension. There was no significant difference with regard to smoking, which is important for changes in the sinuses [22]. The fact that the study was not primarily aimed at investigating the paranasal sinuses makes participation bias unlikely (i.e. those with sinus problems are more likely to participate). Hence, we believe that the cohort is quite representative for the general Norwegian population of that age with regard to the parameters we have studied.

It is a limitation of the study that from the outset investigation the paranasal sinuses were not the main aim; hence MRI parameters may not be optimal for this purpose. All sinuses were completely visualized on 3D Volume T1WI with coronal, sagittal and axial reconstruction. If opacifications were seen on T1WI, but not covered by the T2WI (e.g. in the floor of the maxillary sinus), these participants were excluded. In addition, fluid can in some rear cases be present without a high signal on T2WI, or a distinct air-fluid level [23]. This

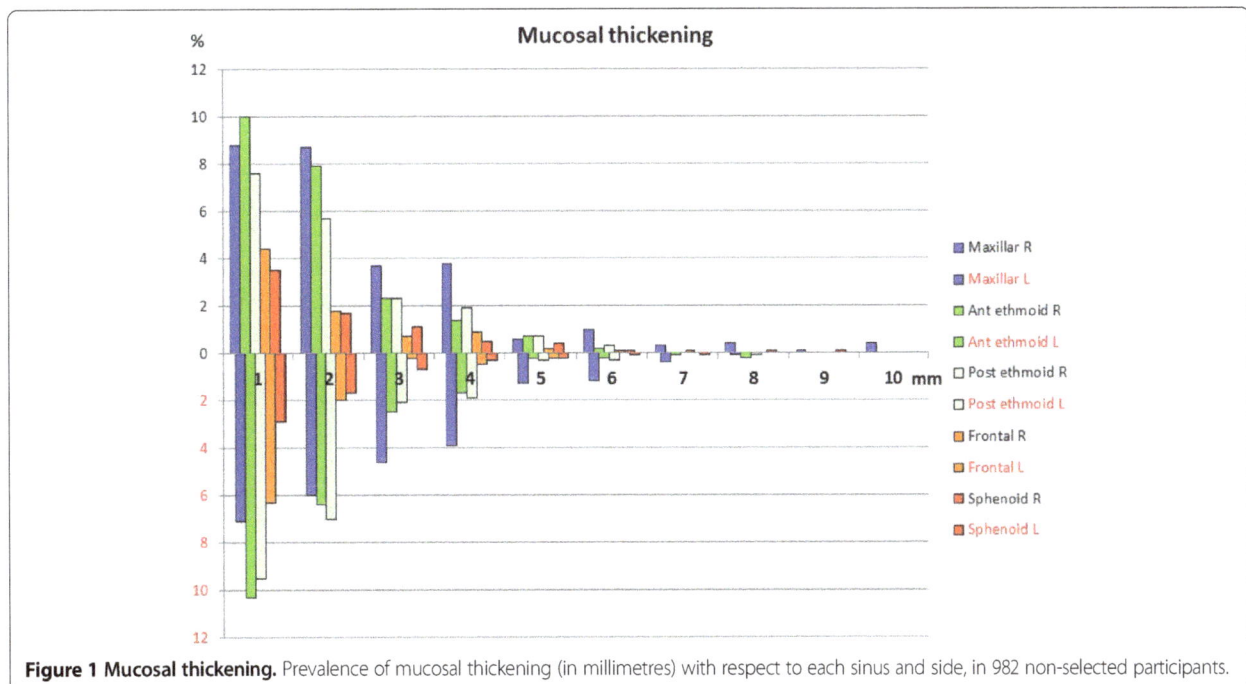

Figure 1 Mucosal thickening. Prevalence of mucosal thickening (in millimetres) with respect to each sinus and side, in 982 non-selected participants.

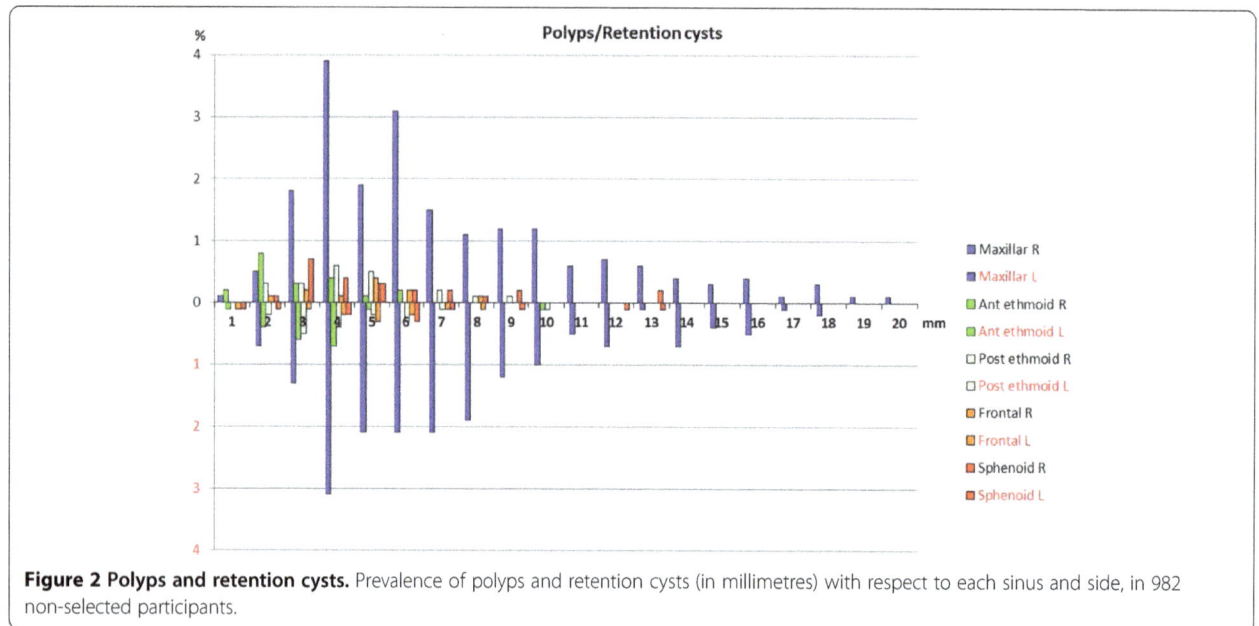

Figure 2 Polyps and retention cysts. Prevalence of polyps and retention cysts (in millimetres) with respect to each sinus and side, in 982 non-selected participants.

can be a pus filled sinus, or allergic fungal sinusitis, and could have been missed with our definition of fluid. Although we hardly encountered such cases in this un-selected material, the prevalence of opacification could be somewhat underestimated.

Also, the participants' age did not represent the entire population; hence extrapolation of the results to other age groups must be done with caution. In addition, there were no data on sinonasal symptoms at the time of the MRIs, so we were unable to relate findings to current symptoms.

In the literature, reports on incidental sinus opacification vary, depending on patient selection and methodology used [5,6,8,17]. Results have often been reported with pre-defined cut-offs, where definitions of a normal mucosal thickening ranges from <2 mm [13] to ≤4 mm [5]. Other studies have used the Lund-Mackay scoring system [14], modified Lund Mackay scoring systems [15], or have defined "minimal mucosal thickening" as normal without specifying a size range [17]. Still, there is no clear definition of normal or abnormal findings in the paranasal sinuses [5]. Furthermore, several studies only reported the most pronounced opacification in each sinus [5,6]. This can potentially lead to an underestimation of findings, since one sinus may contain combinations of mucosal thickening, polyps, cysts, and fluid. In

this study, we counted all visible opacifications that measured at least 1 mm, and there were no predefined cut-off values, which ensures that all findings that can give rise to problems in clinical practice are included.

In our study, the maxillary sinuses frequently showed thickening of mucosa (36% when both sides were considered together), and the majority of these were no larger than 4 mm, which accords with findings in other studies [2,11,12]. In Table 3, we present alternative cut off values and methods, as described by Gordts et al. [6] and Tarp et al. [5] for comparison of results. Gordts et al. [6] (MRI of n = 99), using a cut-off of >3 mm, found opacification in maxillary sinuses in 40% of the study participants. Similarly, Tarp et al. (MRI of n = 404), using a cut-off value of >4 mm, found a similar result (33.7%) [5]. Using the same cut-off values, our figures were lower, possibly reflecting that the other studies were performed in patients. In the other sinuses the differences were smaller (see Table 3).

Polyps and retention cysts were also more frequently seen in the maxillary sinuses (32%), which is in accordance with previous studies [2,5,11,12,24]. They were also of similar size and location as in the previous studies. In a comparable age group, Moon et al. [24] found a lower prevalence of polyps and retention cysts, but higher average cyst size (16–17 mm).

Table 3 Prevalences (%) of paranasal sinus opacifications in 982 non-selected adult participants on MRI, using alternative cut-off values for mucosal thickening*

Cut-off	Maxillary	Anterior ethmoid	Posterior ethmoid	Frontal	Sphenoid
>3 mm*	26	4	4	2	3.5
>4 mm*	25	3	2.8	1.4	3.2

Prevalence of opacifications with respective cut-offs for mucosal thickening, and with polyps/retention cysts and fluid if >0 mm.

Tarp *et al.* [5] reported polyps and cysts in 15% of participants, the majority located in the maxillary sinuses. The higher frequency found in our study can be explained by the fact that we measured polyps and retention cysts even when opacifications of either of the other two groups were present, whereas Tarp *et al.* noted only the most pronounced abnormality.

Fluid was an infrequent finding in our study (6%), comparable to the findings by Gordts *et al.* (<5%) [11], Patel *et al.* (4%) [13], and Rak *et al.* (3%) [8].

Men had a significantly higher prevalence of mucosal thickening and polyps/retention cysts in this study. This is in agreement with most previous studies [5,12,25]. An exception is Maly *et al.* [7], who found opacification more frequently in women.

No clear seasonal variation was observed in this study. In a previous study, Tarp *et al.* [5] found a significantly higher degree of pathology during winter, whereas other studies have not shown significant seasonal variations [12,25]. We chose the seasons mainly due to the climatic conditions in the area from which the participants were recruited, where the costal climate provides an early spring and late autumn. Nevertheless month-by-month comparisons did not show any significant variation.

Conclusions

Our study shows that mucosal thickening, polyps, and retention cysts in the paranasal sinuses are frequent incidental findings on MRIs of the head in the general population. This study contributes to the knowledge of incidental findings in the paranasal sinuses due to its large participant sample from a general population. The results are important because opacifications in the paranasal sinuses challenges physicians and can have impact on clinical practice.

Abbreviations
MRI: Magnetic resonance imaging; MPRAGE: Magnetization prepared rapid acquisition gradient echo; FLAIR: Fluid attenuated inversion recovery; TOF: Time of flight, mm: millimeter.

Competing interests
The authors declare that they have no competing interests.
This research received no specific grant from any funding agency in the public, commercial, or not-for-profit sectors.

Authors' contributions
AGH contributed in conception and design, acquisition of data, analysis and interpretation of data, writing, and drafting the article, revising it critically for important intellectual content. AH contributed in conception and design, acquisition of data, analysis and interpretation of data, drafting the article and revising it critically. LJS contributed in conception and design, acquisition of data, analysis and interpretation of data, drafting the article and revising it critically. ASH contributed in conception and design, analysis and interpretation of data, drafting the article and revising it critically. VB contributed in conception and design, analysis and interpretation of data, drafting the article and revising it. HBE contributed in conception and design, acquisition of data, analysis and interpretation of data, writing, and drafting the article and revising it. SN contributed in conception and design, analysis and interpretation of data, drafting the article and revising. MG

contributed in conception and design, acquisition of data and revising the article. All authors read and approved the manuscript.

Authors' information
AGH is a resident in ENT and a research fellow.
ASH is RN and researcher.
SN is an otolaryngologist and professor.
VB is an otolaryngologist and associate professor.
LJS is a neurologist and professor.
AKH is a professor in medical imaging.
MG is a medical physicist.
HBE is a radiologist.

Acknowledgements
This work was provided as collaboration between the Norwegian Institute of Public Health, the Faculty of Medicine at the Norwegian University of Science and Technology (NTNU), Nord-Trøndelag County Council and the ENT Department, St. Olavs Hospital, Norway. We thank Irina Kazakova who helped providing the figures on behalf of NTNU.

Author details
[1]Department of Ear, Nose and Throat, Head and Neck Surgery, St. Olavs Hospital NTNU, Trondheim, Norway. [2]Department of Public Health and General Practice, NTNU, Trondheim, Norway. [3]Department of Neuroscience, St. Olavs hospital NTNU, Trondheim, Norway. [4]Department of Diagnostic Imaging, Levanger Hospital, Levanger, Norway. [5]Department of Radiology and Nuclear Medicine, Oslo University Hospital, Oslo, Norway.

References
1. Borretzen I, Lysdahl KB, Olerud HM: Diagnostic radiology in Norway trends in examination frequency and collective effective dose. *Radiat Prot Dosimetry* 2007, 124(4):339–347.
2. Wani MK, Ruckenstein MJ, Parikh S: Magnetic resonance imaging of the paranasal sinuses: incidental abnormalities and their relationship to patient symptoms. *J Otolaryngol* 2001, 30(5):257–262.
3. Rege IC, Sousa TO, Leles CR, Mendonça EF: Occurrence of maxillary sinus abnormalities detected by cone beam CT in asymptomatic patients. *BMC Oral Health* 2012, 12:30.
4. Gutmann A: Ethics: the bioethics commission on incidental findings. *Science* 2013, 342(6164):1321–1323.
5. Tarp B, Fiirgaard B, Christensen T, Jensen JJ, Black FT: The prevalence and significance of incidental paranasal sinus abnormalities on MRI. *Rhinology* 2000, 38(1):33–38.
6. Gordts F, Clement PA, Buisseret T: Prevalence of paranasal sinus abnormalities on MRI in a non-ENT population. *Acta Otorhinolaryngol Belg* 1996, 50(3):167–170.
7. Maly PV, Sundgren PC: Changes in paranasal sinus abnormalities found incidentally on MRI. *Neuroradiology* 1995, 37(6):471–474.
8. Rak KM, Newell JD II, Yakes WF, Damiano MA, Luethke JM: Paranasal sinuses on MR images of the brain: significance of mucosal thickening. *AJR Am J Roentgenol* 1991, 156(2):381–384.
9. Lesserson JA, Kieserman SP, Finn DG: The radiographic incidence of chronic sinus disease in the pediatric population. *Laryngoscope* 1994, 104(2):159–166.
10. Hill M, Bhattacharyya N, Hall TR, Lufkin R, Shapiro NL: Incidental paranasal sinus imaging abnormalities and the normal Lund score in children. *Otolaryngol Head Neck Surg* 2004, 130(2):171–175.
11. Gordts F, Clement PA, Buisseret T: Prevalence of sinusitis signs in a non-ENT population. *ORL J Otorhinolaryngol Relat Spec* 1996, 58(6):315–319.
12. Cooke LD, Hadley DM: MRI of the paranasal sinuses: incidental abnormalities and their relationship to symptoms. *J Laryngol Otol* 1991, 105(4):278–281.
13. Patel K, Chavda SV, Violaris N, Pahor AL: Incidental paranasal sinus inflammatory changes in a British population. *J Laryngol Otol* 1996, 110(7):649–651.
14. Oyinloye OI, Akande JH, Alabi BS, Afolabi OA: Incidental paranasal sinus abnormality on cranial computed tomography in a Nigerian population. *Ann Afr Med* 2013, 12(1):62–64.

15. Lim WK, Ram B, Fasulakis S, Kane KJ: **Incidental magnetic resonance image sinus abnormalities in asymptomatic Australian children.** *J Laryngol Otol* 2003, **117**(12):969–972.

16. Seki A, Uchiyama H, Fukushi T, Sakura O, Tatsuya K: **Incidental findings of brain magnetic resonance imaging study in a pediatric cohort in Japan and recommendation for a model management protocol.** *J Epidemiol* 2010, **20**(Suppl 2):S498–S504.

17. Jones RL, Crowe P, Chavda SV, Pahor AL: **The incidence of sinusitis in patients with multiple sclerosis.** *Rhinology* 1997, **35**(3):118–119.

18. Krokstad S, Langhammer A, Hveem K, Holmen TL, Midthjell K, Stene TR, Bratberg G, Heggland J, Holmen J: **Cohort profile: the HUNT study, Norway.** *Int J Epidemiol* 2013, **42**(4):968–977.

19. Honningsvag LM, Linde M, Håberg A, Stovner LJ, Hagen K: **Does health differ between participants and non-participants in the MRI-HUNT study, a population based neuroimaging study? The Nord-Trondelag health studies 1984–2009.** *BMC Med Imaging* 2012, **12**:23.

20. Muller TB, Sandvei MS, Kvistad KA, Rydland J, Håberg A, Vik A, Gårseth M, Stovner LJ: **Unruptured intracranial aneurysms in the Norwegian HUNT-study: risk of rupture calculated from data in a population-based cohort study.** *Neurosurgery* 2013, **73**(2):256–616.

21. Eggesbo HB, Søvik S, Dølvik S, Eiklid K, Kolmannskog F: **CT characterization of developmental variations of the paranasal sinuses in cystic fibrosis.** *Acta Radiol* 2001, **42**(5):482–493.

22. Uhliarova B, Adamkov M, Svec M, Calkovska A: **The effect of smoking on CT score, bacterial colonization and distribution of inflammatory cells in the upper airways of patients with chronic rhinosinusitis.** *Inhal Toxicol* 2014, **26**(7):419–425.

23. Eggesbo HB: **Radiological imaging of inflammatory lesions in the nasal cavity and paranasal sinuses.** *Eur Radiol* 2006, **16**(4):872–888.

24. Moon IJ, Lee JE, Kim ST, Han DH, Rhee CS, Lee CH, Min YG: **Characteristics and risk factors of mucosal cysts in the paranasal sinuses.** *Rhinology* 2011, **49**(3):309–314.

25. Havas TE, Motbey JA, Gullane PJ: **Prevalence of incidental abnormalities on computed tomographic scans of the paranasal sinuses.** *Arch Otolaryngol Head Neck Surg* 1988, **114**(8):856–859.

Ear, nose and throat injuries at Bugando Medical Centre in northwestern Tanzania: a five-year prospective review of 456 cases

Japhet M Gilyoma[1,2] and Phillipo L Chalya[2*]

Abstract

Background: Injuries to the ear, nose and throat (ENT) regions are not uncommon in clinical practice and constitute a significant cause of morbidity and mortality in our setting. There is dearth of literature on this subject in our environment. This study was conducted to describe the causes, injury pattern and outcome of these injuries in our setting and proffer possible preventive measures.

Methods: This was a descriptive prospective study of patients with ear, nose and throat injuries managed at Bugando Medical Centre between May 2007 and April 2012. Ethical approval to conduct the study was sought from relevant authorities. Statistical data analysis was performed using SPSS computer software version 17.0.

Results: A total of 456 patients were studied. The median age of patients at presentation was 18 years (range 1 to 72 years). The male to female ratio was 2:1. The commonest cause of injury was foreign bodies (61.8%) followed by road traffic accidents (22.4%). The ear was the most common body region injured accounting for 59.0% of cases. The majority of patients (324, 71.1%) were treated as an outpatient and only 132(28.9%) patients required admission to the ENT wards after definitive treatment. Foreign body removal and surgical wound debridement were the most common treatment modalities performed in 61.9% and 16.2% of cases respectively. Complication rate was 14.9%. Suppurative otitis media (30.9%) was the commonest complication in the ear while traumatic epistaxis (26.5%) and hoarseness of voice (11.8%) in the aero-digestive tract were commonest in the nose and throat. The overall median length of hospital stay for in-patients was 8 days (range 1 to 22 days). Patients who developed complications and those who had associated injuries stayed longer in the hospital (P < 0.001).
Mortality rate related to isolated ENT injuries was 1.3% (6 deaths). The majority of patients (96.9%) were treated successfully and only 3.1% of cases were discharged with permanent disabilities.

Conclusion: Injuries to the ENT regions are not uncommon in our environment and foreign bodies constitute a significant cause of injury. Majority of these injuries can be prevented through public enlightenment campaigns.

Keywords: ENT injuries, Causes, Injury patterns, Outcome, Tanzania

Background

Injuries to the ear, nose and throat (ENT) regions are not uncommon in clinical practice and constitute a significant cause of morbidity and mortality resulting from increased costs of care and varying degrees of physical, functional and cosmetic disfigurement [1,2]. Studies have shown that ENT injuries are avoidable cause of death and disability [3-5]. In Bugando Medical Centre, ENT injuries are a single most common cause of ENT admissions and contribute significantly to high morbidity and mortality [6,7].

The causes and mechanism of ENT injuries have been reported to vary with age and geographic distribution [3,4,7]. ENT injuries occur in all age groups; however the mechanisms and causes differ between children and adults [3,4,8]. Injuries such as foreign body in the ear, nose and throat remain the commonest and tend to occur more in children with serious complications [9].

* Correspondence: drphillipoleo@yahoo.com
[2]Department of Surgery, Catholic University of Health and Allied Sciences, Mwanza, Tanzania
Full list of author information is available at the end of the article

In adults, the common etiologies of ENT injuries, across the world, are road traffic accidents, assaults, falls and sports [4]. The types of injury in the sub-Saharan region are different from those in the developed countries [8]. Road traffic accident is reported to be the leading cause of ENT injuries in developing countries, while interpersonal violence is the leading cause in developed countries [4]. Injuries to the ear, nose and throat can occur as an isolated injury or may be associated with multiple injuries to the head, chest, abdominal, spinal and extremities [1,9].

ENT injuries have various mechanisms of injury, blunt traumas such as blows and slaps to the ears represent a different spectrum of injuries [10]. Domestic violence and abuse from law enforcement agents are implicated causes of traumatic tympanic membrane perforation [10].

Most tympanic perforations, besides, penetrating and open injuries to the throat are often life threatening with more dramatic presentations [11]. The less dramatic the injury, the longer it takes for the patient to present to a health facility. However, trauma to the nose with epistaxis or foreign body in the esophagus and airway tend to present as emergencies because of either airway obstruction or dysphagia [8,12].

While foreign bodies in the ear and nose can be easily removed under vision in the clinic [13], those in the throat often present as emergency and are removed in the theatre [12]. However, in developing countries, patients with foreign bodies in the ears and nose often present late after having been attempted by an unskilled health worker and this may often end up with complications which require hospitalization. More often than not this poses more challenges to the otolaryngologist practicing in these countries [13].

In the developing countries like Tanzania, the morbidity and mortality associated with ENT injuries remain a significant but neglected problem. Little work has been done on this subject in our local environment despite increase in the number of admissions of this condition. It is on this background that this study, seeks to examine the causes, pattern and outcome of injuries to the ear, nose and throat regions as seen in our institution and to have a baseline for future comparison.

Methods
Study area and design
This was a descriptive prospective study of patients with ENT injuries that were managed in the ENT/Surgery department of Bugando Medical Centre (BMC) from May 2007 to April 2012. BMC is a consultant, tertiary care and teaching hospital for the Catholic University of Health and Allied Sciences-Bugando (CUHAS-Bugando) and has 1000 beds. BMC is one of the four largest referral hospitals in the country and serves as a referral

centre for tertiary specialist care for a catchment population of approximately 13 million people from all regions in the northwestern Tanzania. Department of Ear, Nose and Throat is one of the hospital departments with services, covering the above mentioned region in terms of patients' coverage. There is no trauma centre or established advanced pre-hospital care in Mwanza city as a result all trauma patients are referred to BMC for expertise management.

Study population
Subjects for the study included all patients of ENT injuries of all age groups and gender irrespective of injury severity who was managed at BMC during the study period and who consented for the study. Patients who died before initial assessment and unconscious patients who had no relative to consent for the study on their behalf were excluded from the study. Recruitment of patients to participate in the study was done at the A & E department. Patients were screened for inclusion criteria and those who met the inclusion criteria were, after informed consent to participate in the study, consecutively enrolled into the study.

All study patients were first resuscitated in the A & E department according to Advanced Trauma Life Support (ATLS). Patients with minor injuries and those with foreign bodies in the ears and nose were treated as outpatients were treated as an outpatient and only patients with moderate to severe injuries and those with foreign bodies in the throat and associated injuries required admission to the ENT wards after definitive treatment in theatre. The severity of injury was determined using the Kampala trauma score II (KTS II) [14]. Severe injury consisted of a KTS II ≤ 6, moderate injury 7–8, and mild injury 9–10.

Depending on the type of injury, the patients were treated either conservatively or by surgery. All patients were followed up till discharged or death. This information was collected using a pre-tested questionnaire. Included in the questionnaire were socio-demographic data, mechanism of injury, pre-hospital care, injury-arrival interval, type and pattern of injury, trauma scores (KTS II), body region injured (ENT), presence or absence of associated injuries, treatment offered, complications of treatment. Outcome variables were length of hospital stay, mortality and disability. The term disability was defined according to the World Health Organization as *any restriction or lack (resulting from any impairment) of ability to perform an activity in the manner or within the range considered normal for a human being".

Statistical data analysis
Statistical data analysis was done using SPSS software (Statistical Package for the Social Sciences, version 17.0,

SPSS Inc, Chicago, Ill, USA). Data was summarized in form of proportions and frequent tables for categorical variables. Continuous variables were summarized using range and median. P-values were computed for categorical variables using Chi-square ($\chi2$) test and Fisher's exact test depending on the size of the data set. Independent student t-test was used for continuous variables. Multivariate logistic regression analysis was used to determine predictor variables that are associated with outcome. A p-value of less than 0.05 was considered to constitute a statistically significant difference.

Ethical considerations

The study was carried out after the approval by the department of surgery and BMC/CUHAS-Bugando ethics review board. An informed written consent was sought from patients or relatives.

Results
Demographic profile

During the study period, a total of 530 patients with ENT injuries were managed at Bugando Medical Centre. Of these, 456 patients met the inclusion criteria and these were analyzed. The age of patients at presentation ranged from 1 year to 72 years with a median age of 18 years. The modal age incidence was 1–10 years accounting for 202 (44.3%) patients. There were 302 (66.2%) males and 154 (33.8%) females with a male to female ratio of 2: 1. The majority of patients, 321 (70.4%) came from the urban areas located in Mwanza City.

Circumstances of injury

Regarding the time of injury, 351 (77.0%) patients sustained injury during the day, 55 (12.1%) at night and in 50 (10.9%), the time was not specified. The commonest cause of injury was foreign bodies (61.8%) followed by road traffic accidents (22.4%) (Table 1). Injuries from foreign bodies in the present were found to be commonest

Table 1 Distribution of the cause of injury versus site of injury

Cause of injury/ site of injury	Ear (N/%)	Nose (N/%)	Throat (N/%)	Total (N/%)
Foreign bodies	160(35.1)	40(8.8)	82(18.0)	282 (61.9)
Road traffic accidents	68(14.9)	34(7.5)	-	102(22.4)
Falls	20(4.4)	5(1.1)	-	25(5.5)
Assault	13(2.9)	5(1.1)	2(0.4)	20(4.4)
Burns	5(1.1)	5(1.1)	-	10(2.2
Animal bite	3(0.7)	7(1.5)	-	10(2.2)
Iatrogenic	-	2(0.4)	5(1.1)	7(1.5)
Total	**269(59.0)**	**98(21.5)**	**89(19.5)**	**456(100)**

in the pediatric population. Most of injuries occurred at home (288, 63.2%) and on the road (102, 22.4%). This was followed by school and recreation in 20(4.4%) and 14 (3.7%) patients respectively. The place of injury was not documented in 32 (7.0%) patients. The majority of injuries, 429(94.1%) were unintentional and the remaining 27 (5.9%) injuries were intentional mainly due to assault and suicidal attempt.

There were no cases of indeterminate intent. In this study, only 23 (5.7%) patients received pre-hospital care. The vast majority of patients, 368 (80.7%) reported to the A & E department late (i.e. more than 24 hours after injury) with only 88(19.3%) presenting within 24 hours of injury. The injury-arrival time, defined as the time interval taken from injury and reception at the A& E Department ranged from 1 hour to 8 days with a mean of 18 hours. The median waiting time (i.e. time interval taken from reception at the A& E Department and reception of treatment) was 4 hours (range 1–6 h). The majority of patients, 404(88.6%) were attended to within 1–4 hours of arrival to the A & E department. The remaining 52 (11.4%) patients had delayed definitive treatment.

Injury characteristics/clinical presentations

In this study, foreign body insertion and blunt injuries were the most frequent mechanism of injury in all sites (ENT) and accounted for 382 (83.8%) patients. The remaining 74 (16.2%) patients had either penetrating or combined (blunt and penetrating) injuries. The ear was the most common body region injured accounting for 59.0% of cases. In the ear, foreign body insertion and blunt trauma such as blows and slaps was the highest form of injury. The nose and throat injuries were recorded in 21.5% and 19.5% of patients respectively (Table 1). Coins were the most common type of foreign body in the throat occurring in 54 (65.9%) patients, whereas groundnuts and beans were the most common type of foreign body in the ear and the nose in 140 (87.5%) and 38 (70.0%) patients respectively. Isolated ENT injuries were reported in 402(88.2%) patients while 54 (11.8%) patients had multiple injuries. Associated injuries were reported in 54(11.8%) patients. Of these, head and musculoskeletal injuries were the most common associated injuries accounting for 30 (55.6%) and 10 (18.1%) respectively. Other associated injuries included chest, abdominal and spinal injuries. Generally, according to Kampala trauma score II (KTS II), the majority of patients (328, 71.9%) had mild injuries and the remaining 128 (28.1%) patients had moderate to severe injuries. As shown in Table 2, foreign body insertion/ ingestion was the most frequent clinical presentation of patients.

Table 2 Distribution of patients according to clinical presentation

Anatomical site	Clinical presentation	Frequency	Percentage
Ear	Foreign body insertion	160	35.1
	Hearing loss	34	7.5
	Otalgia	30	6.6
	Mucoid otorrheoa	30	6.6
	Tinnitus	24	5.3
	Lacerations/cuts of the pinna	20	4.4
	Bleeding	17	3.7
	Burns	5	1.1
Nose	Foreign body insertion	40	8.8
	Traumatic epistaxis	24	5.3
	Rhinorrhoea	18	3.9
	Lacerations/cuts	17	3.7
	Anosmia	5	1.1
	Burns	5	1.1
	Nasal obstruction	4	0.9
Throat	Foreign body ingestion/aspiration	82	18.0
	Odynophagia	23	5.0
	Open neck wounds	2	0.4
	Aphonia	2	0.4

Admission pattern and treatment modalities

The majority of patients (324, 71.1%) were treated as an outpatient and the remaining 132(28.9%) patients required admission to the ENT wards after definitive treatment. Most of patients with foreign bodies in the ear and nose and those with minor ENT injuries were treated as outpatients. Associated injuries were treated accordingly. Foreign body removal and surgical wound debridement were the most common treatment modalities performed in 61.9% and 16.2% of cases respectively. Table 3 shows treatment modalities for both isolated and associated injuries.

Outcome and follow up of patients

Complications related to isolated ENT injuries were recorded in 68(14.9%) patients. Generally, the ear had the highest number of complications (86.8%), of which suppurative chronic otitis media was the most common complication accounting for 30.9% of cases (Table 4).

The overall length of hospital stay for in-patients ranged from 1 to 22 days with a median of 8 days. Patients who developed complications and those who had associated injuries stayed longer in the hospital ($p < 0.001$).

In this study, thirty-one patients died giving an overall mortality rate of 6.8%. Mortality rate was higher in

patients with ENT injuries associated with multiple injuries (25 deaths, 80.6%) than in those with isolated ENT injuries (6 deaths, 19.4%). This difference was statistically significant ($p = 0.011$). Generally, the overall mortality rate related to isolated ENT injuries was 1.3% (6 deaths).

The follow up periods ranged between 3–6 months as the case warranted. Out of 425 survivors, 412 (96.9%) were discharged well and the remaining 13 (3.1%) were discharged with permanent disabilities related to loss of pinna and permanent tracheostomy due to traumatic laryngeal stenosis.

Discussion

Injuries to the ear, nose and throat regions are a common but neglected form of trauma and constitute a significant cause of morbidity and mortality worldwide [1,2,7]. In this review, ENT injuries were found to be most common in the first decade of life and tended to affect more males than females. Similar demographic observation was also reported by other authors [1,5].

This could be explained by the fact that these were the active and assertive age group that can be involved in high risk activities such as insertion/ingestion of foreign bodies, fights, climbing or jumping from heights.

In our study, males were more affected than females with a male to female ratio of 2:1 which is in agreement with other studies [1,5,7,8,12]. The reasons for the male preponderance in our series may be attributed to the overactive nature of males as compared to their female counterparts.

Most of the patients in the present study came from the urban areas located in Mwanza City. Similar observation was also reported by Aremu et al. [1], but at variant with Singh et al. [2] who reported that most of patients were from rural areas. The reason for high number of patients from urban areas in our study may

Table 3 Treatment modalities for both isolated ENT and associated injuries

Treatment modality	Frequency	Percentage
Foreign body removal	282	61.9
Surgical wound debridement/wound dressing	74	16.2
Adrenaline nasal packs/epistaxis catheters	10	2.2
Plastic surgery of the pinna (pinnaplasty)	10	2.2
Nasal deformity reconstruction (rhinoplasty)	9	2.0
Treatment of fractures	9	2.0
Exploratory laparotomy	4	0.9
Craniotomy ± barr holes	3	0.7
Tracheostomy	2	0.4

Table 4 Complications associated with ENT injuries (N = 68)

Anatomical site	Complications	Frequency	Percentage
Ear		**(59)**	**(86.8)**
	Chronic otitis media	21	30.9
	Sensorineural hearing loss	16	23.5
	Loss pinna	12	17.6
	Perforated tympanic membrane	6	8.8
	Facial palsy	4	5.9
Nose		**(31)**	**(45.6)**
	Traumatic epistaxis	18	26.5
	Nasal deformity	8	11.8
	Septal abscess	5	7.4
Throat		**(9)**	**(13.3)**
	Hoarseness of voice	8	11.8
	Laryngeal stenosis	1	1.5

be attributed to the fact that our hospital is located in the urban area in Mwanza city.

The commonest cause of injury in our study was foreign bodies followed by road traffic accidents. Injuries from foreign bodies in the present were found to be commonest in the pediatric population. Similar etiological pattern of ENT injuries was also reported by others [3,5,12], but in contrast to other authors [8,15] who reported fall and trauma during playing to be the commonest mode of injuries.

More than sixty percent of injuries in our series occurred at home which is in agreement with other studies [7,8,12]. The home remains a dangerous place especially for children as lack of enough supervision may result in ENT injures such as ingestion/insertion of foreign bodies and other injuries. High percentage of home occurrence ENT injuries in our study reflects lack of coordination and unawareness of dangerous substances especially in children, poor supervision and lack of domestic safety measures.

The pre-hospital care of trauma patient has been reported to be the most important factor in determining the ultimate outcome after the injury [16,17]. In this study, only 5.7% patients received pre-hospital care. Similar observations have been noted in other studies in developing countries [7,8]. The lack of advanced pre-hospital care in our environment coupled with ineffective ambulance system for transportation of patients to hospitals are a major challenges in providing care for trauma patients including ENT trauma.

More than eighty percent of patients reported to the A & E department later than 24 hours after injury which is in keeping with other study done elsewhere [3,8]. Late

presentation in the present study may be attributed to delay in referral from private and public clinics, dispensaries and health centers, self-treatment at home, consultation with traditional healers and transport costs. Delayed presentation following trauma increases the likelihood of death, complications as well as prolonged hospital stay.

In agreement with other studies [3,5], the ear was the most common body region injured. This is at variant with Arif & Saatea [8] who reported nasal trauma as the commonest type of injury. In the ear, foreign body insertion was the highest form of injury which is in contrast with Matilda in Nigeria [18] who reported blows and slaps as the most common cause of otologic injuries.

The clinical presentations depend on the region involved. In this study, clinical presentations did not differ significantly from other studies [3,5]. The presentation was more dramatic in the airway with presentation of dyspnea and stridor. However, patients with foreign bodies in the throat were less dramatic, presenting with dysphagia, odynophagia as the common features.

The presence of associated injuries is an important determinant of the outcome of injuries including ENT patients [15]. ENT injuries are commonly associated with other injuries and these may complicate the management and affect the outcome [1,9]. In the present study, the presence of associated injuries was found to be significantly associated with both mortality and length of hospital stay (morbidity). Early recognition and treatment of associated injuries is important in order to reduce mortality and morbidity associated with ENI injuries.

In this study, more than 70% of patients with foreign bodies in the ear and nose and those with minor ENT injuries were treated as outpatients were treated as an outpatient and only 28.9% of patients required admission to the ENT wards after definitive treatment. Foreign body removal and surgical wound debridement were the most common treatment modalities performed. All the foreign bodies in the ear and nose were successfully removed, that is 100% treatment success rate. This treatment pattern was also reported elsewhere by others [3,5,8]. The reasons for the low rate of ENT admissions in this study may be attributed to the fact that the majority of our patients presented with minor injuries that did not require admission following definitive treatment. Only patients with moderate to severe injuries and those with associated and multiple injuries were admitted.

The presence of complications has an impact on the final outcome of patients presenting with ENT injuries as supported by the present study. The pattern of complications in the present study is similar to what was reported by others [3,8,9]. In our study, suppurative otitis media was the commonest complication in the ear while traumatic epistaxis and hoarseness of voice were the commonest complications in the nose and throat respectively. Of interest, some of complications in the ear and nose resulted from foreign bodies that have been tampered with by the unqualified health personnel and ended up with perforated tympanic membrane and traumatic epistaxis. This observation is more common in most centres in developing countries such as Tanzania and poses more challenges to the otolaryngologist in these countries [7]. The high number of patients with suppurative otitis media following traumatic tympanic membrane perforation was due to the common habit of instilling ear drops into the external auditory canals and meticulous cleaning of blood from the external auditory canal following these injuries. These habits delay the healing of the tympanic membrane thus making the middle ear more prone to infections [3,13]. Early recognition and management of complications following ENT injuries is of paramount in reducing the morbidity and mortality resulting from these injuries.

The length of hospital stay (LOS) has been reported to be an important measure of morbidity among trauma patients. Prolonged hospitalization is associated with an unacceptable burden on resources for health and undermines the productive capacity of the population through time lost during hospitalization and disability [19]. The overall median LOS in this study was relatively higher compared to that reported in Nigeria [1]. Patients who developed complications and those who had associated injuries in our study contributed significantly to prolonged LOS.

The overall mortality rate related to isolated ENT injuries in the present study was 1.3%, a figure which is relatively high compared with Matilda *et al.* [3] who reported no mortality in their series. This low mortality rate in our study may be attributed to the large number of patients with mild injuries.

Generally, the outcome of patients in this study was satisfactory as more than 95 percent of patients were treated successively and discharge well with no permanent disabilities. Late presentation and exclusion of large number of patients from the study were the major limitation in this study. However, despite these limitations, the study has provided local data that can be utilized by health care providers to plan for preventive strategies as well as establishment of management guidelines for patients with ENT injuries.

Conclusion
Injuries to the ear, nose and throat constitute a major cause of ENT admissions in this environment with foreign body as the commonest cause of injury. The young adults that represent the workforce are the population mainly affected. Most of patients in our local setting present late with increased risk of complications. Majority of

these injuries can be prevented through public enlightenment campaigns. Early recognition and treatment of ENT injuries is important in order to reduce mortality and morbidity associated with these injuries.

Competing interests
The authors declare that they have no competing interests.

Authors' contributions
JMG conceived the study and did the literature search, coordinated the write-up, editing. PLC participated in the literature search, writing of the manuscript, editing and submission of the article. All the authors read and approved the final manuscript.

Acknowledgements
We are most grateful to the patients who participated in this study and we wish to thank the Senior House Officers (SHO) in the departments of ENT and surgery for their tireless effort in data collection and care of our study patients.

Author details
[1]Otorhinolaryngology unit, Bugando Medical Centre, Mwanza, Tanzania. [2]Department of Surgery, Catholic University of Health and Allied Sciences, Mwanza, Tanzania.

References
1. Aremu SK, Alabi BS, Segun-Busari SW, Omotoso SW: **Audit of Pediatric ENT Injuries.** *Int J Biomed Sci* 2011, 7:218–221.
2. Singh I, Gathwala G, Gathwala L, Yadav SPS, Wig U: **Ear, Nose and Throat injuries in children.** *Pak J Otolaryngol* 1993, 9:133–135.
3. Matilda I, Lucky O, Chibuike N: **Ear, nose and throat injuries in a tertiary institution in Niger delta region Nigeria.** *J Med Res Prac* 2012, 1:59–62.
4. Arif RK, Naseem U, Inayat U, Shah ED, Noor SK: **Causes and complications of ear, nose and throat injuries in children. A study of 80 cases.** *J Med Sc* 2006, 14(1):57–59.
5. Sogebi OA, Olaosun AO, Tobih JE, Adedeji TO, Adebola SO: **Pattern of ear, nose and throat injuries in children at Ladoke Akintola University of technology teaching hospital, Osogbo, Nigeria.** *Afric J. Pediatr Surg.* 2006, 3:61–63.
6. Bugando Medical Centre (BMC): *Medical record database, 2010/2011.*
7. Gilyoma JM, Chalya PL: **Endoscopic procedures for removal of foreign bodies of the aerodigestive tract: The Bugando Medical Centre experience.** *BMC Ear, Nose Throat Disorders* 2011, 11:2.
8. Arif RK, Saatea A: **Ear, nose and throat injuries in children.** *Ayub med Coll Abbottabad* 2005, 17:54–56.
9. Figueiredo RR, Azevedo AA, Kos AO, Tomita S: **Complications of Ear, nose and throat foreign bodies.** *Braz J Otorhinolaryngol* 2008, 74:7–15.
10. Orji FT: **Non-explosive blast injury of the tympanic membrane in Umuahia, Nigeria.** *Nig J Med* 2009, 18:365–369.
11. Okoye BC, Oteri AJ: **Cut throat injuries in Port Harcourt.** *Sahel Medical J* 2001, 4:207–209.
12. Endican S, Garap JP, Dubey SP: **Ear, nose and throat foreign body in Melanesian children: an analysis of 1037 cases.** *Int J Pediatr Otorhinolaryngol* 2006, 70:1539–1545.
13. Okoye BC, Onotai LO: **Foreign body in the nose.** *Niger J Med* 2006, 15:301–304.
14. Mutooro SM, Mutakooha E, Kyamanywa P: **A comparison of Kampala trauma score II with the new injury severity score in Mbarara University Teaching Hospital in Uganda.** *East Cent Afr J Surg* 2010, 15:62–70.
15. Synders LC, Jian VN, Saltzman DA, Strate RG, Perry JE, Leonard AS: **Blunt Trauma in Adults and Children, a comparative analysis.** *J Trauma* 1990, 30:1239–1245.
16. Trunkey Donald D, Maull Kimball I: **Prehospital Trauma care.** In *Current Therapy of Trauma.* 4th edition. Edited by Trunkey Donald D, Lewis Frank R. Philadelphia: Mosby; 1999:121–122.
17. Liberman M, Mulder D, Lavoie A, Denis R, Sampalis JS: **Multicenter Canadian study of prehospital trauma care.** *Ann Surg* 2003, 237(2):153–160.

Cortisol suppression and hearing thresholds in tinnitus after low-dose dexamethasone challenge

Veerle L Simoens[1,2,3] and Sylvie Hébert[3,4,5*]

Abstract

Background: Tinnitus is a frequent, debilitating hearing disorder associated with severe emotional and psychological suffering. Although a link between stress and tinnitus has been widely recognized, the empirical evidence is scant. Our aims were to test for dysregulation of the stress-related hypothalamus-pituitary adrenal (HPA) axis in tinnitus and to examine ear sensitivity variations with cortisol manipulation.

Methods: Twenty-one tinnitus participants and 21 controls comparable in age, education, and overall health status but without tinnitus underwent basal cortisol assessments on three non-consecutive days and took 0.5 mg of dexamethasone (DEX) at 23:00 on the first day. Cortisol levels were measured hourly the next morning. Detection and discomfort hearing thresholds were measured before and after dexamethasone suppression test.

Results: Both groups displayed similar basal cortisol levels, but tinnitus participants showed stronger and longer-lasting cortisol suppression after DEX administration. Suppression was unrelated to hearing loss. Discomfort threshold was lower after cortisol suppression in tinnitus ears.

Conclusions: Our findings suggest heightened glucocorticoid sensitivity in tinnitus in terms of an abnormally strong glucocorticoid receptor (GR)-mediated HPA-axis feedback (despite a normal mineralocorticoid receptor (MR)-mediated tone) and lower tolerance for sound loudness with suppressed cortisol levels. Long-term stress exposure and its deleterious effects therefore constitute an important predisposing factor for, or a significant pathological consequence of, this debilitating hearing disorder.

Keywords: Cortisol, Hearing sensitivity, Hearing threshold, HPA axis, Low-dose dexamethasone suppression test, Stress, Tinnitus

Background

Subjective tinnitus ("tinnitus") is the perception of sound in the ears or head in the absence of an external sound and difficult to treat. Individuals with tinnitus can experience severe emotional distress, depression, anxiety, and insomnia [1-5]. A recent study in 14,278 adults reported an overall prevalence of 25.3% for any experience of tinnitus in the previous year and 7.9% for frequent or constant (at least once a day) tinnitus [6]. Prevalence increases with age, peaking at 31.4% and 14.3% from age 60 to 69 years for these two tinnitus frequencies, respectively [6]. The increasing prevalence with age is not surprising, because hearing loss is

known to be an associated risk factor for tinnitus [7]. With increasing life expectancy, and because hearing loss and noise exposure are increasingly affecting military personnel [8,9] and youth [10], tinnitus has become a significant public health issue.

Hearing loss predicts tinnitus presence, but not severity [11,12]. Conversely, individuals with hearing loss do not necessarily experience tinnitus. There is therefore a need to determine other factors for this debilitating hearing disorder and its consequences for health in order to better prevent and treat it. One likely candidate is stress. Because stress has long been identified as a trigger or co-morbidity of tinnitus, based mainly on anecdotal and retrospective reports, this idea has been taken for granted in classical teachings on tinnitus [13]. In addition, recent large population studies have established that emotional exhaustion and long-term stress

* Correspondence: Sylvie.hebert@umontreal.ca
[3]BRAMS, International Laboratory for Brain, Music, and Sound research, Montreal, Canada
Full list of author information is available at the end of the article

are predictors of hearing disorders, including tinnitus [14,15]. Functional and electroencephalographic brain imaging studies have also shown aberrant links between limbic (involved in emotions) and auditory system structures [16-18]. Structural brain differences (i.e., grey matter decrease) in tinnitus involving parts of the limbic system have also been reported. More specifically, less grey matter in the nucleus accumbens [18,19] and the left hippocampus [20] suggests a depletion that could be related to long-term exposure to stress, among other factors.

Another line of research has focused on the hypothalamus-pituitary-adrenal (HPA) axis functioning responsible for the stress response via the stress hormone cortisol. In a first study, overall or chronic basal cortisol levels (secreted naturally in a circadian pattern) were higher in a subsample of tinnitus participants when levels were considered over a one-week period, although diurnal levels were similar to those of age-matched controls [21,22]. In a further study [23], tinnitus participants were submitted to the Trier Social Stress Test [24]. They showed delayed and blunted cortisol response to the stressor despite similar psychological stress levels to age-matched controls. This response is similar to that of patients with chronic fatigue syndrome [25], suggesting an exhausted stress response due to long-term stress in tinnitus participants. The apparent contradiction between these two studies could be explained by the fact that basal cortisol levels and stress responsiveness are modulated by two distinct feedback systems. Circulating glucocorticoids are released by the HPA axis and bind with two kinds of receptors: the high-affinity mineralocorticoid receptor (MR) and the lower-affinity glucocorticoid receptor (GR). The HPA axis is a closed-loop system that is subjected to a tight negative feedback control mediated by these two receptor types. HPA axis tone, assessed in basal cortisol levels, is regulated by the MR receptors [26]. Stress responsiveness is determined by the GR receptors, which are more critical for terminating the HPA axis stress response, and are located in many brain areas such as the hypothalamus, brain stem, hippocampus, amygdala, and pituitary gland, as well as the inner ear.

A noninvasive way to test for exhausted HPA axis hypothesis in tinnitus participants is to examine the sensitivity of the HPA axis negative feedback response to glucocorticoids. The Dexamethasone (DEX) suppression test is a pharmacological challenge that is widely used to test for HPA axis dysregulation in clinical populations such as patients with depression or post-traumatic stress disorder. Dexamethasone is a synthetic glucocorticoid with high GR receptor affinity that does not cross the blood-brain barrier [27-29]. Because the pituitary gland is located outside the blood-brain barrier, DEX selectively activates the pituitary GR, leaving the pituitary MR and the MR and GR in other brain tissues unaffected [30,31]. Once the pituitary GRs are activated, they downregulate cortisol production further down the HPA axis in the adrenal cortex. The DEX suppression test is therefore a direct test for an altered effect of GR activation in the pituitary on cortisol secretion [32], and it indicates the sensitivity of the HPA axis negative feedback response to glucocorticoids. Depressed patients often show HPA axis hyperactivity and nonsuppression of HPA axis cortisol secretion after DEX administration [33]. In contrast, patients suffering from post-traumatic stress disorder often display cortisol *hyper*suppression. Hypersuppression is detected by using a lower dose of DEX (0.5 mg instead of 1 mg) to better discriminate HPA axis feedback sensitivity between patients and controls [34].

In the present study, both basal cortisol and HPA axis response to the low-dose DEX test were measured in tinnitus participants and controls comparable in age, education, and overall health status. By assessing MR-mediated (basal) as well as GR-mediated (cortisol suppression after DEX administration) feedback in the same participants, both feedback systems were assessed simultaneously to gain a more global insight into HPA axis anomalies in tinnitus participants. If tinnitus participants display greater sensitivity to HPA axis negative feedback (GR-mediated), they should display hypersuppression after DEX administration compared to age-matched controls, despite normal basal (MR-mediated) cortisol levels.

In addition, hearing thresholds were assessed before and after pharmacological challenge to examine the effects of cortisol manipulation on both detection and discomfort thresholds. Glucocorticoid receptors (GR) have been found in abundance in the human inner ear [35], but their function remains unclear. Although no studies have examined the effects of experimental manipulation of cortisol *suppression* on hearing detection thresholds in humans, there is some evidence that cortisol *increase* exerts a direct influence on hearing. For instance, patients with adrenal cortical insufficiency (a quasi-total absence of cortisol secretion, such as in Addison's disease) had more acute auditory detection sensitivity and lower discomfort threshold than matched controls [36]. When corticosteroid levels were restored to normal via administration of exogenous glucocorticoids, auditory measures reverted to normal. This effect has been replicated in rats [37]. Experimentally increased cortisol concentrations in normal adults have resulted in reduced auditory sensitivity at high frequencies [38]. The opposite effect was recently reported in rats, however, although the cortisol increase was induced by a stressful stimulus and not cortisol administration: rats exposed to a rodent acoustic repellent showed higher cortisol levels but lower hearing thresholds [39]. To our knowledge, the effects of cortisol manipulation on hearing discomfort thresholds have never been assessed in human participants with tinnitus. Yet, it is estimated that increased hearing sensitivity is present in 80% of patients with tinnitus [40]. Discomfort thresholds have also been found to predict tinnitus prevalence and severity in the general population [12]. Based on human studies, it was thus hypothesized that detection and discomfort thresholds in both tinnitus and control participants would be lower after cortisol suppression, and possibly to a greater extent in tinnitus than in control ears due to their greater sensitivity to cortisol manipulation.

Methods

Participants

Twenty-one participants (11 men and 10 women) with chronic tinnitus for at least six months (mean duration of tinnitus was 16.6 years, $SD = 15.7$) and 21 controls without tinnitus (10 men and 11 women) were recruited through newspaper advertisements, word of mouth, and a self-help local tinnitus association. Thirteen tinnitus participants had bilateral (perceived in both ears or the head) and eight had unilateral (perceived in one ear only) tinnitus. Groups were similar in age, educational level, and body mass index (see Table 1). All participants were in good physical and mental health. Stringent exclusion criteria were used: taking medication that interferes with the HPA axis (e.g., beta-blockers, antidepressants), having a disease that interferes with the HPA axis (e.g., diabetes, uncontrolled hypo-or hypertension, lupus), having jet lag or having undergone surgery in the past six months, smoking, wearing a hearing aid, and having a BMI of 30 or more. All women were postmenopausal, and two (one in each group) were taking hormone replacement therapy.

Questionnaires

All participants were tested for symptoms of depression using the Beck Depression Inventory II [41], with similar scores for the two groups (see Table 1). Subjective tinnitus severity was assessed in tinnitus participants with

the French version of the Tinnitus Reaction Questionnaire [42].

Cortisol assessment and manipulation

To assess basal cortisol levels, five saliva samples per day were collected at home for three days on Day 1, 3, and 5 at awakening, 30 minutes after awakening, before lunch, before dinner, and before going to bed. One day of rest (Day 4) was provided between basal cortisol sampling days.

To assess HPA axis reactivity to DEX, all participants took 0.5 mg of DEX at home at 23:00 on Day 1. Saliva samples were taken in the lab at 8:00, 9:00, 10:00, 11:00, and 12:00 the following day (Day 2). Post-DEX cortisol assessment was always performed between Day 1 and Day 3 so that post-DEX days were consistently timed across participants. Figure 1 presents a schematic diagram of the procedure.

Participants took saliva samples at home for Day 1, 3, and 5 using a Salivette (Sarstedt Inc., Nümbrecht, Germany) and stored them in the refrigerator. When returned to the lab, all samples were stored at -20°C. Saliva samples taken in the lab (Day 2) were stored the same day at -20°C. All samples were recoded for blind analysis before being sent to Trier University (Germany), where cortisol levels were determined with a time-resolved fluorescence immunoassay. The inter-assay coefficient of variation was < 50%.

Hearing assessment

Hearing detection and discomfort thresholds were measured on Days 0 and 2 at the same time of day in a soundproof booth at the laboratory, meaning for instance that if participants came at 10:00 on Day 0, hearing detection and discomfort thresholds were assessed at 10:00 also on Day 2. Detection thresholds were assessed for half-octave frequency steps from 250 to 8,000 Hz using an adaptive psychophysical automated procedure (-5, +3, -1, +1). The threshold was determined as the mean of the last 8 reversals. Hearing discomfort thresholds were assessed for frequencies 1 kHz, 2 kHz, and 4 kHz using the methods of limits in 5 dB intensity steps. Threshold was determined as the level at which the sound was judged too loud [43]. Trains of

Table 1 Sociodemographic and questionnaire data on the Tinnitus and Control groups

	Tinnitus (N = 21)	Controls (N = 21)	P value
Age (SD)	65.7 (7.1)	65.7 (8.7)	1.0
Education (SD)	14.2 (2.8)	15.3 (3.3)	.48
Body Mass Index (SD)	24.1 (2.6)	23.4 (3.6)	.23
Beck Depression Inventory (SD)	5.2 (5.2)	4.2 (4.2)	.52
Tinnitus Reaction Questionnaire (SD)	11.5 (9.97)	–	–

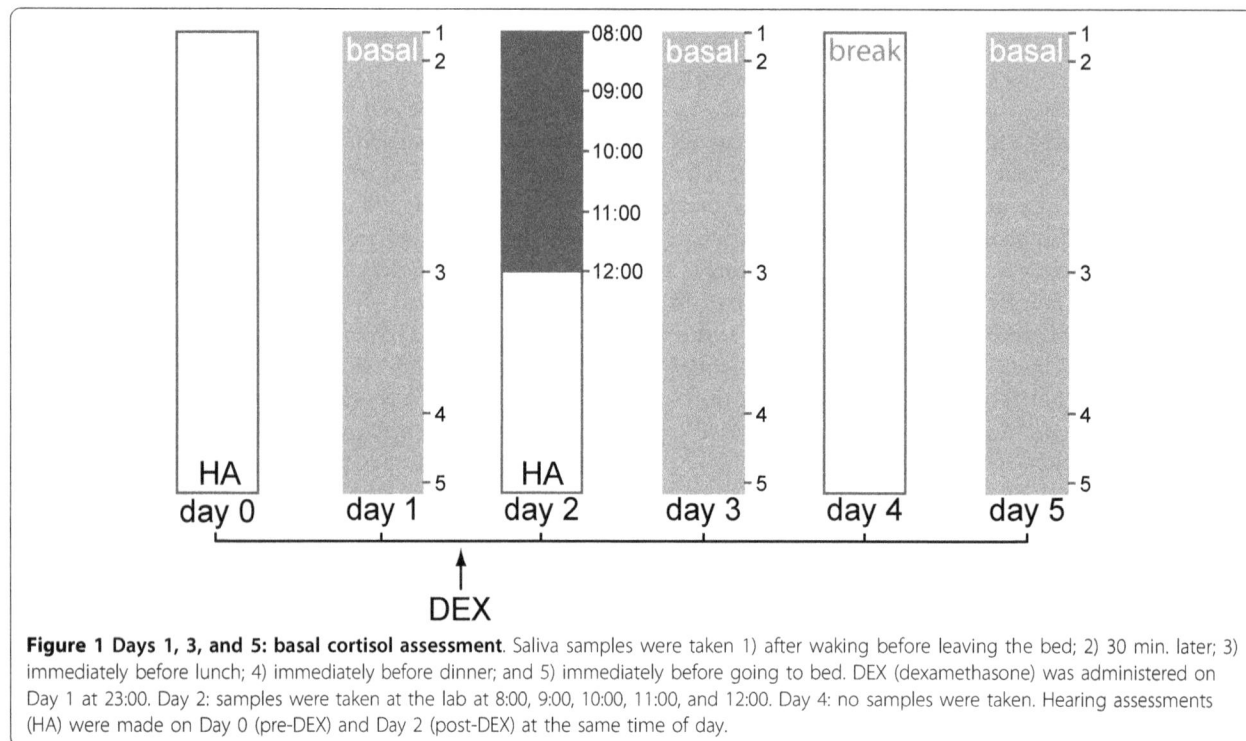

Figure 1 Days 1, 3, and 5: basal cortisol assessment. Saliva samples were taken 1) after waking before leaving the bed; 2) 30 min. later; 3) immediately before lunch; 4) immediately before dinner; and 5) immediately before going to bed. DEX (dexamethasone) was administered on Day 1 at 23:00. Day 2: samples were taken at the lab at 8:00, 9:00, 10:00, 11:00, and 12:00. Day 4: no samples were taken. Hearing assessments (HA) were made on Day 0 (pre-DEX) and Day 2 (post-DEX) at the same time of day.

three pure tones of 300 ms, each separated by 300 ms of silence (20 ms rise and fall), were used in both tasks. The entire procedure was automated and programmed with Matlab using a real-time signal processing system (Tucker Davis Technology-3) under Sennheiser HD265 headphones calibrated with a Larson-Davis sound level meter combined with an artificial ear AEC101 and a 2559 model microphone.

The experiment was approved by the institutional ethics committee of the *Institut Universitaire de Gériatrie de Montréal* and was conducted with the understanding and consent of each participant. All tests were conducted in accordance with the Declaration of Helsinki.

Data analysis
Basal cortisol
Basal cortisol measurements were analyzed in two different ways: area under the curve (AUC) per day and diurnal cycle [44]. AUC was calculated for each of the three basal cortisol assessment days (Days 1, 3, and 5): the minimum number of minutes for each group between the first and fifth (last) sample on the same day was determined (635 min or 10 h 35 min) and taken as the cutoff point for the AUC calculation for all three days for all participants. New data points were interpolated based on the curve slope at 635 min from the first sample.

On the post-DEX day (Day 2), participants took saliva samples every hour throughout the morning only. In order to compare cortisol values on the post-DEX day with basal cortisol values, a new variable was computed (AUC2) from all AUC values recalculated with a cutoff time point of 226 min (3 h 46 min), or the minimum number of minutes between the first and last sample on the post-DEX day for all participants.

Diurnal cortisol values indicate the change in cortisol level throughout the day. The diurnal cortisol measure is the mean cortisol level at each time of day across the three basal cortisol assessment days.

Cortisol suppression
Percent suppression after DEX administration was calculated as 100 - ((AUC2 post-DEX/mean basal AUC) * 100), where AUC2 post-DEX is the area under the curve of the post-DEX day, cut off at 226 min, and mean basal AUC is the mean area under the curve of the basal cortisol assessment of Day 1 and Day 5 (averaged), also cut off at 226 min. Extreme outliers (> 3× interquartile range) were determined for each group and excluded from further analysis.

Hearing measures
The frequencies for which hearing detection thresholds were determined were combined into three groups: Low (250 Hz, 354 Hz, 500 Hz), Mid (707 Hz, 1000 Hz, 1414 Hz, 2000 Hz, 2828 Hz), and High (4000 Hz, 5657 Hz, 8000 Hz). Missing values were not replaced. Extreme outliers (> 3× interquartile range) were determined separately by ear group (control and tinnitus ears) and excluded from further analysis.

Statistical analysis

The statistical analysis was performed with PASW Statistics 18.0 and IBM SPSS 19.0. On cortisol data (AUC and AUC2), ANOVAs were run with Group (Tinnitus vs. Control) as a between-subject factor and Day of basal cortisol assessment (Days 1 vs. 3 vs. 5) as a within-subject factor. On diurnal data, an ANOVA was run with Group (Tinnitus vs. Control) as a between-subject factor and Time of Day (samples 1 to 5) as a within-subject variable (averaged across Day 1 and 5). Independent sample t-tests were used to compare sociodemographic, questionnaire, and percent suppression variables. An analysis of covariance (ANCOVA) on percent suppression was run to adjust for hearing thresholds in mid and high frequencies, which were used as covariables. Correlations were run between TRQ scores, years of tinnitus, and percent suppression in the Tinnitus group.

On hearing data, ANOVAs with Day (pre- vs. post-DEX) as a within-subject factor and Ear (Tinnitus vs. Control) as a between-subject factor were performed separately, with the hearing threshold test (low vs. mid vs. high frequencies) and the loudness discomfort threshold test (1 kHz vs. 2 kH vs. 4 kHz) as within-subject variables. Non-tinnitus ears in participants with unilateral tinnitus (N = 8) were excluded from this analysis. T-tests were run for simple effects. All tests were two-tailed and p-value was set at 0.05.

Results

Basal cortisol

On AUC data, the interaction between Group and Day was significant, $F(2, 78) = 4.11$, $p = .020$ (see Figure 2). The Tinnitus group showed a difference in AUC across the three days, $F(2, 38) = 5.48$, $p = .008$. A highly

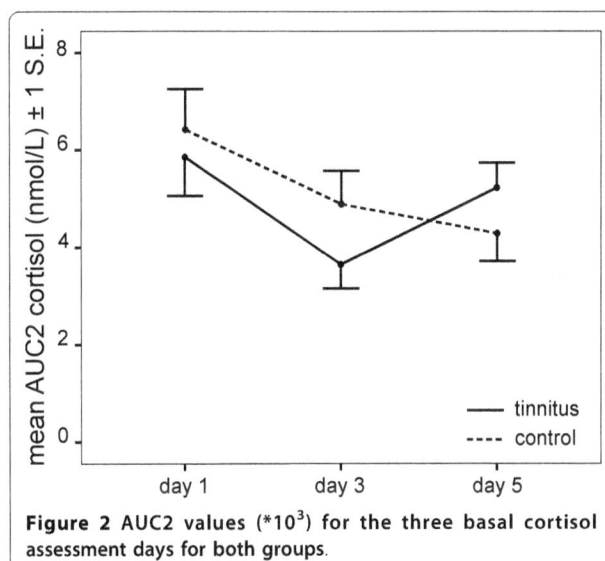

Figure 2 AUC2 values ($*10^3$) for the three basal cortisol assessment days for both groups.

significant quadratic trend was found in AUC across days, $F(1, 19) = 8.88$, $p = .008$, with lowest mean AUC on Day 3 of basal cortisol assessment and higher mean AUC on Day 1 and Day 5. AUC did not differ between days in Controls, $F < 1$. Neither the main effect of Day, $F(2,78) = 1.26$, $p = .289$, nor the effect of Group, $F < 1$, was significant.

On AUC2 data, the interaction between Day and Group just failed to reach significance, $F(2, 78) = 2.51$, $p = .08$. However the quadratic trend was again highly significant in the Tinnitus group, $F(1, 19) = 13.02$, $p = .002$, but not in the Control group, $F < 1$, suggesting a long-lasting carryover effect of the DEX challenge in the Tinnitus group. In order to test the possibility of an ever more delayed dex effect, we ran an ANOVA on each group separately with Days of basal cortisol assessment (Day 1, 3, and 5) as a within-subject factor. In Controls, pairwise comparisons (with Bonferroni correction for multiple comparisons) indicated that Days 3 and 5 did not differ significantly ($p = .95$), and neither did Day 1 and Day 3 ($p = .14$), suggesting that by Day 3 cortisol levels had returned to normal values. In contrast, in Tinnitus, Days 3 and 5 differed from one another ($p = .015$), and so did Days 1 and 3 ($p = .03$), but not Days 1 and 5 ($p = 1.00$), suggesting that by Day 5 cortisol levels had returned to normal levels, but not by Day 3. Because of this potentially confounding influence on basal cortisol levels in Tinnitus participants, Day 3 was excluded from further analyses of basal cortisol measures.

Diurnal cortisol showed a normally expected circadian pattern throughout the day (higher values in the morning, peaking at 30 min after waking up, and decreasing gradually thereafter) in both groups, as shown by a highly significant effect of Time of day, $F(4, 160) = 70.61$, $p < .001$, all $ps < .001$, for the different measurement times. There was no effect of Group or any interaction between Time and Group, both $Fs < 1$ (see Figure 3).

DEX suppression test

Suppression (% suppression) was strong in both groups, but significantly stronger in Tinnitus participants than Controls, with means of 95.9% and 93.8%, respectively, $t(33) = -2.19$, $p = .036$ (see Figure 4). Importantly, this suppression effect was still significant after adjusting for detection thresholds in the Mid and High frequencies averaged across ears, $F(1, 31) = 5.84$, $p = .022$. The % suppression in the Tinnitus group was outside the 95% confidence interval of the Controls (91.9%-95.6%), as well as the more stringent 99% confidence interval (91.7%-95.7%). In the Tinnitus group, % suppression was not correlated with subjective tinnitus-related distress ($p = .43$) or tinnitus duration in years ($p = .97$).

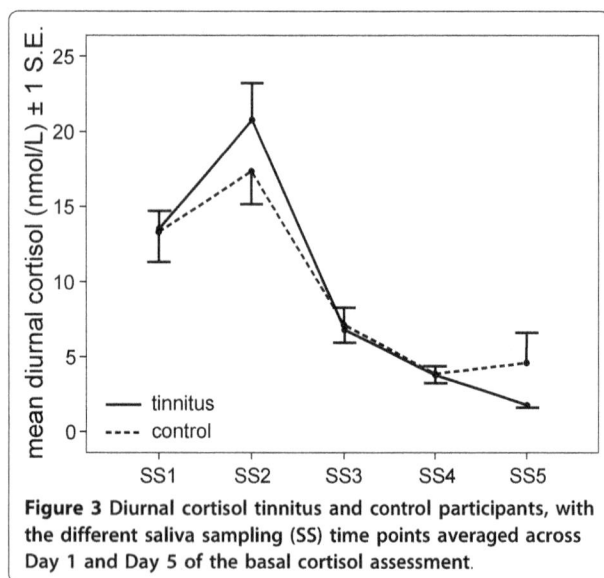

Figure 3 Diurnal cortisol tinnitus and control participants, with the different saliva sampling (SS) time points averaged across Day 1 and Day 5 of the basal cortisol assessment.

Hearing measures

Figure 5 shows detection and discomfort thresholds before and after DEX challenge. On detection thresholds, the interaction between Ear and Frequency was significant F (2, 146) = 33.82, p < .001. Unsurprisingly, Tinnitus ears had higher thresholds than Control ears in Mid and High frequencies, t < 1, t(76) = -5.04, p < .001, and t(81) = -5.18, p < .001 for Low, Mid, and High frequencies, respectively. In both groups, hearing thresholds (SD) for Mid frequencies, where sensitivity is optimal, were lower than for Low and High frequencies, with means of 31.5, 23.4, and 47.7 for Low, Mid and High frequencies, respectively (all ps < .001). The main

effect of DEX was in the expected direction but not significant, with means of 33.9 and 33.2 for pre- and post-DEX, respectively, F (1, 73) = 2.27, p = .14. There was no interaction between DEX and any other factor, all Fs < 1. Looking at detection thresholds for frequencies 1 kHz, 2 kHz, and 4 kHz only, the same pattern of results was found.

On discomfort thresholds, there was a trend for the main effect of DEX towards significance, F (1, 74) = 2.94, p = .09, with more sensitive (lower) post- than pre-DEX thresholds (means of 93.9 and 95.3, respectively). Although the interaction between Ear and DEX just failed to reach significance, F (1, 74) = 3.28, p = .07 (Figure 5), the effect of DEX was driven by the lower threshold in Tinnitus ears post-DEX than pre-DEX, t (33) = 2.29, p = .029 (means = 93.3 vs. 96.2, respectively), whereas Control ears differed only slightly, t < 1 (means = 94.0 vs. 93.8 dB, respectively). The main effect of Frequency was significant, F (2, 164) = 14.99, p = .001. Thresholds differed significantly, with means of 92.2, 94.3, and 96.4 for 1 kHz, 2 kHz, and 4 kHz, respectively, all ps < .02. The DEX factor did not interact significantly with any other factor, all Fs < 1.

Discussion

We report three novel findings that establish differences between tinnitus participants and controls in terms of cortisol hypersuppression, longer-lasting effects of the DEX test on basal cortisol levels, and hearing discomfort threshold. The first novel finding is that tinnitus participants had more strongly suppressed cortisol levels than controls after pharmacological challenge, despite similar basal cortisol levels. This is consistent with the normal

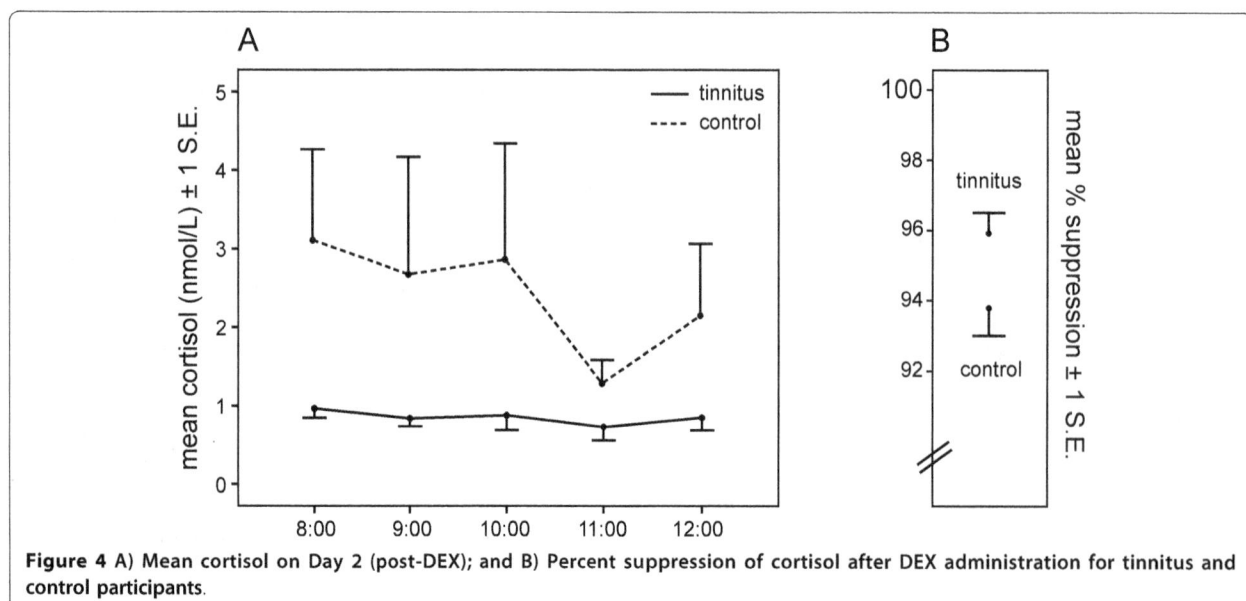

Figure 4 A) Mean cortisol on Day 2 (post-DEX); and B) Percent suppression of cortisol after DEX administration for tinnitus and control participants.

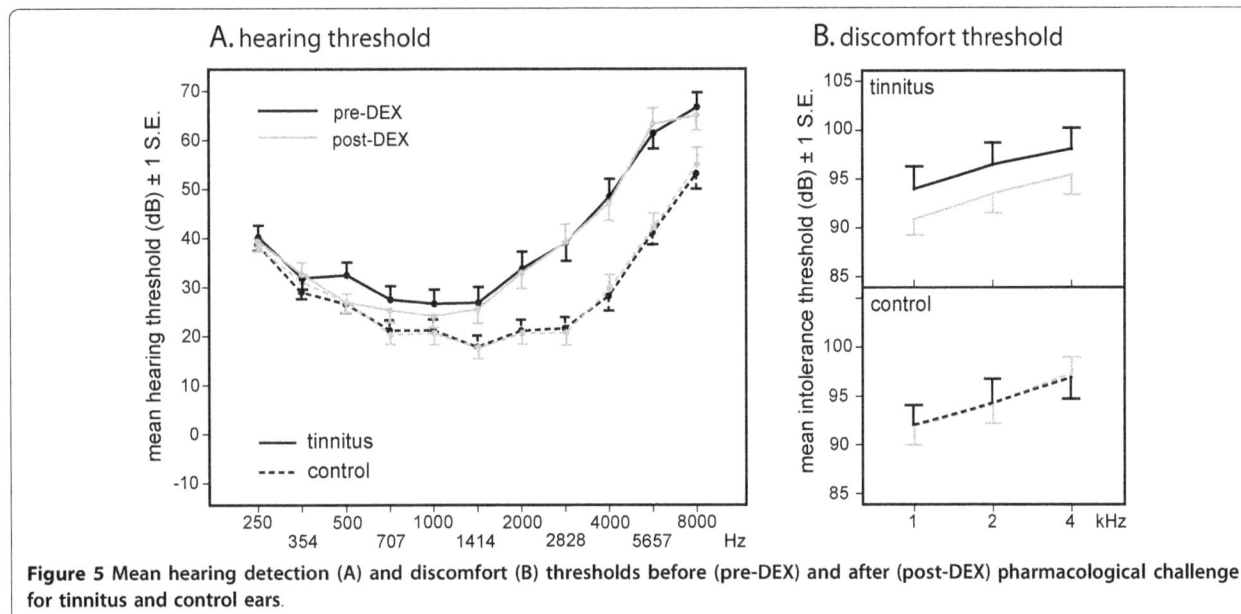

Figure 5 Mean hearing detection (A) and discomfort (B) thresholds before (pre-DEX) and after (post-DEX) pharmacological challenge for tinnitus and control ears.

diurnal and blunted response to psychosocial stress in tinnitus participants described in a previous study [23], and supports the hypothesis that tinnitus participants have greater sensitivity to HPA axis negative feedback. Hypersuppression in the presence of normal or near-normal basal cortisol levels has also been found in other clinical populations, such as patients with chronic fatigue syndrome [45-47] and burnout [48]. All these findings are consistent with the notion that basal cortisol and post-DEX cortisol suppression are mediated by two separate receptor feedback systems. More importantly, the suppression effect was independent of hearing loss. This is a key finding, because these factors are difficult to disentangle in tinnitus studies [19,23], and it argues for a true effect of tinnitus in addition to, but unrelated to, hearing loss. Our findings therefore directly link tinnitus to a stress-related disorder, and not just to a hearing-related disorder, as some recent population studies suggest [12,49].

The second important finding is that tinnitus participants showed a long-lasting carryover effect of cortisol manipulation. They had lower basal cortisol the day after the post-DEX day assessment compared to the two other basal cortisol assessment days, indicating not only cortisol hypersuppression, but also a longer-lasting effect of DEX administration. Although it cannot be excluded that these findings could be related to slower DEX clearance in these patients, this possibility is unlikely, because there is no rationale for altered liver function in this particular group, which moreover did not differ from controls in terms of age, BMI, or physical or mental health. Furthermore, the carryover effect was observed in the tinnitus participants approximately 36

hours after DEX administration, whereas cortisol and DEX levels should return to baseline 24 hours after oral administration of 0.5 mg DEX [50]. A likely interpretation is that the carryover effect might have been due to HPA axis homeostatic vulnerability, and that hypersuppression might have been caused by increased glucocorticoid sensitivity.

The third original finding is an association between cortisol suppression and cortisol-induced hearing discomfort in humans. When cortisol levels were suppressed, sound loudness tolerance decreased. Because the dB scale is logarithmic, a 3 dB reduction in level corresponds to a 50% decrease in sound pressure. At high sound levels, sound level tolerance therefore decreases markedly. This effect was more pronounced in tinnitus ears, which appeared to be more sensitive to cortisol manipulation, supporting a direct effect of glucocorticoid action on the inner ear cells in addition to the well-known systemic anti-inflammatory or immuno-suppressive effect, as suggested in previous studies [35,51,52]. A much smaller (statistically non-significant) dB change was observed for the sound detection threshold, but the effect of cortisol manipulation was in a concordant direction (i.e., lower threshold after cortisol suppression). One likely explanation is that at such low sound levels the sensory organs operate at maximal sensitivity, possibly resulting in a floor effect, given the highly sensitive adaptive procedure used in this study. The changes found in the discomfort threshold are consistent with previous human studies showing that restored cortisol levels in individuals with cortisol depletion increased hearing threshold and discomfort level [36]. They are also consistent with a recent study showing that discomfort threshold and emotional exhaustion are strong predictors of both tinnitus presence and prevalence [12]. Future studies could corroborate and extend these findings by examining dose-response relationships between cortisol manipulations and changes in hearing thresholds using auditory brainstem responses, for instance.

A strength of our study is that the same participants were tested for both basal cortisol and responsiveness to pharmacological challenge, which allowed examining both receptor types and consolidating previous findings. Because all participants were also rigorously screened for health status, greater HPA axis disturbance could be found in participants with more comorbid conditions. In addition, the very small variation in post-DEX cortisol levels in tinnitus participants could indicate a ceiling effect. An even lower dose of DEX (i.e., 0.25 mg) could be used to investigate whether tinnitus participants display even greater suppression [53]. Although these differences in cortisol suppression document for the first time HPA axis disturbance at the pituitary level in tinnitus, a limitation of our study is that no information is provided on how negative feedback inhibition occurs in the tinnitus brain. Practical reasons prevented us from performing blood and cerebrospinal fluid punctures, so adrenocorticotropic hormone (ACTH, secreted by the anterior pituitary) and corticotropin-releasing factor (CRF, released from the parvocellular neurons of the parventricular nucleus of the hypothalamus) levels were not assessed. CRF is the most dominant trigger of the HPA axis response. CRF also serves as a transmitter to modulate anxiety-related behaviour, cognitive function, and sleep, and it projects to the limbic nuclei and the brainstem. Therefore, further pharmacological challenges using combined DEX/CRF tests should be undertaken to more precisely identify the locus of the dysregulation. In the absence of any relevant data, and given the rarity of these anomalies in clinical populations, our working hypothesis is that tinnitus patients have anomalies in the negative feedback sensitivity system. This is a valuable finding in itself, especially given the deleterious consequences of HPA axis disturbance on health (e.g., on the immune system, pain, and fatigue). However, whether these alterations are a consequence of suffering from this chronic phantom sound in the ears, or instead a predisposition for the disorder, is unknown. Due to the cross-sectional design, the relationship between HPA axis disturbance and tinnitus is an association, not a causality, and we cannot conclude whether stress precedes, maintains, or is a consequence of tinnitus. Intuitively, we may posit a causal relationship (i.e., that tinnitus produces the abnormal stress response). However, in a recent tinnitus model, Rauschecker and colleagues [54] suggested that a limbic system dysfunction would actually *trigger* tinnitus by blocking its inhibitory input to the thalamus. That is, a tinnitus signal would originate from the lesion-induced plasticity of the auditory pathways (i.e., some degree of peripheral damage is assumed to be always present, even when not measurable in the audiogram [55]). Normally, this signal would be tuned out by feedback connections from limbic regions, which would prevent tinnitus from reaching the auditory cortex. In the presence of limbic damage, this "noise-cancellation" would collapse and chronic tinnitus would result. This could explain why some individuals with hearing loss do not experience tinnitus. Our results would therefore show that stress is a predisposing factor for tinnitus, and not just a consequence. Stress has also been suggested as a predisposing factor for CFS [56]. Future studies should examine this possibility by following up large cohorts with and without hearing loss over time to determine which individuals develop tinnitus in relation to various stress-related factors.

In any case, considering tinnitus as a stress-related disorder by demonstrating HPA axis disturbance can open up new research avenues. For instance, studies of similar disorders show the same anomalies. There is a great need for new pharmacological targets in tinnitus [57], and a deeper understanding of HPA disturbance could lead to the development of pharmacotherapy targeting the HPA axis [58] as well as monitoring tools to assess the efficacy of tinnitus treatments and therapies.

Conclusions

Our findings suggest heightened glucocorticoid sensitivity in tinnitus in terms of an abnormally strong GR-mediated HPA-axis feedback (despite a normal MR-mediated tone) and lower tolerance for sound loudness with suppressed cortisol levels. Long-term stress exposure and its deleterious effects therefore constitute an important predisposing factor for, or a significant pathological consequence of, this debilitating hearing disorder.

Acknowledgements
The authors thank Dr. Rémi Rabasa-Lhoret for his help in patient screening. This research was supported by a salary granted by the *Fonds de la recherche en Santé du Québec* (FRSQ) to SH and by a studentship granted by the Finnish Graduate School of Functional Imaging in Medicine to VS.

Author details
[1]Cognitive Brain Research Unit, Cognitive Science, Department of Behavioural Sciences, University of Helsinki, Helsinki, P.O. Box 9 00014, Finland. [2]Finnish Centre of Excellence in Interdisciplinary Music Research, Department of Music, University of Jyväskylä, Jyväskylä, Finland. [3]BRAMS, International Laboratory for Brain, Music, and Sound research, Montreal, Canada. [4]École d'orthophonie et d'audiologie, Faculté de médecine, Université de Montréal, Canada, and Centre de recherche de l'Institut universitaire de gériatrie de Montréal, Montréal, Canada. [5]Université de Montréal BRAMS, Pavillon 1420, Mont-Royal C.P. 6128, succ. Centre-ville, Montréal, QC H3C 3J7, Canada.

Authors' contributions

VS participated in design and coordination, carried out the testing, organized the final data file, partly ran statistical analysis, and drafted the manuscript. SH conceptualized and designed the study, performed statistical analysis, and revised the manuscript. Both VS and SH read and approved the final manuscript.

Competing interests

The authors report no conflicts of interest. The authors alone are responsible for the content and writing of the paper.

References

1. Bartels H, Middel BL, van der Laan BF, Staal MJ, Albers FW: **The additive effect of co-occurring anxiety and depression on health status, quality of life and coping strategies in help-seeking tinnitus sufferers.** *Ear Hear* 2008, **29(6)**:947-956.
2. Langguth B, Kleinjung T, Fischer B, Hajak G, Eichhammer P, Sand PG: **Tinnitus severity, depression, and the big five personality traits.** *Prog Brain Res* 2007, **166**:221-225.
3. Hesser H, Andersson G: **The role of anxiety sensitivity and behavioral avoidance in tinnitus disability.** *Int J Audiol* 2009, **48(5)**:295-299.
4. Langguth B, Landgrebe M, Kleinjung T, Sand PG, Hajak G: **Tinnitus and depression.** *The World Journal of Biological Psychiatry* .
5. Hebert S, Fullum S, Carrier J: **Polysomnographic and quantitative electroencephalographic correlates of subjective sleep complaints in chronic tinnitus.** *J Sleep Res* 2011, **20(1 Pt 1)**:38-44.
6. Shargorodsky J, Curhan GC, Farwell WR: **Prevalence and characteristics of tinnitus among US adults.** *Am J Med* 2010, **123(8)**:711-718.
7. Eggermont JJ, Roberts LE: **The neuroscience of tinnitus.** *Trends Neurosci* 2004, **27(11)**:676-682.
8. Mrena R, Savolainen S, Kiukaanniemi H, Ylikoski J, Makitie AA: **The effect of tightened hearing protection regulations on military noise-induced tinnitus.** *Int J Audiol* 2009, **48(6)**:394-400.
9. Nageris BI, Attias J, Shemesh R: **Otologic and audiologic lesions due to blast injury.** *J Basic Clin Physiol Pharmacol* 2008, **19(3-4)**:185-191.
10. Shargorodsky J, Curhan SG, Curhan GC, Eavey R: **Change in prevalence of hearing loss in US adolescents.** *Jama* 2010, **304(7)**:772-778.
11. Holgers KM, Erlandsson SI, Barrenas ML: **Predictive factors for the severity of tinnitus.** *Audiology* 2000, **39(5)**:284-291.
12. Hébert S, Canlon B, Hasson D: **Emotional exhaustion as a predictor of tinnitus prevalence and severity.** *Psychotherapy and Psychosomatics* .
13. **Tinnitus handbook.** Edited by: Tyler RS. San Diego: Singular; 2000:.
14. Hasson D, Theorell T, Wallen MB, Leineweber C, Canlon B: **Stress and prevalence of hearing problems in the Swedish working population.** *BMC Publ Health* 2011, **11**:130.
15. Hasson D, Theorell T, Westerlund H, Canlon B: **Prevalence and characteristics of hearing problems in a working and non-working Swedish population.** *J Epidemiology Community Health* 2010, **64(5)**:453-460.
16. Lockwood AH, Salvi RJ, Coad ML, Towsley ML, Wack DS, Murphy BW: **The functional neuroanatomy of tinnitus: evidence for limbic system links and neural plasticity.** *Neurology* 1998, **50(1)**:114-120.
17. Vanneste S, Plazier M, van der Loo E, Van de Heyning P, Congedo M, De Ridder D: **The neural correlates of tinnitus-related distress.** *NeuroImage* 2010, **52(2)**:470-480.
18. Leaver AM, Renier L, Chevillet MA, Morgan S, Kim HJ, Rauschecker JP: **Dysregulation of limbic and auditory networks in tinnitus.** *Neuron* 2011, **69(1)**:33-43.
19. Muhlau M, Rauschecker JP, Oestreicher E, Gaser C, Rottinger M, Wohlschlager AM, Simon F, Etgen T, Conrad B, Sander D: **Structural brain changes in tinnitus.** *Cereb Cortex* 2006, **16(9)**:1283-1288.
20. Landgrebe M, Langguth B, Rosengarth K, Braun S, Koch A, Kleinjung T, May A, de Ridder D, Hajak G: **Structural brain changes in tinnitus: grey matter decrease in auditory and non-auditory brain areas.** *NeuroImage* 2009, **46(1)**:213-218.
21. Hebert S, Paiement P, Lupien SJ: **A physiological correlate for the intolerance to both internal and external sounds.** *Hear Res* 2004, **190(1-2)**:1-9.
22. Heinecke K, Weise C, Schwarz K, Rief W: **Physiological and psychological stress reactivity in chronic tinnitus.** *J Behav Med* 2008, **31(3)**:179-188.
23. Hebert S, Lupien SJ: **The sound of stress: blunted cortisol reactivity to psychosocial stress in tinnitus sufferers.** *Neurosci Lett* 2007, **411(2)**:138-142.
24. Kirschbaum C, Pirke KM, Hellhammer DH: **The 'Trier Social Stress Test'-a tool for investigating psychobiological stress responses in a laboratory setting.** *Neuropsychobiology* 1993, **28(1-2)**:76-81.
25. Cleare AJ: **The neuroendocrinology of chronic fatigue syndrome.** *Endocr Rev* 2003, **24(2)**:236-252.
26. de Kloet ER, Schmidt M, Meijer OC: **Corticosteroid receptors and HPA-axis regulation.** In *Handbook of stress and the brain. Volume 15.* Edited by: Steckler T, Kalin N, Reul J. Amsterdam: Elsevier; 2005:265-294.
27. Ueda K, Okamura N, Hirai M, Tanigawara Y, Saeki T, Kioka N, Komano T, Hori R: **Human P-glycoprotein transports cortisol, aldosterone, and dexamethasone, but not progesterone.** *J Biol Chem* 1992, **267(34)**:24248-24252.
28. Schinkel AH, Wagenaar E, van Deemter L, Mol CA, Borst P: **Absence of the mdr1a P-Glycoprotein in mice affects tissue distribution and pharmacokinetics of dexamethasone, digoxin, and cyclosporin A.** *J Clin Invest* 1995, **96(4)**:1698-1705.
29. Meijer OC, de Lange EC, Breimer DD, de Boer AG, Workel JO, de Kloet ER: **Penetration of dexamethasone into brain glucocorticoid targets is enhanced in mdr1A P-glycoprotein knockout mice.** *Endocrinology* 1998, **139(4)**:1789-1793.
30. de Kloet ER, van der Vies J, de Wied D: **The site of the suppressive action of dexamethasone on pituitary-adrenal activity.** *Endocrinology* 1974, **94(1)**:61-73.
31. Miller AH, Spencer RL, Pulera M, Kang S, McEwen BS, Stein M: **Adrenal steroid receptor activation in rat brain and pituitary following dexamethasone: implications for the dexamethasone suppression test.** *Biol Psychiatry* 1992, **32(10)**:850-869.
32. Cole MA, Kim PJ, Kalman BA, Spencer RL: **Dexamethasone suppression of corticosteroid secretion: evaluation of the site of action by receptor measures and functional studies.** *Psychoneuroendocrinology* 2000, **25(2)**:151-167.
33. Holsboer F: **The corticosteroid receptor hypothesis of depression.** *Neuropsychopharmacology* 2000, **23(5)**:477-501.
34. Yehuda R, Southwick SM, Krystal JH, Bremner D, Charney DS, Mason JW: **Enhanced suppression of cortisol following dexamethasone administration in posttraumatic stress disorder.** *Am J Psychiatry* 1993, **150(1)**:83-86.
35. Rarey KE, Curtis LM: **Receptors for glucocorticoids in the human inner ear.** *Otolaryngol Head Neck Surg* 1996, **115(1)**:38-41.
36. Henkin RI, Daly RL: **Auditory detection and perception in normal man and in patients with adrenal cortical insufficiency: effect of adrenal cortical steroids.** *J Clin Invest* 1968, **47(6)**:1269-1280.
37. Siaud P, Maurel D, Lucciano M, Kosa E, Cazals Y: **Enhanced cochlear acoustic sensitivity and susceptibility to endotoxin are induced by adrenalectomy and reversed by corticosterone supplementation in rat.** *Eur J Neurosci* 2006, **24(12)**:3365-3371.
38. Beckwith BE, Lerud K, Antes JR, Reynolds BW: **Hydrocortisone reduces auditory sensitivity at high tonal frequencies in adult males.** *Pharmacol Biochem Behav* 1983, **19(3)**:431-433.
39. Mazurek B, Haupt H, Joachim R, Klapp BF, ver T, Szczepek AJ: **Stress induces transient auditory hypersensitivity in rats.** *Hear Res* 2010, **259(1-2)**:55-63.
40. Dauman R, Bouscau-Faure F: **Assessment and amelioration of hyperacusis in tinnitus patients.** *Acta Otolaryngol* 2005, **125(5)**:503-509.
41. Beck AT: *Beck Depression Inventory II* Toronto, ON: The Psychological Corporation; 1997.
42. Wilson PH, Henry J, Bowen M, Haralambous G: **Tinnitus reaction questionnaire: psychometric properties of a measure of distress associated with tinnitus.** *J Speech Hear Res* 1991, **34(1)**:197-201.
43. Allen JB, Hall JL, Jeng PS: **Loudness growth in 1/2-octave bands (LGOB)-a procedure for the assessment of loudness.** *J Acoust Soc Am* 1990, **88(2)**:745-753.
44. Smyth JM, Ockenfels MC, Gorin AA, Catley D, Porter LS, Kirschbaum C, Hellhammer DH, Stone AA: **Individual differences in the diurnal cycle of cortisol.** *Psychoneuroendocrinology* 1997, **22(2)**:89-105.

45. Gaab J, Huster D, Peisen R, Engert V, Schad T, Schurmeyer TH, Ehlert U: Low-dose dexamethasone suppression test in chronic fatigue syndrome and health. *Psychosom Med* 2002, **64(2)**:311-318.
46. Van Den Eede F, Moorkens G, Hulstijn W, Van Houdenhove B, Cosyns P, Sabbe BGC, Claes SJ: Combined dexamethasone/corticotropin-releasing factor test in chronic fatigue syndrome. *Psychol Med* 2008, **38(7)**:963-973.
47. Papadopoulos A, Ebrecht M, Roberts ADL, Poon L, Rohleder N, Cleare AJ: Glucocorticoid receptor mediated negative feedback in chronic fatigue syndrome using the low dose (0.5 mg) dexamethasone suppression test. *J Affective Disorders* 2009, **112(1-3)**:289-294.
48. Pruessner JC, Hellhammer DH, Kirschbaum C: Burnout, perceived stress, and cortisol responses to awakening. *Psychosom Med* 1999, **61(2)**:197-204.
49. Baigi A, Odens A, Almlid-Larsen V, Barrenas ML, Holgers KM: Tinnitus in the General Population With a Focus on Noise and Stress: A Public Health Study. *Ear Hear* .
50. Loew D, Schuster O, Graul EH: Dose-dependent pharmacokinetics of dexamethasone. *Eur J Clin Pharmacol* 1986, **30(2)**:225-230.
51. Canlon B, Meltser I, Johansson P, Tahera Y: Glucocorticoid receptors modulate auditory sensitivity to acoustic trauma. *Hear Res* 2007, **226(1-2)**:61-69.
52. Tahera Y, Meltser I, Johansson P, Bian Z, Stierna P, Hansson AC, Canlon B: NF-kappaB mediated glucocorticoid response in the inner ear after acoustic trauma. *J Neurosci Res* 2006, **83(6)**:1066-1076.
53. Yehuda R, Boisoneau D, Lowy MT, Giller EL: Dose-response changes in plasma cortisol and lymphocyte glucocorticoid receptors following dexamethasone administration in combat veterans with and without posttraumatic stress disorder. *Arch Gen Psychiatry* 1995, **52(7)**:583-593.
54. Rauschecker JP, Leaver AM, Mühlau M: Tuning out the noise: limbic-auditory interactions in tinnitus. *Neuron* 2010, **66(6)**:819-826.
55. Weisz N, Hartmann T, Dohrmann K, Schlee W, Norena A: High-frequency tinnitus without hearing loss does not mean absence of deafferentation. *Hear Res* 2006, **222(1-2)**:108-114.
56. Van Houdenhove B, Van Den Eede F, Luyten P: Does hypothalamic-pituitary-adrenal axis hypofunction in chronic fatigue syndrome reflect a 'crash' in the stress system? *Medical Hypotheses* 2009, **72(6)**:701-705.
57. Langguth B, Salvi R, Elgoyhen AB: Emerging pharmacotherapy of tinnitus. *Expert Opin Emerg Drugs* 2009, **14(4)**:687-702.
58. Ben-Zvi A, Vernon SD, Broderick G: Model-based therapeutic correction of hypothalamic-pituitary-adrenal axis dysfunction. *PLoS Computational Biology* 2009, **5(1)**:e1000273.

Posterior laryngitis: a disease with different aetiologies affecting health-related quality of life: a prospective case–control study

Hillevi Pendleton[1,6*], Marianne Ahlner-Elmqvist[2], Rolf Olsson[3], Ola Thorsson[4], Oskar Hammar[5], Magnus Jannert[1] and Bodil Ohlsson[5]

Abstract

Background: Laryngo-pharyngeal reflux (LPR) is assumed to be the most common cause of posterior laryngitis (PL). Since LPR is found in healthy subjects, and PL patients are not improved by acid-reducing therapy, other aetiologies to PL must be considered. The aims of this study in PL were to investigate the prevalence of acid reflux in the proximal oesophagus and functional gastrointestinal symptoms, to analyse motilin levels in plasma, and to assess health-related quality of life (HRQOL) before and after treatment.

Methods: Forty-six patients (26 women), with verified PL, median age 55 (IQR 41–68) years, were referred to oesophago-gastro-duodenoscopy and 24-h pH monitoring. Plasma motilin was analysed. The 36-item Short-Form questionnaire was completed at inclusion and at follow-up after 43±14 months, when also the Visual Analogue Scale for Irritable Bowel Syndrome was completed. Values were compared to controls. Treatment and relief of symptoms were noted from medical records.

Results: Thirty-four percent had proximal acid reflux and 40% showed signs of distal reflux. Ninety-four percent received acid-reducing treatment, with total relief of symptoms in 17%. Patients with reflux symptoms had lower plasma motilin levels compared to patients without reflux symptoms (p = 0.021). The HRQOL was impaired at inclusion, but improved over time. Patients, especially men, had more functional gastrointestinal symptoms than controls.

Conclusions: This study indicates that a minority of patients with PL has LPR and is cured by acid-reducing therapy. Disturbed plasma motilin levels and presence of functional gastrointestinal symptoms are found in PL. The impaired HRQOL improves over time.

Keywords: Posterior laryngitis, Laryngo-pharyngeal reflux, Motilin, Functional gastrointestinal disorder, Health-related quality of life

Background

Posterior laryngitis (PL) is defined as an inflammation involving the most posterior part of the glottic region, and sometimes involving the oesophageal inlet, in conjunction with symptoms such as chronic cough, hoarseness, a sensation of having a lump in the throat (globus), excessive throat clearing, excessive phlegm, voice fatigue, throat pain and dysphagia [1-4]. The

pathogenesis of inflammation is multifactorial and smoking, alcohol abuse, viral or bacterial infections, allergy, chronic sinusitis, voice abuse, and laryngo-pharyngeal reflux (LPR) can be the underlying causes.

LPR is defined as a back flow of gastric contents into the laryngo-pharynx and can be established by objective measurements [5]. A previous study indicate that 4%–10% of the patients who visit a Department of Oto-Rhino-Laryngology have complaints related to LPR [2]. One study showed that as many as 50% of patients affected by laryngeal and voice disorders have a pH-documented reflux [1]. Although the exact mechanism is unknown, reflux is associated with oesophageal

* Correspondence: Hillevi.Pendleton@med.lu.se
[1]Department of Clinical Sciences, Division of Oto-Rhino-Laryngology, Skåne University Hospital, Malmö, Lund University, Lund, Sweden
[6]Department of Oto-Rhino-Laryngology, Lasaretts gatan 21, Skåne University Hospital, SE-22185 Lund, Sweden
Full list of author information is available at the end of the article

dysmotility in 50%–60% of cases and reduced pressure of the lower oesophageal sphincter (LOS) in the majority of cases [6-8]. The influences on the function of the LOS are numerous. Motilin is an intestinal hormone, which regulates the migrating motor complex (MMC) of the ventricle and affects the pressure of the LOS. The hormone is found in enterochromaffin cells in the duodenum and jejunum, and ingestion of fat and gastric acid stimulates secretion of motilin into the bloodstream [9,10]. Patients with reflux have been shown to have altered motilin levels [11].

Patients with PL are at risk of being over-diagnosed as having extra-oesophageal acid reflux, as LPR is the most often assumed aetiology of PL [12,13]. Consequently, an inappropriate use of proton pump inhibitors (PPIs) are prescribed even though the symptoms and the findings are not related to acid reflux [14]. It has recently been shown that patients with PL, despite treatment with sufficient doses of PPI over many years, still suffer from their initial symptoms and complaints, with impaired health-related quality of life (HRQOL) as a result [15].

Apart from acid reflux, functional heartburn, functional dyspepsia and functional oesophageal disease may lead to oesophageal complaints [16]. An overlap and comorbidity between different functional disorders often exists. This also applies to functional gastrointestinal disorders (FGID), one of the most common being irritable bowel syndrome (IBS) [17]. The reason to functional disturbances is unclear, but may depend on altered central processing of visceral afferent information [18], where patients with FGID are thought to have a heightened perception of normal visceral stimuli, called visceral hypersensitivity [19-21]. The same functional aetiology has also been suggested in the case of PL [13,15].

Aim

The primary aim of the present study of PL was to investigate how many of the patients who had acid reflux in the proximal part of the oesophagus. Secondary aims were to examine motilin levels in plasma; to determine whether PL was associated with symptoms of FGID; and to register the HRQOL before and after treatment.

Methods

This study was performed according to the Helsinki declaration, and was approved by the Regional Ethics Review Board at Lund University. Informed, written consent was obtained from the participants.

Subjects

All consecutive patients, >18 years of age, from the Department of Oto-Rhino-Laryngology, Skåne University Hospital, Malmö, were invited during the period June 2007 to May 2011 to participate in the study when the

diagnosis PL was made by fibre optic laryngoscopy of an examiner not blinded to the patients symptoms. The diagnosis criteria for PL [1-4], and thereby the criteria for inclusion in the study, were the thickening and/or oedema of the posterior part of the glottic region *in combination* with one or several of the following symptoms: chronic cough, hoarseness, a sensation of having a lump in the throat (globus), excessive throat clearing, excessive phlegm, voice fatigue, throat pain and dysphagia. Patients with signs of PL but no symptoms were not enrolled in the study. Additional exclusion criteria were inflammatory bowel disease (IBD), coeliac disease, pregnancy, serious illness such as severe heart, lung, liver or kidney diseases and mental illness. Patients with Hepatitis B, C and HIV/AIDS were not included.

Study design

At the time of inclusion, age, symptoms and findings typical of the diagnosis PL, duration of symptoms, previous treatment for acid-related disease and symptoms, and tobacco and alcohol habits were registered. The patients were asked to fill in the 36-item Short-Form questionnaire (SF-36) to evaluate HRQOL. All patients were referred to a single-probe, 24-h pH monitoring in the proximal part of the oesophagus and an oesophago-gastro-duodenoscopy (OGD). An instant test for *Helicobacter Pylori* was made at OGD when clinically indicated. Blood samples were collected for the analysis of motilin.

At follow-up 43 ± 14 months later, a letter including the questionnaire SF-36 and the Visual Analogue Scale for Irritable Bowel Syndrome (VAS-IBS) was sent to the patients. Medical records were scrutinized and information such as choice of treatment (kind of drug, dosage and duration of treatment) and the extent of relief of symptoms were noted.

Ambulatory 24-h pH monitoring

All participants were instructed to cease their PPI therapy seven days before, and other acid inhibitors 16 h before the monitoring. They were asked to avoid acid beverages, e.g. fruit juice, during the 24-h duration of the pH monitoring and to fast 4 h before the catheter was introduced. The positioning of the catheter was performed in the Diagnostic Centre of Imaging and Functional Medicine, with the aid of fluoroscopy (Philips Multidiagnost Eleva, CA, USA). The catheter was introduced through the nose and under fluoroscopic control positioned in the proximal part of the oesophagus, 5 cm below the upper oesophageal sphincter.

Ambulatory pH monitoring for proximal reflux was performed for 24 h. Oesophageal pH monitoring was performed using an antimony pH electrode with an internal reference electrode (Versaflex, Sierra Scientific Instruments, Los Angeles, Ca, USA). Before each study, the pH-probe was calibrated in buffer solutions of pH 7 and 1. An episode of acid reflux was defined as a decrease in oesophageal pH to below 4 for more than 10 s. Previously established upper limits of normal acid exposure in clinical studies, with pH < 4 for 1% of total time, were used in the analysis of the data [22,23]. The data were stored on a portable digital recorder (Digitrapper pH400, Synectics Medical, Stockholm, Sweden) and were analysed with commercially available software (Polygram NET, SynMed Medical, Stockholm, Sweden).

Measurements of motilin

After fasting for at least 9 h, blood samples were taken at the time of the OGD. All blood samples consisted of 8.0 ml whole blood drawn into heparinised tubes. The plasma was separated and frozen at –20°C within 1 h of collection. Plasma motilin was measured as previously described by a radioimmunoassay (RIA) using a rabbit antiserum (R-8423), raised against highly purified, porcine motilin. The antiserum is directed to the NH2-terminal of motilin (amino acids 1–9). The coefficient of variation, intra-assay CV, was < 8% for controls at 140 pmol/l [24].

Questionnaires

The 36-item short-form questionnaire

SF-36 is an extensively used HRQOL instrument, which provides reproducible, reliable data on large populations, and has been shown to be useful as a global health monitor in clinical practice [25]. It is available in Swedish [26], and Swedish reference data are available for many different conditions. The SF-36 questionnaire is divided into eight subscales of general health, arranged according to the degree to which they measure physical vs. mental health. These subscales are physical functioning (PF), role functioning-physical (RP), bodily pain (BP), general health (GH), vitality (VT), social functioning (SF), role functioning-emotional (RE), and mental health (MH). Two additional dimensions can be calculated, physical (PCS) and emotional health (MCS), based on the weighting of the importance of the other eight subscales. The raw data were recoded at the time of analysis; the maximum score is 100, the higher score the better the HRQOL.

The visual analogue scale for irritable bowel disease

The VAS-IBS questionnaire is designed to measure the symptoms, the response to the treatment, and well-being in patients suffering from IBS. It was previously developed and validated for patients with gastrointestinal symptoms without organic causes [27]. Patients estimated seven different aspects of their gastrointestinal condition on a visual analogue scale (VAS) from 0–100 mm, where 0 represents very severe problems and 100 represents absence of problems. The aspects are abdominal pain, diarrhoea, constipation, bloating and flatulence, vomiting and nausea, perception of psychological well-being and the intestinal symptoms' influence on daily life. It also contains two additional questions concerning the patient's sense of urgency to defecate and the feeling of incomplete evacuation after defecation, which can be answered by "yes" or "no".

Statistical analyses

The data were analysed using the statistical software package SPSS for Windows© (Release 20.0; IBM). Distribution among the study population was tested by the Kolmogorov-Smirnov test and differed significantly from a normal distribution (p < 0.001) regarding age, VAS-IBS, and motilin levels. Results are given as means and the standard error of the mean (SEM) or median and interquartile range (IQR). Differences between groups were calculated, when appropriate by the Mann–Whitney U-test. Fisher's exact test was used for categorical variables and Spearman rank correlation test was used for correlations. The one-sample t-test was used to compare data from the SF-36 questionnaire with the Swedish reference values. Values were compared with the norm values of the general, and the Swedish female and male population, corrected for age [26]. As the patient group was older than the controls for VAS-IBS, the VAS variables were age-standardized using a linear regression model into which age was added as a covariate (independent). The dependent variables abdominal pain, diarrhoea, constipation, bloating and flatulence, vomiting, nausea, perception of psychological well-being, and the intestinal symptoms' influence on daily life were expressed as z-scores. As symptoms differ between gender [28], the results for women and men were calculated separately. Logistic regression analysis, adjusted for age (divided into 5-year intervals) and gender, was used to calculate odds ratios with 95% confidence intervals (OR with 95% CI) for the prevalence of the patient's sense of urgency to defecate and whether the bowel was totally emptied after defecation. The level of statistical significance was set to p ≤ 0.050.

Results

At inclusion

Patient characteristics

Forty-six out of 60 invited patients with verified PL (26 women), median age 55 (IQR 41–68) years, accepted to participate and were included in the study. Fourteen patients did not want to participate, the majority declining without giving a reason. Thirty-five patients tolerated the 24-h pH monitoring, 37 patients agreed to give blood samples for analysis of motilin, 42 patients were examined by OGD, and 44 patients filled in the SF-36 questionnaire (Figure 1). The mean duration of the disease was 13.5 (range 0–180) months. The most common symptoms

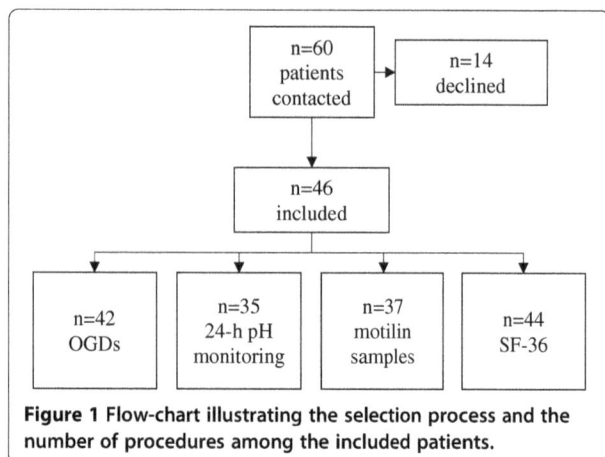

Figure 1 Flow-chart illustrating the selection process and the number of procedures among the included patients.

registered were globus (61%), excessive phlegm (48%), hoarseness (37%), voice fatigue (26%), and heartburn (26%) (Table 1). At fibre laryngoscopy, signs of PL such as inter-arytenoid pachydermia (76%), arytenoid oedema (56%), post-cricoid oedema (22%), and erythema of the vocal folds (11%) were found. Seventeen (11%) of the patients were smokers and 14 (9%) had been treated for dyspepsia, gastro-oesophageal reflux disease (GORD) or ulcer before their visit to the ear, nose and throat specialist. Five patients had a previously found hiatal hernia. Information about drinking habits was lacking in the majority of the cases.

Ambulatory 24-h pH monitoring and OGD

Thirty-four percent, 12 of the 35 patients examined (6 women), median age 55 (IQR 30–70) years, had a pathological reflux to the proximal oesophagus. Voice problems were associated with a pathological 24-h pH monitoring result (p = 0.050).

No ulcerations or tumours were found at OGD, but seven suffered from oesophagitis, 10 from Barrett's

Table 1 The prevalence of the various symptoms in the patients with posterior laryngitis (n=46)

Symptoms[a]	Number and percentage of patients
Globus	28 (61)
Excessive phlegm	22 (48)
Hoarseness	17 (37)
Heartburn	12 (26)
Voice fatigue	12 (26)
Acid regurgitation/reflux	11 (24)
Coughing	11 (24)
Excessive throat clearing	11 (24)
Dysphagia	9 (20)
Breathing difficulties	1 (2)

[a]More than one symptom for each patient was registered.

oesophagus, 14 from hiatal hernia and 14 had normal OGDs. Of the 12 patients complaining of voice problems, 11 were examined by OGD. The results of this procedure showed that these patients suffered from one or several of the following findings: five patients had a hiatal hernia, three suffered from Barrett's metaplasia, two had oesophagitis and one patient was positive for *Helicobacter Pylori*. Two patients had normal OGDs.

Measurements of motilin

Thirty-seven patients (20 women), median age 55 (IQR 40–67) years, gave blood samples for the analysis of motilin. Twenty-one healthy volunteers (14 women), median age 43 (IQR 36–53) years, served as controls. The motilin levels showed no correlations with age (r_s = 0.180, p = 0.287). There were no differences in plasma levels of motilin between patients and controls (p = 0.517), but the motilin levels differed between patients reporting typical reflux symptoms, i.e. heartburn and/or regurgitations (median 61 (IQR 52–68) pmol/l), compared to those without reflux symptoms (median 71 (IQR 64–85) pmol/l) (p = 0.021). There were no differences in plasma levels of motilin between patients with a positive or negative 24-h pH monitoring result (p = 0.057) or between patients with a pathological or normal OGD (p = 0.441).

SF-36

The women had significantly lower scores for all sub-scales, except PF that did not differ from the Swedish female population (p = 0.264) or the general Swedish population (p = 0.116) (Figure 2). In men, no differences in scores were found compared to the general Swedish population (Figure 2). The score for MH was significantly lower in the PL group compared to the Swedish male population (p = 0.050). The total PL population (n = 44)

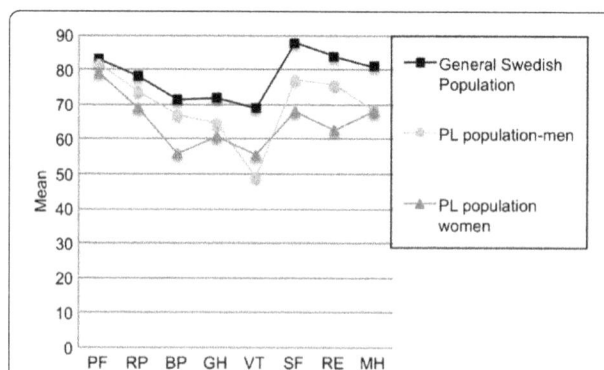

Figure 2 Analysis of the SF-36 questionnaire at inclusion in the population of men and women with posterior laryngitis (PL) and the general Swedish population. Gender- and age-matched values are presented as mean values. PF = physical functioning, RP = role-physical, BP = bodily pain, GH = general health, VT = vitality, SF = social functioning, RE = role-emotional, ME = mental health. One-sample t-test. P ≤ 0.050 was considered statistically significant.

had significantly lower scores for all subscales except PF and RP, compared to the general Swedish population (data not shown).

Treatment results

Forty-three patients (94%) received acid-reducing treatment. The most common treatment prescribed was PPIs alone or in combination with alginic acid (Table 2). The preferred choice of dose and duration of treatment was 20 mg PPI twice daily for 2–3 months. About one-fifth of the patients were treated for 8 weeks or less and 16% were treated for 4 weeks or less. At the clinical follow-up, more than half of the patients were better, but only 17% were asymptomatic (Table 2). An appointment with the physician, with a renewed fibre optic examination of the larynx was the most common mode of follow-up (52%), whereas 44% of the patients were followed by a telephone consultation. Two patients had no follow-up.

Follow-up

At study follow-up, 40 patients (22 women), median age 61 (IQR 44–72) years, completed both SF-36 and VAS-IBS.

SF-36

The women had a significantly lower score for the subscale GH compared to the general Swedish population (p = 0.046) (Figure 3), but no significant difference was noted compared to the Swedish female population (data not shown). In men, no differences in scores were found compared to the general Swedish population (Figure 3) or to the Swedish male population (data not shown). The total PL population had significantly lower scores in the subscales RP (p = 0.047), GH (p = 0.016), and VT (p = 0.028) compared to the general Swedish population.

Table 2 Medical treatment and results of treatment (n = 46)

	Patients n (%)
Medical treatment[a]	
Proton pump inhibitor	41 (89)
Alginic acid	13 (28)
Histamine receptor blocker	2 (4)
Aluminum dihydroxide	0 (0)
Missing information	3 (7)
Relief of symptoms	
Complete lack of symptoms	8 (17)
Improved	26 (57)
No change	9 (20)
Worse	1 (2)
Missing information	2 (4)

[a]Some patients were treated with more than one drug.

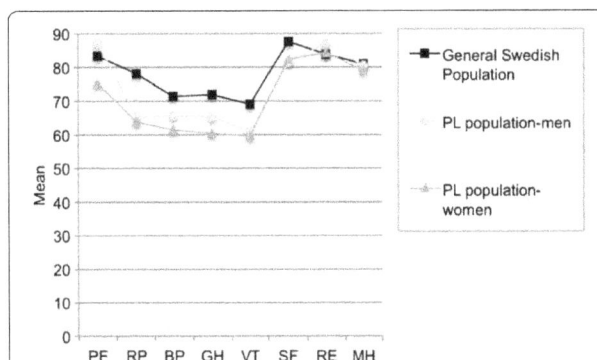

Figure 3 Analysis of the SF-36 questionnaire at follow-up in the population of men and women with posterior laryngitis (PL) and the general Swedish population. Gender- and age-matched values are presented as mean values. PF = physical functioning, RP = role-physical, BP = bodily pain, GH = general health, VT = vitality, SF = social functioning, RE = role-emotional, ME = mental health. One-sample t-test. P ≤ 0.050 was considered statistically significant.

Visual analogue scale for irritable bowel syndrome

Eighty-three volunteers (65 women), median age 39 (IQR 35–44) years, not suffering from PL or severe organic disease, served as controls for the VAS-IBS questionnaire. Women in the PL group registered significantly lower scores than the controls concerning abdominal pain (AP) (p = 0.001). The men in the PL group rated their symptoms as more severe than the controls, with a significant difference concerning abdominal pain (AP) (p<0.001), bloating and flatulence (BF) (p = 0.042), perception of psychological well-being (PW) (p = 0.024), and their intestinal symptoms' influence on daily life (IDL) (p = 0.020) (Figure 4). A positive correlation was found between emotional health (MCS) and perception of psychological well-being (WB) (r_s = 0.542, p = 0.001) and intestinal symptoms' influence on daily life (IDL) (r_s = 0.423, p = 0.009). There was no correlation between physical health (PCS) and the VAS-IBS (data not shown).

There was no significant difference between the PL group and the controls concerning the patient's sense of urgency to defecate (OR = 1.497, 95% CI = 0.233–9.605, p = 0.670) or the feeling of incomplete evacuation after defecation (OR = 1.494, 95% CI = 0.340–6.569, p = 0.595).

Discussion

The majority of the patients with PL in the present study had been prescribed acid-reducing treatment. However, only a minority of the patients were asymptomatic at clinical follow-up. Although the patients were perceived as having LPR-induced inflammation, only 34% of the patients with typical signs and symptoms of PL had a proximal acid reflux and associated voice problems. At

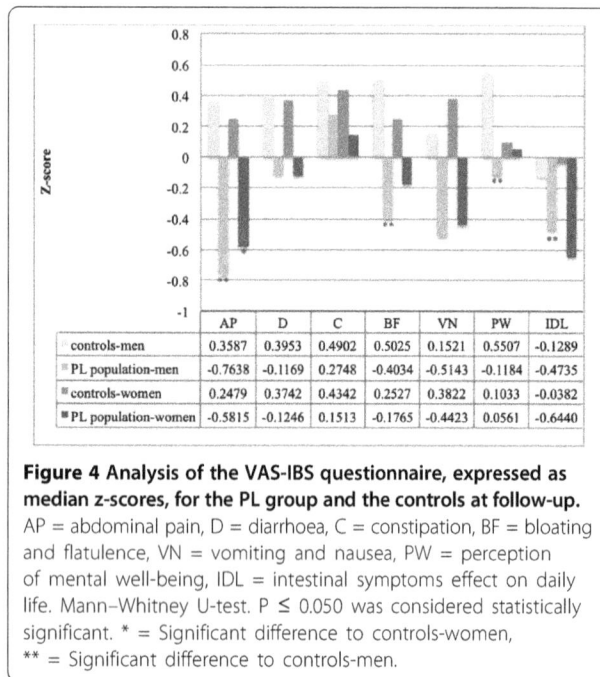

Figure 4 Analysis of the VAS-IBS questionnaire, expressed as median z-scores, for the PL group and the controls at follow-up.
AP = abdominal pain, D = diarrhoea, C = constipation, BF = bloating and flatulence, VN = vomiting and nausea, PW = perception of mental well-being, IDL = intestinal symptoms effect on daily life. Mann–Whitney U-test. P ≤ 0.050 was considered statistically significant. * = Significant difference to controls-women, ** = Significant difference to controls-men.

	AP	D	C	BF	VN	PW	IDL
controls-men	0.3587	0.3953	0.4902	0.5025	0.1521	0.5507	-0.1289
PL population-men	-0.7638	-0.1169	0.2748	-0.4034	-0.5143	-0.1184	-0.4735
controls-women	0.2479	0.3742	0.4342	0.2527	0.3822	0.1033	-0.0382
PL population-women	-0.5815	-0.1246	0.1513	-0.1765	-0.4423	0.0561	-0.6440

OGD, approximately 40% displayed signs of distal reflux. There was no difference in plasma levels of motilin between patients and controls, but patients with reflux symptoms had lower motilin levels compared to those without these symptoms. The total PL population's HRQOL was improved during the study, and the women's HRQOL improved more than the men's. The PL group, especially the men, experienced functional symptoms from the gastrointestinal tract to a greater extent than controls.

The terminology concerning PL and LPR is unclear and the terms are used synonymously. Patients included in studies are defined to have LPR when they actually have signs and symptoms of PL and vice versa [29,30]. Laryngo-pharyngeal reflux has been observed in healthy subjects without any association to typical symptoms of PL [31-34]. Further, Ylitalo et al. [35] could not prove a significant difference in the occurrence of any specific pharyngeal or laryngeal symptom or finding between the patients with and without extra-oesophageal reflux in patients with chronic heartburn. Although LPR has been shown to be more prevalent in PL patients than in controls, LPR does not render specific laryngeal symptoms [32]. This indicates an incomplete concordance between symptoms, objective findings and reflux in PL, and that the diagnosis cannot be based on symptoms alone [5,32]. Nevertheless, it is assumed that most patients suffering from PL have reflux of gastric content into the pharynx and larynx, LPR.

In the current study, all patients included displayed typical findings and symptoms of PL, but only 34% of the patients had a pathological 24-h pH value. Still, the majority of our patients received anti-reflux treatment with PPIs. Only 17% of the patients reported disappearance of symptoms at the clinical follow-up. Almost half of the patients were followed by a consultation by telephone. As a previous study has displayed that symptoms of PL treated with PPI resolve before laryngeal lesions heal, we assumed that a telephone consultation after 2–3 months of treatment is a sufficient mode of follow-up in the majority of cases [36]. At the telephone consultation, if the treatment has failed to improve the patient's symptoms, a new evaluation should be performed and additional aetiologies of PL, e.g. allergy, voice abuse, viral or bacterial infection, insufficient doses of PPI or functional disease should be considered.

Patients suffering from functional oesophageal disease are known to display typical reflux symptoms (heartburn/regurgitations) in spite of a normal acid exposure time and a normal oesophageal mucosa [19]. This is considered to be due to visceral hypersensitivity, i.e. an enhanced perception of normal physiological signals arising from the oesophagus. Different functional disorders often overlap, and patients may suffer from more than one such disorder [37]. These patients have a poorer response to acid suppressive therapy [3,19], which also applies to acid-suppressing therapy to patients with PL [15]. In accordance with patients affected by functional oesophageal disease, patients diagnosed with PL might suffer from functional pharyngeal-laryngeal disease. Patients with FGID are known to have a comorbidity of affective disturbances, e.g. depression and anxiety [38], which also has been noted in patients with PL [30]. The likelihood of a functional component is further strengthened by the expression of serum antibodies against gonadotropin-releasing hormone in patients both with PL and IBS [39,40].

The men had lower scores concerning abdominal pain, bloating and flatulence compared to the controls, whereas women only had lower scores for abdominal pain, indicating that patients with PL suffer from more gastrointestinal symptoms than the controls. Women have more gastrointestinal symptoms than men in the general population [28,41]. On the contrary, Sadik et al. [42] found in a group of patients with severe unexplained gastrointestinal symptoms, that gastrointestinal transit abnormalities were more common in men. The VAS-IBS results in our study are in agreement with these results [42], and suggest that the prevalence of gastrointestinal disorders may not differ that much between genders, when efforts are made to objectively assess the complaints.

The present study could not prove a difference in plasma levels of motilin between patients and controls, but patients with reflux symptoms had lower levels of motilin compared to those without these symptoms.

Altered plasma levels of motilin have been observed in patients with GORD, and motilin has in vitro been shown to elicit contractions of the LOS [10,11]. Patients with GORD, defective LOS pressure, and oesophageal dysmotility have been found to have lower plasma motilin levels than patients with normal peristalsis, and the motilin levels, LOS pressure and oesophageal dysmotility were normalised after anti-reflux surgery [43]. We have recently shown in a group of diabetic patients that plasma motilin concentrations vary with abnormalities in oesophageal motility [44], and the results of the present study raise the hypothesis that motilin might be of importance for the LOS function and oesophageal motility in LPR-induced PL. Basal and peak plasma levels of motilin, 24-h combined multi-channel intra-luminal impedance and pH testing (MII-pH) or 24-h pH monitoring with dual probes, would be of interest to further determine the role of motilin in patients with PL.

Siupsinskiene et al. [30] reported a significant deterioration in HRQOL in PL patients. Carrau et al. [29] also demonstrated, by using the SF-36 questionnaire, that patients with symptoms of LPR have a significantly inferior HRQOL than the general U.S. population.

In the present study, HRQOL was improved at the follow-up after 43 months, compared to the initial assessment. The absence of correlation between physical health (PCS) and the physical items of the VAS-IBS confirms that the impaired HRQOL in our patients with PL are not due to FGID, but due to PL. The lower HRQOL of women at the start of the study might reflect the propensity of women to complain about their symptoms [28,41,45]. Subsequent normalisation of their HRQOL at follow-up might be due to adequate treatment, receiving a diagnosis and information about the nature of their disease, or being taken care of. Bengtsson et al. [46] have shown that being taken care of, and information/education, improves women's quality of life when suffering from functional diseases.

One limitation of this study is the small group of patients studied. Also, we have not excluded the possibility that our patients might suffer from weakly acidic, gaseous or non-acidic reflux, as we have registered their reflux only by pH monitoring with a single probe, and not with combined multi-channel intra-luminal impedance and pH testing (MII-pH) or 24-h pH double probe monitoring. Our controls for motilin and VAS-IBS were entirely or partly recruited from hospital staff, who may be healthier than the average individual, and our control and study groups might have gained from being better matched. We have tried to compensate for this shortcoming by statistical adjustments of the data.

Conclusion

This study indicates that patients with typical findings and symptoms of PL to a lesser extent have LPR, and

that PL, in a subgroup of patients, may be due to functional disease. Voice problems were associated with pathological 24-h pH values. The plasma level of motilin is affected among PL patients with typical reflux symptoms, suggesting that this hormone is important in the pathogenesis of LPR. The HRQOL of the patients, especially the women, was low initially, but improved over time. It is highly probable that there are subgroups within PL, where some patients may have LPR, some display dysmotility of the oesophagus, and some patients have a functional disease.

Abbreviations
FGID: Functional gastrointestinal disorders; GORD: Gastro-oesophageal reflux disease; HRQOL: Health-related quality of life; LOS: Lower oesophageal sphincter; LPR: Laryngo-pharyngeal reflux; OGD: Oesophago-gastro-duodenoscopy; PL: Posterior laryngitis; PPI: Proton pump inhibitor; SF-36: 36-item Short-Form questionnaire; VAS-IBS: Visual analogue scale for irritable bowel syndrome.

Competing interests
The authors declare that they have no competing interests.

Authors' contributions
HP, BO, MJ and MAE together designed the study. HP has substantial contribution to study conception, acquisition of data and for mainly drafting the manuscript. HP and BO are mainly responsible for analysis and interpretation of data. RO collected the data from Medical Radiology, Diagnostic Centre of Imaging and Functional Medicine. OT collected the data from Nuclear Medicine, Diagnostic Centre of Imaging and Functional Medicine. OH collected data concerning the controls for VAS-IBS from the Department of Internal Medicine. All authors contributed to the manuscript with constructive criticism, and read and approved the final manuscript.

Acknowledgements
This study was performed with grants from the Swedish ACTA Otolaryngologica Foundation, Ruth and Richard Julins Foundation and the Development Foundation of Region Skane.

Author details
[1]Department of Clinical Sciences, Division of Oto-Rhino-Laryngology, Skåne University Hospital, Malmö, Lund University, Lund, Sweden. [2]Department of Health Sciences, Lund University, Lund, Sweden. [3]Divison of Medical Radiology, Diagnostic Centre of Imaging and Functional Medicine, Skåne University Hospital, Malmö, Lund University, Lund, Sweden. [4]Division of Nuclear Medicine, Diagnsotic Centre of Imaging and Functional Medicine, Skåne University Hospital, Malmö, Lund University, Lund, Sweden. [5]Department of Clinical Sciences, Divison of Internal Medicine, Skåne University Hospital, Malmö, Lund University, Lund, Sweden. [6]Department of Oto-Rhino-Laryngology, Lasaretts gatan 21, Skåne University Hospital, SE-22185 Lund, Sweden.

References
1. Koufman JA, Amin MR, Panetti M: **Prevalence of reflux in 113 consecutive patients with laryngeal and voice disorders.** *Otolaryngol Head Neck Surg* 2000, 123(4):385–388.
2. Hopkins C, Yousaf U, Pedersen M: **Acid reflux treatment for hoarseness.** *Cochrane Database Syst Rev* 2006, 25(1):CD005054.
3. Pearson JP, Parikh S, Orlando RC, Johnston N, Allen J, Tinling SP, Belafsky P, Arevalo LF, Sharma N, Castell DO, *et al*: **Review article: reflux and its consequences--the laryngeal, pulmonary and oesophageal manifestations. Conference held in conjunction with the 9th International Symposium on Human Pepsin (ISHP) Kingston-upon-Hull, UK, 21–23 April 2010.** *Aliment Pharm Ther* 2011, 33(Suppl 1):1–71.

4. Watson MG: Review article:laryngopharyngeal reflux-the ear, nose and throat patient. *Aliment Pharm Ther* 2011, **33**(Suppl 1):53–57.

5. Bove MJ, Rosen C: Diagnosis and management of laryngopharyngeal reflux disease. *Curr Opin Otolaryngol Head Neck Surg* 2006, **14**(3):116–123.

6. Kahrilas PJ: Anatomy and physiology of the gastroesophageal junction. *Gastroenterol Clin North Am* 1997, **26**(3):467–486.

7. Diener U, Patti MG, Molena D, Fisichella PM, Way LW: Esophageal dysmotility and gastroesophageal reflux disease. *J Gastrointestinal Surg* 2001, **5**(3):260–265.

8. Ho SC, Chang CS, Wu CY, Chen GH: Ineffective esophageal motility is a primary motility disorder in gastroesophageal reflux disease. *Dig Dis Sci* 2002, **47**(3):652–656.

9. Mitznegg P, Bloom SR, Christofides N, Besterman H, Domschke W, Domschke S, Wunsch E, Demling L: Release of motilin in man. *Scand J Gastroenterol Suppl* 1976, **39**:53–56.

10. Tomita R, Tanjoh K, Munakata K: The role of motilin and cisapride in the enteric nervous system of the lower esophageal sphincter in humans. *Surg Today* 1997, **27**(11):985–992.

11. Perdikis G, Wilson P, Hinder RA, Redmond EJ, Wetscher GJ, Saeki S, Adrian TE: Gastroesophageal reflux disease is associated with enteric hormone abnormalities. *Am J Surg* 1994, **167**(1):186–191. discussion 191–182.

12. Vakil N: The frontiers of reflux disease. *Dig Dis Sci* 2006, **51**(11):1887–1895.

13. Kotby MN, Hassan O, El-Makhzangy AM, Farahat M, Milad P: Gastroesophageal reflux/laryngopharyngeal reflux disease: a critical analysis of the literature. *Eur Arch Otorhinolaryngol* 2010, **267**(2):171–179.

14. Barry DW, Vaezi MF: Laryngopharyngeal reflux: More questions than answers. *Cleve Clin J Med* 2010, **77**(5):327–334.

15. Pendleton H, Ahlner-Elmqvist M, Jannert M, Ohlsson B: Posterior laryngitis: a study of persisting symptoms and health-related quality of life. *Eur Arch Otorhinolaryngol* 2013, **270**(1):187–195.

16. Sifrim D, Zerbib F: Diagnosis and management of patients with reflux symptoms refractory to proton pump inhibitors. *Gut* 2012, **61**(9):1340–1354.

17. Hungin AP, Whorwell PJ, Tack J, Mearin F: The prevalence, patterns and impact of irritable bowel syndrome: an international survey of 40,000 subjects. *Aliment Pharm Ther* 2003, **17**(5):643–650.

18. Ringel Y, Drossman DA, Leserman JL, Suyenobu BY, Wilber K, Lin W, Whitehead WE, Naliboff BD, Berman S, Mayer EA: Effect of abuse history on pain reports and brain responses to aversive visceral stimulation: an FMRI study. *Gastroenterol* 2008, **134**(2):396–404.

19. Kahrilas PJ, Hughes N, Howden CW: Response of unexplained chest pain to proton pump inhibitor treatment in patients with and without objective evidence of gastro-oesophageal reflux disease. *Gut* 2011, **60**(11):1473–1478.

20. Richter JE, Barish CF, Castell DO: Abnormal sensory perception in patients with esophageal chest pain. *Gastroenterol* 1986, **91**(4):845–852.

21. Silverman DH, Munakata JA, Ennes H, Mandelkern MA, Hoh CK, Mayer EA: Regional cerebral activity in normal and pathological perception of visceral pain. *Gastroenterol* 1997, **112**(1):64–72.

22. Dobhan R, Castell DO: Normal and abnormal proximal esophageal acid exposure: results of ambulatory dual-probe pH monitoring. *Am J Gastroenterol* 1993, **88**(1):25–29.

23. Postma GN: Ambulatory pH monitoring methodology. *Ann Otol Rhinol Laryngol Suppl* 2000, **184**:10–14.

24. Sjolund K, Ekman R, Lindgren S, Rehfeld JF: Disturbed motilin and cholecystokinin release in the irritable bowel syndrome. *Scand J Gastroenterol* 1996, **31**(11):1110–1114.

25. Winstead W, Barnett SN: Impact of endoscopic sinus surgery on global health perception: an outcomes study. *Otolaryngol Head Neck Surg* 1998, **119**(5):486–491.

26. Sullivan MKJ, Taft C: SF-36: Swedish manual and interpretation guide. 2nd edition. Gothenburg: Sahlgrenska University Hospital; 2002.

27. Bengtsson M, Ohlsson B, Ulander K: Development and psychometric testing of the Visual Analogue Scale for Irritable Bowel Syndrome (VAS-IBS). *BMC Gastroenterol* 2007, **7**:16.

28. Simren M, Abrahamsson H, Svedlund J, Bjornsson ES: Quality of life in patients with irritable bowel syndrome seen in referral centers versus primary care: the impact of gender and predominant bowel pattern. *Scand J Gastroenterol* 2001, **36**(5):545–552.

29. Carrau RL, Khidr A, Crawley JA, Hillson EM, Davis JK, Pashos CL: The impact of laryngopharyngeal reflux on patient-reported quality of life. *Laryngoscope* 2004, **114**(4):670–674.

30. Siupsinskiene N, Adamonis K, Toohill RJ: Quality of life in laryngopharyngeal reflux patients. *Laryngoscope* 2007, **117**(3):480–484.

31. Belafsky PC, Postma GN, Koufman JA: The validity and reliability of the reflux finding score (RFS). *Laryngoscope* 2001, **111**(8):1313–1317.

32. Ylitalo R, Lindestad PA, Ramel S: Symptoms, laryngeal findings, and 24-hour pH monitoring in patients with suspected gastroesophago-pharyngeal reflux. *Laryngoscope* 2001, **111**(10):1735–1741.

33. Andersson O, Ylitalo R, Finizia C, Bove M, Magnus R: Pharyngeal reflux episodes at pH 5 in healthy volunteers. *Scand J Gastroenterol* 2006, **41**(2):138–143.

34. Sun G, Muddana S, Slaughter JC, Casey S, Hill E, Farrokhi F, Garrett CG, Vaezi MF: A new pH catheter for laryngopharyngeal reflux: Normal values. *Laryngoscope* 2009, **119**(8):1639–1643.

35. Ylitalo R, Lindestad P, Hertegard S: Pharyngeal and laryngeal symptoms and signs related to extraesophageal reflux in patients with heartburn in gastroenterology practice: a prospective study. *Clin Otolaryngol* 2005, **30**(4):347–352.

36. Belafsky PC, Postma GN, Koufman JA: Laryngopharyngeal reflux symptoms improve before changes in physical findings. *Laryngoscope* 2001, **111**(6):979–981.

37. North CS, Downs D, Clouse RE, Alrakawi A, Dokucu ME, Cox J, Spitznagel EL, Alpers DH: The presentation of irritable bowel syndrome in the context of somatization disorder. *Clin Gastroenterol Hepatol* 2004, **2**(9):787–795.

38. Elsenbruch S, Rosenberger C, Enck P, Forsting M, Schedlowski M, Gizewski ER: Affective disturbances modulate the neural processing of visceral pain stimuli in irritable bowel syndrome: an fMRI study. *Gut* 2010, **59**(4):489–495.

39. Pendleton H: Antibodies Against Gonadotropin-Releasong Hormone in Patients with Posterior Laryngitis. *Drug Targets Insights* 2013, **7**:1–8.

40. Ohlsson B, Sjoberg K, Alm R, Fredrikson GN: Patients with irritable bowel syndrome and dysmotility express antibodies against gonadotropin-releasing hormone in serum. *Neurogastroenterol Motil* 2011, **23**(11):1000–1006. e1459.

41. Dimenas E, Carlsson G, Glise H, Israelsson B, Wiklund I: Relevance of norm values as part of the documentation of quality of life instruments for use in upper gastrointestinal disease. *Scand J Gastroenterol Suppl* 1996, **221**:8–13.

42. Sadik R, Stotzer PO, Simren M, Abrahamsson H: Gastrointestinal transit abnormalities are frequently detected in patients with unexplained GI symptoms at a tertiary centre. *Neurogastroenterol Motil* 2008, **20**(3):197–205.

43. Gardenstätter M: Alterations of Gut Neuropeptides in Gastroesophageal Reflux Disease Are Resolved after Antireflux Surgery. *Am J Surg* 2000, **180**:483–487.

44. Pendleton H, Ekman R, Olsson R, Ekberg O, Ohlsson B: Motilin concentrations in relation to gastro intestinal dysmotility in diabetes mellitus. *Eur J Intern Med* 2009, **20**(6):654–659.

45. Tibblin G, Bengtsson C, Furunes B, Lapidus L: Symptoms by age and sex. The population studies of men and women in Gothenburg, Sweden. *Scand J Prim Health Care* 1990, **8**(1):9–17.

46. Bengtsson M, Ulander K, Borgdal EB, Christensson AC, Ohlsson B: A course of instruction for women with irritable bowel syndrome. *Patient Educ Couns* 2006, **62**(1):118–125.

Association of the 4 g/5 g polymorphism of plasminogen activator inhibitor-1 gene with sudden sensorineural hearing loss. A case control study

Seong Ho Cho[1,2*], Haimei Chen[1], Il Soo Kim[1], Chio Yokose[1], Joseph Kang[1], David Cho[1], Chun Cai[3], Silvia Palma[4], Micol Busi[5], Alessandro Martini[5] and Tae J Yoo[3]

Abstract

Background: The 5 G/5 G genotype of PAI-1 polymorphism is linked to decreased plasminogen activator inhibitor-1 (PAI-1) levels and it has been suggested that lower PAI-1 levels may provide protective effects on inflammation, local microcirculatory disturbance, and fibrotic changes, which are likely associated with development of sudden sensorineural hearing loss (SSNHL).

Methods: The association of the 4 G/5 G PAI-1 polymorphism with the development and clinical outcome of SSNHL is evaluated *via* a case control study. 103 patients with SSNHL and 113 age and sex-matched controls were enrolled at University of Ferrara, Italy and hearing loss outcome was measured at least 3 months after the onset of hearing loss. DNA was isolated from peripheral blood using the QIAamp kit and the 4 G/5 G polymorphism in the −675 promoter region was genotyped with an allele-specific PCR. Genotype distribution was tested in patients and compared to controls by chi-square and odd-ratio analysis. The codominant and recessive models were used for the multiple logistic regression analyses of the PAI-1 gene allele.

Results: In this population, 5 G/5 G genotype had a two-time lower frequency in SSNHL patients compared to healthy controls (15.5% vs 30.1%) and was associated with decreased odds compared to 4 G/5 G genotype (OR 0.37, 95% CI 0.19-0.75, $p = 0.005$). In addition, the patients with 5 G/5 G genotype showed a trend of more than 2 times higher ratio of hearing recovery (> 20 dB) after systemic corticosteroid treatment compared to 4 G/5 G genotype (OR 2.3, 95% CI 0.32 - 16.83, $p = 0.39$), suggesting a better clinical outcome.

Conclusions: The 5 G/5 G genotype of PAI-1 may be associated with a reduced risk of SSNHL in the Italian population.

Keywords: Sudden hearing loss, Plasminogen activator inhibitor-1, 4 G/5 G polymorphism

Background

Sudden sensorineural hearing loss (SSNHL) is defined as a rapid onset sensorineural hearing loss occurring over a 72-hour period with a decrease in hearing of > 30 decibels (dB) affecting at least 3 consecutive frequencies [1]. The majority of patients with SSNHL have no identifiable

causes and are thus classified as "idiopathic" [2]. SSNHL affects 5 to 20 persons for each 100,000 individuals annually and can be devastating because they can lose their hearing permanently. The etiology of SSNHL is still unclear although the most recent studies suggest viral infection, vascular impairment, intracochlear membrane rupture, and autoimmune process as possible causes [3,4]. Several studies have been reported on the association between cardiovascular risk factors and SSNHL, showing that high concentrations of cholesterol, fibrinogen, and homocysteine were risk factors [5-9]. Other reports evaluated the association between SSNHL and genetic

---
* Correspondence: seong-cho@northwestern.edu
[1]Division of Allergy-Immunology, Department of Medicine, Northwestern University Feinberg School of Medicine, 676 N. St Clair street #14028, Chicago, IL 60611, USA
[2]Kyung Hee University, College of Medicine, Seoul, Korea
Full list of author information is available at the end of the article

polymorphisms of thromboembolic factors, mainly factor V Leiden and prothrombin G20210A variant, with controversial results [10-13].

Plasminogen activator inhibitor-1 (PAI-1) is the principal inhibitor of tissue plasminogen activator (tPA) and urokinase-type plasminogen activator (uPA), which actively facilitate plasminogen, and hence fibrinolysis. PAI-1 is a key molecule for thrombus formation and inflammation [14]. Elevation in plasma levels of PAI-1 has been reported to be associated with many diseases, such as cardiovascular diseases [14], stroke [15] and asthma [16-18]. Marcucci et al. [6] also reported that plasma levels of PAI-1 were significantly higher in patients with SSNHL compared to control subjects. One of most probable causes of SSNHL appears to be impaired cochlear blood circulation involving the pathogenic micro-thrombotic mechanism [19,20]. Cochlear function is very sensitive to changes in blood supply which is mainly derived from the labyrinthine artery. Vascular compromise of the cochlea caused by reduced blood flow, vasospasm, thrombosis or embolus, may result in SSNHL [13,21]. Our previous case report demonstrated the effectiveness of fibrinolytic therapy for sudden hearing loss with an improvement of 50 dB using a recombinant tPA, which appeared to improve the microcirculation of the inner ear [20]. These findings suggest that PAI-1 is a possible risk factor and a potential therapeutic target for SSNHL.

The PAI-1 gene has variation in the promoter region on the basis of a single guanosine insertion-deletion (5 G or 4 G) [16]. Previous studies on healthy subjects show the PAI-1 genotype distribution of 4G4G, 4G5G and 5G5G were 36.4%, 50.5% and 12.9% for a German population [11], 27.4%, 47.0%, and 25.6% for an Italian population [22], 28.7%, 42.5%, and 28.7% for a Turkish population [19], and 27.5%, 52.5% and 20.0% for a Spanish population [23] respectively. It has been reported that the subjects with 4 G/4 G have increased plasma PAI-1 levels and the ones with 5 G/5 G have decreased plasma levels, while the ones with 4 G/5 G have intermediate plasma levels [24]. Increased PAI-1 levels facilitate the inhibition of the fibrinolytic system [16], which may impair cochlear blood circulation and thus predispose the development of SSNHL [6,20]. It has been reported that the 4 G/5 G polymorphism of PAI-1 gene is associated with cardiovascular and thromboembolic diseases [16,25]. Rudack, Yildiz, and their coworkers also investigated the association between PAI-1 4 G/5 G polymorphism and SSHNL in the German [11] and Turkish [19] populations although the results were not conclusive.

In this study we investigated the 4 G/5 G polymorphism of PAI-1 gene in the Italian patients with SSNHL to see if this polymorphism is a risk factor in developing

SSNHL and can be used as a prognostic indicator for clinical outcome in patients with this disease. We demonstrated a significant contribution of 5 G/5 G polymorphism to lowering the risk of developing SSNHL and a trend of improved hearing recovery in follow up evaluation after treatment of SSNHL.

Methods
Patients and controls
One hundred and three patients, 54 females and 49 males (age range, 23–83; female mean age 54.1, male mean age 55.7), were evaluated at the Department of Audiology at the University of Ferrara and Modena with a diagnosis of SSNHL and gave their consent to participate in the study. They were referred to the department from January 2005 to December 2009. All the patients underwent audiological examinations including pure tone audiometry, speech recognition threshold, immittance measurements such as tympanogram and acoustic reflex; other audiometric tests for the differential diagnosis of cochlear vs retrocochlear pathologies were performed in selected cases. Auditory brainstem response (ABR) was always performed except when hearing loss exceeded 80 dB in the acute frequencies. Audiometric inclusion criterion was a decrease in hearing of at least 30 dB in 3 contiguous frequencies. The following scale of hearing loss degree was used: mild, $\geq$ 30 to < 40 dB hearing loss; moderate, $\geq$ 40 to < 70 dB hearing loss; severe, $\geq$ 70 to < 90 dB hearing loss; and profound, $\geq$ 90 dB hearing loss. Patients did not receive vestibular evaluation because exclusion criteria were the presence of vertigo or suspected Meniere's disease. Acoustic neuroma was excluded by performing MRI or by serial audiometry in selected cases. Any participant with a history of head trauma was also excluded from the study.

All the subjects provided their informed consent for the study and blood was taken as usual for routine laboratory exams, in the morning before starting the pharmacological therapy. Medical treatment consisted of betamethasone 4 mg i.m. for 3 days and 1.5 mg i.m. for 3–4 days, and oral prednisone was administered for at least 7 days afterwards, depending on clinical evolution. Pure tone audiometry was repeated daily according the history of the patient. We examined follow-up audiometry at least 6 months after the initial episode of hearing loss and considered a hearing improvement more than 20 dB as a significant recovery. The practice guidelines suggest <10 dB changes as no recovery [2]. Therefore we chose 20 dB as a clear cut-off for significant improvement, which would include partial and complete recovery. The age and sex-matched healthy Italian subjects (n = 113) were enrolled in the same geographical area. Control subjects had no history of hearing loss, circulatory or metabolic diseases, or autoimmune disorders. They were healthy clinic staffs and clinic patients with other otolaryngology disorders, such as allergic rhinitis, who gave their consent for the study. All of them had normal hearing.

DNA extraction
Blood was taken from each patient or control for genomic DNA extraction, which was performed using the QIAamp kit (Qiagen Inc., Valencia, CA) as directed to obtain 3 to 12 μg of DNA from 200 μl whole blood.

PAI-1 genotyping
The PAI-1 4 G/5 G genotype was analyzed with an allele-specific PCR modified from that of Falk et al. [26], using an alternative forward primer (GTCTGGA CACGTGGGGG for the 5 G allele or GTCTGGA CACGTGGGGA for the 4 G allele) with a common reverse primer (TGCAGCCAGCCACGTGATTGTC TAG, designed to minimize primer-dimer formation) and a control reverse upstream primer (AAGCTTT TACC ATGGTAACCCCTGGT). The PCR procedure included a hot-start initial step to avoid primer-dimer artifacts. The PCR mixture was subjected to 30-step cycles of 94°C (1 minute), 60°C (1 minute) and 72°C (1 minute). The PCR reaction was performed in a total volume of 25 μl with 0.5 μg of genomic DNA by using C1000™ Thermal Cycler (Bio-Rad Laboratories, Inc., Hercules, CA). The reaction mixture contained 10 mmol/L Tris–HCl (pH 8.0), 2.5 mmol/L $MgCl_2$, 200 μmol/L deoxyribonucleoside triphosphates, and 25 pmol of each primer. For each PCR, 2.5 U of Taq polymerase (Promega, Madison, MI) was used. Electrophoresis was performed in 2% agarose with 1 x TAE buffer. The gels were photographed after ethidium bromide staining. As a control of this PCR technique, PCR analysis was performed on DNA samples of known genotypes.

Statistical analysis
Genotype distribution and allele frequencies were tested in patients and compared to controls by chi-square test (χ^2) and odd-ratio analysis using GraphPad Prism for Windows version 4.03 (GraphPad Software Inc., San Diego, CA). We also used chi-square test ($\chi 2$) and odd-ratio analysis for the association between genotype distribution and hearing outcome. A p value of less than 0.05 was considered to be statistically significant. All odds ratios (OR) are given with their 95% confidence interval (CI). In the multiple logistic regression analyses for each PAI-1 gene allele, we used multiple inheritance models, including codominant model (the relative hazard differed between subjects with one minor allele and those with two minor alleles) and recessive model (only subjects with two minor alleles were at increased risk of the disease). 5 G was considered the minor allele in our case.

Results
A total of 103 SSNHL patients and 113 healthy controls were analyzed for 4 G and 5 G PAI-1 gene alleles. A typical PAI-1 genotyping experiment is shown in Figure 1. The frequencies of allele 4 G were 48.7% in SSNHL and 47.1% in controls, comparable to those for allele 5 G of 51.3% (SSNHL) and 52.9% (controls). The frequencies of genotypes 4 G/5 G, 4 G/4 G, and 5 G/5 G were 61.2%, 23.3%, and 15.5%, respectively, in SSNHL, and 44.2%, 25.7%, and 30.1% in controls (Table 1). The prevalence of 5 G/5 G genotype in the SSNHL patients (15.5%) was two times lower than that in control (30.1%). The 5 G/5 G genotype appeared to have the risk effect three times lower than that of the 4 G/5 G genotype (OR 0.37, 95% CI 0.19-0.75, $p < 0.005$), which is the most prevalent genotype. When we compared the 5 G/5 G genotype with combined non-5 G/5 G genotypes (4 G/5 G + 4 G/ 4 G), the 5 G/5 G genotype had two times lower risk of developing SSNHL than non-5 G/5 G genotypes. However, the 4 G/4 G genotype did not have significantly increased risk compared to the 4 G/5 G genotype.

We further examined to see if the polymorphism of PAI-1 gene is associated with clinical outcome in patients with SSNHL (Table 2). We were able to obtain follow-up pure tone audiometry from only 34 patients.

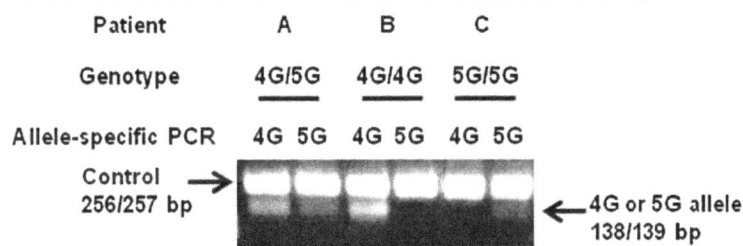

Figure 1 Gel patterns demonstrating the 4 G and 5 G alleles in the promoter region of the PAI-1 gene. PCR products with a forward primer for the 4 G allele or the 5 G allele and a control upstream primer are indicated by 4 G or 5 G, respectively; Lanes 1 and 2 for patient **A** (4 G/5 G genotype); Lanes 3 and 4 for patient **B** (4 G/4 G genotype); and Lanes 5 and 6 for patient **C** (5 G/5 G genotype).

Table 1 Genotype distribution of PAI-1 polymorphism in SSNHL and controls

Model	Genotype	Controls, n = 113 (Frequency)	SSNHL, n = 103 (Frequency)	OR	95 % CI	χ^2	p value
Co-dominant	4 G/5 G	50 (44.2 %)	63 (61.2 %)	1			
	4 G/4 G	29 (25.7 %)	24 (23.3 %)	0.66	0.34 – 1.27	1.59	0.210
	5 G/5 G	34 (30.1 %)	16 (15.5 %)	0.37	0.19 - 0.75	7.83	**0.005**
Recessive	4 G/4 G-4 G/5 G	79 (69.9 %)	87 (84.5 %)	1			
	5 G/5 G	34 (30.1 %)	16 (15.5 %)	0.43	0.22 - 0.83	6.42	**0.011**

SSNHL sudden sensorineural hearing loss; Odds ratios (OR) with 95 % confidence intervals (CI) and results (*p* values) of χ^2 analysis (chi-square test) were calculated for genotype frequencies compared with control.

Of these patients, SSNHL was unilateral in 33 patients and bilateral in 1. Among the unilateral cases, the degree of SSNHL was mild in 6 patients, moderate in 15, severe in 8, and profound in 4; one bilateral case was moderate degree in both side. Among these SSNHL patients, patients with 5 G/5 G genotype showed a tendency to have better outcome with 60% of patients having > 20 dB recovery after treatment, while patients with 4 G/5 G and 4 G/4 G genotypes had only 39.1% and 33.3% recovery rates (> 20 dB improvement), respectively. The genotype 5 G/5 G appeared to have a recovery effect 2.3 times higher than that of 4 G/5 G (OR 2.33; 95% CI 0.32 - 16.83). However, this finding of better clinical outcome in patients with the 5 G/5 G genotype was not statistically significant due to a relatively small number of patients who had received the available follow-up pure tone audiometry.

Discussion

One of most probable mechanisms of SSNHL appears to be impaired cochlear blood circulation involving the pathogenic micro-thrombotic mechanism [20]. There are precedent polymorphism studies on the roles of various prothrombotic risk factors in SSNHL, including GPIa C807T [27], FV 1691 G-A [11,28], MTHFR 677 C-T [12,19], and G20210A [10,29]. It has been known that elevated plasma levels of PAI-1 are associated with SSNHL [6], but the role of the PAI-1 is controversial [6,11]. In this study, we found that the 5 G/5 G genotype of the PAI-1 gene was associated with reduced risk of developing SSNHL.

Table 2 Significant hearing improvement (> 20 dB) in PAI-1 polymorphism

Genotype	4 G/5 G, n = 23 (Frequency)	5 G/5 G, n = 5 (Frequency)	4 G/4 G, n = 6 (Frequency)
No improvement	14 (60.9%)	2 (40.0%)	4 (66.7%)
Improvement	9 (39.1%)	3 (60.0%)	2 (33.3%)
OR (95% CI)	1	2.33 (0.32 - 16.83)	0.78 (0.12 - 5.17)
χ^2; p value		0.73; 0.39	0.068; 0.79

OR odd ratio, *CI* confidence interval.

To investigate the potential contribution of polymorphism within the PAI-1 gene to the development of SSNHL, we recruited SSNHL patients and control subjects from Ferrara and Modena, Italy, from a white, homogeneous population. In this population, we found the frequencies of 5 G allele (51.3%, 52.9%) had no significant difference from those of 4 G allele (48.7%, 47.1%) either in patients or in controls. However, the frequency of the 5 G/5 G genotype was two times lower in the SSNHL group (15.5%) compared to that in the control group (30.2%). This 5 G/5 G genotype showed 2–3 times lower risk effect than 4 G/4 G and 4 G/5 G. In this study, we found the 4 G/4 G genotype had no significant risk ratio in developing SSNHL. However, the 5 G/5 G genotype appeared to have a protective effect against developing SSNHL. Our findings are supported by several previous reports that the patients with 5 G/5 G genotype are known to have lower plasma levels of PAI-1 compared to those with 4 G/4 G [16,24], and lower PAI-1 level can provide protective effects on inflammation, local microcirculatory disturbance, and fibrotic changes, which are likely associated with developing SSNHL [4,6,30]. Our data showing the significance of the 5 G/5 G genotype are different from a previous study on German patients with SSNHL [11], where the 5 G/5 G genotype in the experimental group had no significant difference in frequency compared to the controls. Notably, their study showed the control genotype distribution were 36.4% (4G4G), 50.5% (4G5G), and 12.9% (5G5G), significantly different from our control study with Italian population (25.7%, 44.2%, and 30.1%). Additionally, their study elected only severe SSNHL patients with a loss of 60 dB or more. In contrast, our study recruited patients with a hearing loss of 30 dB or more. It is not clear whether the discrepancy between these two studies is due to different population (Italian vs German) or different severity of the disease.

It has been known that there is no effective treatment of SSNHL other than systemic corticosteroids which is generally used but has limitation to some patients [2]. Our study suggests that lowering plasma levels of PAI-1 may be a strategy to prevent SSNHL, especially in people who are likely to have high plasma levels of PAI-1, such as subjects who are obese, diabetic, or smokers [16,18]. Our study also suggests that the patients with the 5 G/5 G genotype have a tendency of 2–3 times higher ratio of hearing recovery (> 20 dB) compared to those with the 4 G/4 G and 4 G/5 G genotypes, although it was not statistically significant. We defined a change in hearing of > 20 dB as significant improvement, although practice guidelines usually suggest >10 dB improvement as significant, which includes both partial and complete recovery. We had a limited number of long-term follow-up audiometry results, which resulted in a lack of power in our analysis. Collecting more data on long-term follow-up audiometry would provide better insight into the influence of 4 G/5 G genotype on the clinical outcomes of SSNHL. We previously reported a case which showed significant improvement of hearing (> 50 dB) with recombinant tPA treatment two years after the development of SSNHL [20]. This case is an interesting observation that may suggest a link between fibrinolytic treatment and clinical outcome in patients with SSNHL. However, it is too early to suggest tPA use as an alternative treatment for SSNHL.

Conclusions
This study suggests that the individuals with the 5 G/5 G genotype of PAI-1 have less risk of developing SSNHL, and the 5 G/5 G genotype may function as a prognostic factor in recovery from SSNHL. This result may be of clinical significance in diagnosis, treatment, and prognosis for SSNHL patients and may provide a new therapeutic strategy for SSNHL.

Abbreviations
SSNHL: Sudden sensorineural hearing loss; PAI-1: Plasminogen activator inhibitor-1; tPA: Tissue plasminogen activator; uPA: Urokinase-type plasminogen activator.

Competing interests
Authors declare that there is no financial or non-financial competing interests in relation to this manuscript.

Authors' contributions
SC, SP, MB, AM and TY conceived of the study, and participated in its design and coordination and helped to draft the manuscript. HC, CY, DC and JK involved in drafting the manuscript or revising it critically for important intellectual content and performed the statistical analysis. IK and CC carried out the molecular genetic studies, participated in drafted the manuscript. All authors read and approved the final manuscript.

Acknowledgements
Funding sources: ACAAI Young Faculty Support Award and Ernest Bazley Fund to Seong H Cho and Allergy Support Fund of the University of Tennessee to Tae J Yoo.

Author details
[1]Division of Allergy-Immunology, Department of Medicine, Northwestern University Feinberg School of Medicine, 676 N. St Clair street #14028, Chicago, IL 60611, USA. [2]Kyung Hee University, College of Medicine, Seoul, Korea. [3]University of Tennessee, College of Medicine, Memphis, TN, USA. [4]University of Modena, Modena, Italy. [5]University of Ferrara, Ferrara, Italy.

References
1. Stachler RJ: Clinical practice guideline: sudden hearing loss. Otolaryngol Head Neck Surg 2012, 146:S1–S35.
2. Kuhn M, Heman-Ackah SE, Shaikh JA, Roehm PC: Sudden Sensorineural Hearing Loss: A Review of Diagnosis, Treatment, and Prognosis. Trends Amplif 2011, 15:91–105.
3. Chau JK, Lin JR, Atashband S, Irvine RA, Westerberg BD: Systematic review of the evidence for the etiology of adult sudden sensorineural hearing loss. Laryngoscope 2010, 120:1011–1021.
4. Lazarini PR, Camargo AC: Idiopathic sudden sensorineural hearing loss: etiopathogenic aspects. Braz J Otorhinolaryngol 2006, 72:554–561.
5. Cadoni G: Coenzyme Q 10 and cardiovascular risk factors in idiopathic sudden sensorineural hearing loss patients. Otol Neurotol 2007, 28:878–883.
6. Marcucci R, et al: Cardiovascular and thrombophilic risk factors for idiopathic sudden sensorineural hearing loss. J Thromb Haemost 2005, 3:929–934.
7. Capaccio P, et al: Genetic and acquired prothrombotic risk factors and sudden hearing loss. Laryngoscope 2007, 117:547–551.
8. Ballesteros F, et al: Is there an overlap between sudden neurosensorial hearing loss and cardiovascular risk factors? Audiol Neurootol 2009, 14:139–145.
9. Aimoni C, et al: Diabetes, cardiovascular risk factors and idiopathic sudden sensorineural hearing loss: a case–control study. Audiol Neurootol 2010, 15:111–115.
10. Gorur K, Tuncer U, Eskandari G, Ozcan C, Unal M, Ozsahinoglu C: The role of factor V Leiden and prothrombin G20210A mutations in sudden sensorineural hearing loss. Otol Neurotol 2005, 26:599–601.
11. Rudack C, Langer C, Junker R: Platelet GPIaC807T polymorphism is associated with negative outcome of sudden hearing loss. Hear Res 2004, 191:41–48.
12. Cadoni G, et al: Lack of association between inherited thrombophilic risk factors and idiopathic sudden sensorineural hearing loss in Italian patients. Ann Otol Rhinol Laryngol 2006, 115:195–200.
13. Mosnier I, et al: Cardiovascular and Thromboembolic Risk Factors in Idiopathic Sudden Sensorineural Hearing Loss: A Case–control Study. Audiol Neuro-Otol 2011, 16:55–66.
14. Suzuki J, et al: Effects of specific chemical suppressors of plasminogen activator inhibitor-1 in cardiovascular diseases. Expert Opin Investig Drugs 2011, 20:255–264.
15. de Paula Sabino A: Plasminogen activator inhibitor-1 4G/5G promoter polymorphism and PAI-1 plasma levels in young patients with ischemic stroke. Mol Biol Rep 2011, 38:5355–5360.
16. Ma Z, Paek D, Oh CK: Plasminogen activator inhibitor-1 and asthma: role in the pathogenesis and molecular regulation. Clin Exp Allergy 2009, 39:1136–1144.
17. Cho SH, Tam SW, Demissie-Sanders S, Filler SA, Oh CK: Production of plasminogen activator inhibitor-1 by human mast cells and its possible role in asthma. J Immunol 2000, 165:3154–3161.
18. Cho S, et al: Association of elevated plasminogen activator inhibitor 1 levels with diminished lung function in patients with asthma. Ann Allergy Asthma Immunol 2011, 106:371–377.
19. Yildiz Z, Ulu A, Incesulu A, Ozkaptan Y, Akar N: The importance of thrombotic risk factors in the development of idiopathic sudden hearing loss. Clin Appl Thromb Hemost 2008, 14:356–359.
20. Mora R, Mora F, Mora M, Barbieri M, Yoo TJ: Restoration of hearing loss with tissue plasminogen activator. Case report. Ann Otol Rhinol Laryngol 2003, 112:671–674.
21. Schuknecht HF, Kimura RS, Naufal PM: The pathology of sudden deafness. Acta oto-laryngologica 1973, 76:75–97.
22. Gentilini D, et al: Plasminogen activator inhibitor-1 4 G/5G polymorphism and susceptibility to endometriosis in the Italian population. Eur J Obstet Gynecol Reprod Biol 2009, 146:219–221.
23. Garcia-Segarra G, et al: Increased mortality in septic shock with the 4 G/4G genotype of plasminogen activator inhibitor 1 in patients of white descent. Intensive Care Med 2007, 33:1354–1362.
24. Mansfield MW, Stickland MH, Grant PJ: Plasminogen activator inhibitor-1 (PAI-1) promoter polymorphism and coronary artery disease in non-insulin-dependent diabetes. Thromb Haemost 1995, 74:1032–1034.
25. Cho SH, et al: Possible role of the 4 G/5G polymorphism of the plasminogen activator inhibitor 1 gene in the development of asthma. J Allergy Clin Immunol 2001, 108:212–214.

26. Falk G, Almqvist A, Nordenhem A, Svensson H, Wiman B: **Allele-Specific Pcr for Detection of a Sequence Polymorphism in the Promoter Region of the Plasminogen-Activator Inhibitor-1 (Pai-1) Gene.** *Fibrinolysis* 1995, **9:**170–174.

27. Santoso S, Kunicki TJ, Kroll H, Haberbosch W, Gardemann A: **Association of the platelet glycoprotein Ia C807T gene polymorphism with nonfatal myocardial infarction in younger patients.** *Blood* 1999, **93:**2449–2453.

28. Akar N, Yilmaz E, Akar E, Avcu F, Yalcin A, Cin S: **Effect of plasminogen activator inhibitor-1 4 G/5 G polymorphism in Turkish deep vein thrombotic patients with and without FV1691 G-A.** *Thromb Res* 2000, **97:**227–230.

29. Mercier E, *et al*: **The 20210A allele of the prothrombin gene is an independent risk factor for perception deafness in patients with venous thromboembolic antecedents.** *Blood* 1999, **93:**3150–3152.

30. Aso Y: **Plasminogen activator inhibitor (PAI)-1 in vascular inflammation and thrombosis.** *Front Biosci* 2007, **12:**2957–2966.

Laryngopharyngeal reflux disease in the Greek general population, prevalence and risk factors

Nikolaos Spantideas[1*], Eirini Drosou[2], Anastasia Bougea[3] and Dimitrios Assimakopoulos[4]

Abstract

Background: To assess the prevalence of laryngopharyngeal reflux (LPR) in the Greek general population and its risk factors.

Methods: Questionnaire based epidemiological, adult participants' survey. The Reflux Symptom Index (RSI) was used for the assessment of LPR prevalence. The RSI questionnaire was completed by 340 (183 male and 157 female) randomly selected subjects. Subjects with RSI score ≥13 were considered as LPR patients and those with RSI score <13 were considered as non LPR subjects.

Results: The prevalence of LPR in the general Greek population was found to be 18.8 % with no statistically significant difference between the two genders (p > 0.05). The age group of 50–64 years showed the higher prevalence rate. Tobacco smoking and alcohol consumption were found to be related with LPR. No reported concomitant disease or medication was found to be related with LPR.

Conclusions: LPR prevalence in the Greek general population was found to be 18.8 %. Tobacco smoking and alcohol consumption were found to be related with LPR.

Keywords: Reflux, Gastroesophageal reflux, Laryngopharyngeal reflux, Epidemiologic study, Risk factors

Background

LPR is defined as the retrograde movement of gastric contents into the larynx and pharynx leading to a diversity of upper aero digestive tract symptoms [1].

LPR has a significant negative impact on patient's quality of life [2]. LPR is an underdiagnosed entity in otolaryngology and its actual prevalence and predisposing factors in the community have not been established. Potential risk factors and co-morbidities for LPR remain unknown. Data concerning LPR prevalence in Greece are lacking.

In 2002, Belafsky et al developed the Reflux Symptom Index (RSI), a self-administered nine-item questionnaire, designed to assess various symptoms related to LPR. Each item is scaled from 0 (no problem) to 5 (severe problem), with a maximum score of 45 indicating the most severe symptoms. An RSI ≥ 13 is considered abnormal and strongly indicative of LPR [3].

Since the introduction of RSI, many studies have shown the reliability and consistency of the method in various populations throughout the globe, establishing the method as a very useful diagnostic tool in every day practice [4–6]. Feng GJ et al have found that laryngopharyngeal pH monitoring and RSI scoring have the same value in diagnosing laryngopharyngeal reflux disease (LPRD) [7].

The primary aim of this study was to assess the prevalence of LPR in the general adult Greek population using RSI as the diagnostic screening tool. Secondary aims of the study were to identify any predisposing or associated factors for developing LPR.

Methods

The study was carried out in the general Greek population during the period from September to November 2013.

* Correspondence: spandideas@gmail.com
[1]Athens Speech Language and Swallowing Institute, 10 Lontou Street, Glyfada, Athens 16675, Greece
Full list of author information is available at the end of the article

A random sample (n = 1.000) of adults living in Athens (500 people) and in rural Greek areas (500 people) was initially approached through an "alert" telephone. During the communication, the scope of the study was explained and permission to send the questionnaire to the subjects' address was obtained. The participants were randomly selected through the telephone catalogue of Athens City and telephone catalogues of randomly selected rural areas using a Table of random numbers generated for the study. Five different investigators performed the calls ten days before sending the questionnaire. Of the 1000 subjects who were approached, 450 accepted to participate in the study and provided their personal details (name - address). Only one person per family has to fill the sent questionnaire. In the envelope that was sent to the participants a more detailed explanation for the scope of the study, detailed instructions for filling out the questionnaire, an informed consent and a prepaid envelope were included, so that subjects could easily send back the filled-in questionnaire as well as the signed informed consent at no cost for them. Three hundred fifty individuals returned the questionnaires (189 or 54 % from Athens and 161 or 46 % from rural areas).

Data related to LPR symptoms were gathered through a questionnaire containing the validated Greek version of RSI. Additional questions concerning demographic data (age and gender), behavioral characteristics (smoking status and alcohol consumption) concomitant diseases and concurrent medication were also included in the posted questionnaire.

Inclusion criterion for our study was age since the main scope of our study was to asses LPR prevalence in the general adult population. In this regard, only subjects >18 year old were included in the study. Subjects with pre-existing gastro-esophageal reflux and those taking anti-reflux medications were also included in the study. Exclusion criteria for participation in the study were current upper respiratory tract infections and known laryngopharyngeal malignancies.

For the purpose of this study LPR diagnosis was based on RSI score ≥ 13 as proposed by Belafsky et al [3].

The study protocol was approved by the Scientific Committee and Review Board of Athens Speech, Language and Swallowing Institute. Informed consent was obtained from all participants prior to inclusion in the study.

Statistical tests were performed using the IBM SPSS Statistics 20 software.

Variables of the analysis were: Demographic parameters, smoking and alcohol habits, health background (concomitant diseases), concomitant medication and the reflux symptom index.

The independent samples of Student's test were used to compare the RSI values in the patients with LPR

and in subjects without LPR which were used as control group.

The study sample size was calculated based on the assumption that LPR prevalence is higher than 15 %

Statistical tests used for the statistical analysis were:

- Significance level for all hypothesis testing (p-value) was 0.05
- Correlations between the levels of the RSI were performed using the Spearman's Rho correlation coefficient test.
- The prevalence of LPR was estimated using a minimum cut-off score of ≥ 13 on the RSI as proposed by Belafski et al. [3]

We assessed the prevalence of LPR in the general Greek population using the RSI. In this regard, the Greek version of the validated RSI questionnaire was given to 450 subjects from different parts of Greece (50 % from urban areas and 50 % from rural areas) to be completed. Eventually 350 completed questionnaires were collected.

Results

The questionnaire was given to 450 subjects. Three hundred and fifty subjects (response rate 77.8 %) returned completed questionnaires. In 10 out of the 350 returned questionnaires, critical information like gender and age were lacking. Thus 340 (183 male and 157 female) duly completed questionnaires were appropriate for statistical analysis. Demographic data and patients' behavioral characteristics are shown in Table 1. The mean age of the participants was 46.86 ± 14.54 years. Most participants belonged to the age group of 35–49 (131 subjects) while the age groups > 80 and < 20 were poorly represented (3 subjects > 80 year and 2 subjects < 20 year).

One hundred seventy four (51.2 %) participants were smokers with mean number of cigarettes per day 20.5 and mean duration of smoking 18.23 ± 8.6 years for male and 17.02 ± 8.0 years for female, with no statistically significant difference between the two genders (t-test >0,05).

One hundred and one subjects (29.7 %) drank alcohol regularly (68.3 % male and 31.7 % female). Mean alcohol consumption per day was 2.43 ± 1.62 units for males and 2.17 ± 1.32 units for females with no statistical significance between the two genders (t-test > 0.05). The most commonly reported alcoholic drinks were wine (30) followed by beer (21) and whisky (18).

One hundred forty two (41.8 %) participants reported one or more diseases. The reported diseases were: cardiovascular 50 (35.2 %), gastrointestinal 25 (17.6 %), musculoskeletal 15 (10.6 %), respiratory 10 (7.0 %), thyroidopathy 9 (6.3 %), anemia 3 (2.1 %) and other diseases 30 (21.1 %). Among the reported gastrointestinal diseases, 5 cases were

Table 1 Demographic data and behavioral characteristics of study participants

Variable	Group	Number	Percent
Gender	Female	157	46.2
	Male	183	53.8
Total		340	100.0
Age (in years) Mean (±SD): 46.86 (±14.54)	<20	2	0.6
	20–34	71	20.9
	35–49	131	38.5
	50–64	88	25.9
	65–79	45	13.2
	> = 80	3	0.9
Total		340	100.0
Smoking	Yes	174	51.2
	No	166	48.8
Total		340	100
Duration of smoking (years) Mean (±SD): 18.23 (±8.6)	1–5	7	4.1
	5–10	29	17.2
	10–15	39	23.1
	15–20	34	20.1
	20–25	30	17.8
	25–30	9	5.3
	>30	21	12.4
Total		169	100
Number of cigarettes per day Mean (±SD): 20.51 (±11.83)	1–9	18	13.7
	10–19	38	29.0
	20–29	42	32.1
	30–39	17	13.0
	40–49	13	9.9
	50–59	1	0.8
	60+	2	1.5
Total		131	100
Drinker	No	239	70.3
	Yes	101	29.7
Total		340	100
Number of drinks per day	1–2	72	71.3
	3–4	17	16.8
	5–6	11	10.9
	9–10	1	1.0
Total		101	100

gastroesophageal reflux disease (GERD), 13 dyspepsia, 5 gastritis and 2 duodenal ulcers.

One hundred and thirty seven (40.3 %) participants reported use of one or more medication for the concomitant diseases. The reported medications were: antihypertensive 43 (31.4 %), anticholesterol 19 (13.9 %), antiulcerants 19 (13.9 %), [15 PPIs (proton pump inhibitors) and 4 H_2 antagonists], antidiabetics 11 (8.0 %), anti-asthmatics/COPD (chronic obstructive pulmonary disease) 11 (8.0 %), antihypothyroidism 9 (6.6 %), antiosteoporotics 7 (5.1 %) [5 calcium carbonate and 2 bisphosphonates], non steroidal anti-inflammatory drugs 4 (1,2 %) and other medications 18 (13.1 %).

Two hundred sixty six subjects (78.2 %) reported one or more symptoms included in the RSI. The most commonly reported symptoms were No 9 "Heartburn, chest pain, indigestion, or stomach acid coming up" (52 %) and No 2 "Clearing your throat" (48.2 %) (Table 2).

Sixty four subjects (18.8 %) out of the 340 participants of our study presented an RSI ≥13 and were considered as patients with LPR, compared to 276 subjects with an RSI < 13 who were considered to be subjects without LPR. The mean RSI score in patients with LPR was 24.8 ± 8.0 compared to the subjects without LPR the mean RSI of which was 2.3 ± 3.2 ($p < 0.001$) (Table 3).

Spearman's Rho correlations analysis showed that all the pairs between the 9 items of the RSI were correlated, meaning that if a subject responded positively to one item there was a high probability to respond positively to the other item.

Based on the findings of our study the prevalence of LPR in the Greek general population was found to be 18.8 %. The LPR prevalence for males was 19.7 % and for females 17.8 % with no statistically significant difference between the two genders (t-test, p > 0.05).

Most subjects with LPR (RSI ≥13) belonged to the age groups of 50–64 year (40.6 %) and 35–49 (34.4 %). These two age groups represented 75 % of the LPR cases encountered in the general Greek population. No LPR cases reported in ages >80 and <20 but this may be due to the very small sample size of these two particular age groups.

Statistical analysis did not show any relation between LPR and any of the reported diseases nor LPR and

Table 2 Frequency of reported symptoms included in reflux symptom index by the participants of the study

Symptom	Number	Percent
1. Hoarseness or a problem with your voice	131	38,5
2. Clearing your throat	164	48,2
3. Excess throat mucus or postnasal drip	130	38,2
4. Difficulty swallowing food, liquids, or pills	99	29,1
5. Coughing after you ate or after lying down	110	32,3
6. Breathing difficulties or choking episodes	108	31,8
7. Troublesome or annoying cough	105	30,9
8. Sensation of something sticking in your throat or a lump in your throat	138	40,6
9. Heartburn, chest pain, indigestion, or stomach acid coming up	177	52

Table 3 Mean score and standard deviation of the reflux symptom index items in patients with LPR and in non LPR subjects

Group	RSI1	RSI2	RSI3	RSI4	RSI5	RSI6	RSI7	RSI8	RSI9	Total RSI
LPR										
Mean	3,1598	3,6201	2,8217	1,8081	2,1246	3,1041	1,9204	2,8788	3,3224	24,76
SD	1,2624	1,5578	1,1601	1,3196	1,4513	1,3143	1,4723	1,1786	1,5923	8,0032
Non LPR										
Mean	0,2218	0,3832	0,4689	0,2125	0,1987	0,0989	0,1375	0,3137	0,2718	2,3207
SD	0,3726	0,4576	0,7238	0,3806	0,9086	0,8076	0,7178	0,4463	0,6534	3,2261
P valueLPR vs Non LPR	<0,001	< 0,001	< 0,001	< 0,001	< 0,001	< 0,001	< 0,001	< 0,001	< 0,001	< 0,001

RSI1: Hoarseness or a problem with your voice, RSI2: Clearing your throat, RSI3: Excess throat mucus or postnasal drip, RSI4: Difficulty swallowing food, liquids, or pills, RSI5: Coughing after eating or after lying down, RSI6: Breathing difficulties or choking episodes, RSI7: Troublesome or annoying cough, RSI8: Sensations of something sticking in your throat or a lump in your throat, RSI9: Heartburn, chest pain, indigestion, or stomach acid coming up

reported medications (Chi-square test > 0.05 for both cases). The lack of such findings has to be accepted with reservations and not as conclusive due to the limited number of reported diseases and medications, and since the primary aim of this study was not to assess these two parameters.

A correlation was found between LPR and smoking and alcohol consumption. Factor analysis was used to assess a potential association between the Factor's Score and the information available for every person. It was concluded that alcohol drinkers and nondrinkers have a statistically significant difference in their mean factor score, as well as smokers compared to nonsmokers (t-test, p-value < 0.001 and p-value = 0.006 respectively). The direction of this association is shown in the box plots (Figs. 1 and 2).

We should be aware that the smokers of this study tend to consume alcohol more often than non-smokers. For that reason we cannot be sure which of the two, tobacco or alcohol consumption has an effect on increasing the average score of the RSI.

Discussion

LPR remains a controversial topic with inconsistent data concerning its epidemiology, etiology, diagnosis and management [8].

It is difficult to estimate the prevalence of LPR in the general population since there is not an easy and generally accepted diagnostic method available for large scale epidemiological studies [9]. It has been reported that up to 10 % of patients presenting to an otolaryngologist's

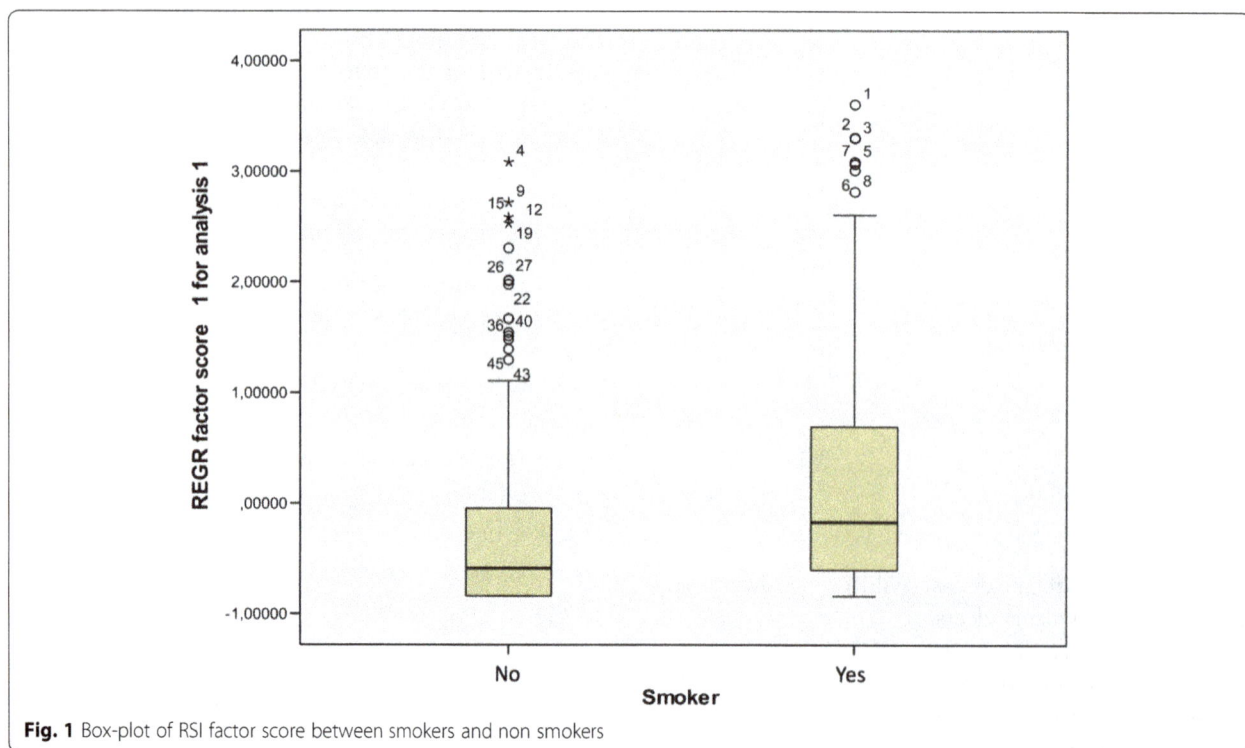

Fig. 1 Box-plot of RSI factor score between smokers and non smokers

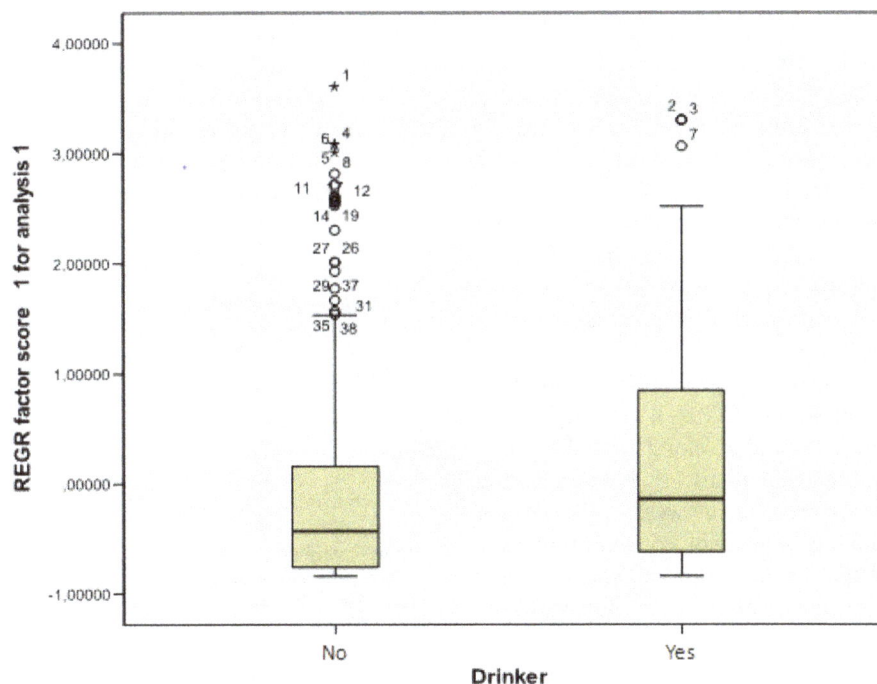

Fig. 2 Box-plot of RSI factor score between drinkers and non drinkers

office and more than 50 % of patients with hoarseness are patients with reflux related disease [10, 11]. LPR episodes have been reported by 30–50 % of the normal control [12, 13] and the prevalence of LPR in the general population has been reported to vary between 7.1 % [14] to 64 % [9]. The big difference in the reported LPR prevalence is mainly attributed to the differences in the methods used by each investigator as well as to the absence of a generally adopted definition of LPR.

The need for an easily administered and generally accepted diagnostic method for early detection of LPR patients is crucial, considering that LPR is better at predicting the presence of esophageal adenocarcinoma than typical gastroesophageal reflux symptoms [15], and that LPR is related to laryngopharyngeal carcinoma [16].

There is not a reliable known prevalence of LPR symptoms in the Greek population and thus the objectives of this study were to use a validated tool, the RSI in Greek, to identify LPR symptoms.

In this study subjects scoring RSI ≥ 13 are presumed to be LPR patients and those with RSI < 13 were presumed to be LPR free subjects.

According to the findings of this study, the prevalence of LPR in the general Greek population was found to be 18.8 %. No significant difference was observed between males and females in the prevalence of LPR. The age group where LPR prevalence was reported more frequently was 50–64 (40.2 %). Lowden et al demonstrated that 26.5 % of patients attending a general practice in

UK had an RSI >10 [17]. Kamani T et al. have shown that 30 % of the UK general population have an RSI > 10 [18]. A study conducted in Greece using the RSI as a diagnostic tool for LPR has found the prevalence of LPR to be 8.5 % in the Greek population. However, that study did not refer to the general population since the participants were mainly ambulatory patients who were visiting primary care centers for various chronic diseases or patients' escorts [19]. Another drawback of the previously mentioned study was the exclusion of subjects with certain diseases like irritable bowel syndrome (IBS), peptic ulcer disease, major psychiatric illnesses and those using non steroidal anti-inflammatory drugs (NSAIDs), conditions that are all well known to have a higher LPR prevalence [18, 20]. In addition, the gender make-up was not well balanced and male participants represented only 36.3 % of the study population vs 63.7 % female. Although this study did not find a significant difference in LPR prevalence between men and women in agreement with finding from other studies [18, 21], some other investigators have found LPR prevalence to be much higher in males [22, 23]. The different LPR prevalence rate obtained by the above mentioned studies, which used RSI as diagnostic tool for LPR diagnosis, reflects the different methodology each investigator used regarding LPR definition and population selection.

It is important to mention the high frequency of LPR related symptoms reported by the participants of our study. Two hundred sixty out of the total 340 (78.2 %)

reported one or more symptom included in the RSI. Most common reported symptoms were RSI9 "Heartburn, chest pain, indigestion, or stomach acid coming up" (52 %) and RSI2 "Clearing your throat" (48.2 %). The high frequency of RSI9, especially in the middle aged people of the general population, is also in line with the findings of other investigators [18, 24].

No relation between LPR and reported diseases nor LPR and medication was found. However these findings could not be considered as conclusive due to the small number of reported concomitant diseases and to the small number of medications.

A correlation was found between LPR and smoking and alcohol consumption. Lin CC et al reported a correlation between total RSI and smoking as well as alcohol drinking with certain RSI items [4]. Kamani T et al did not find any association between LPR related symptoms and smoking or alcohol consumption [18]. It should be noted that in our study the smokers tend to consume alcohol more often than non-smokers. That's why we cannot be sure which of the two, smoking or alcohol habits, has an effect on increasing the average score of the RSI nor which causes the other. Kamani T et al have found alcohol not to be a risk factor for LPR-related symptoms [18]. Controversy regarding the effect of alcohol exists not only for LPR, but also for GERD, as the results of different studies are diverse and contradictory. Despite the controversies regarding the effect of smoking and drinking on LPR, the recommendation of lifestyle modifications for the treatment of LPR include smoking cessation and limiting alcohol intake [25].

To the best of our knowledge, our study is the first that has been designed to assess the prevalence of LPR in the general population using the RSI score of ≥13 as the criterion for LPR diagnosis. Similar studies coming from different countries and populations can give us a more clear view on LPR prevalence. So that the findings of future studies are comparable we propose the cut-off point of RSI ≥13 to be the base for LPR diagnosis and the sample to refer to pure general population.

A limitation of this study could be the lack of comparison between the applied method and a method with higher specificity (flexible endoscopy or ambulatory 24-h double-probe pH monitoring), but on one hand these methods are invasive and costly and are not suitable for large scale epidemiological studies and on the other hand this comparison has already been done in other studies and has proved similar validity of the two methods [7]. Another limitation of the study could be the small sample size of concomitant diseases and medications that did not permit us to reach a confident conclusion regarding the relationship between LPR and the above mentioned factors.

Conclusions

LPR prevalence in the general Greek population assessed by RSI was found to be 18.8 %. Tobacco smoking and alcohol consumption were found to be related with LPR. RSI is an easy and useful tool in daily clinical practice not only for the diagnosis and management of LPR but also for epidemiological studies.

Abbreviations
LPR: Laryngopharyngeal reflux; LPRD: Laryngopharyngeal reflux disease; GERD: Gastroesophageal reflux disease; RSI: Reflux symptom index; PPIs: Proton pump inhibitors; COPD: Chronic obstructive pulmonary disease; IBS: Irritable bowel syndrome; NSAIDs: Non steroidal anti-inflammatory drugs.

Competing interests
The authors declare that there is no competing of interests regarding the publication of this paper.

Authors' contributions
NS. Conception and design, acquisition of data, analysis and interpretation of data, drafting the manuscript, final approval of the version to be published. ED. Conception and design, acquisition of data, analysis and interpretation of data, drafting the manuscript, final approval of the version to be published. AB. Conception and design, acquisition of data, analysis and interpretation of data, drafting the manuscript, final approval of the version to be published. DA. Conception and design, acquisition of data, analysis and interpretation of data, drafting the manuscript, final approval of the version to be published. All authors read and approved the final manuscript.

Acknowledgment
None.

Funding
This research received no specific grant from any funding agency, commercial or not-for-profit sectors.

Author details
[1]Athens Speech Language and Swallowing Institute, 10 Lontou Street, Glyfada, Athens 16675, Greece. [2]Athens Speech Language and Swallowing Institute, 37 Oinois Street, Glyfada, Athens 16674, Greece. [3]Athens Speech and Language Institute, 1 Griva Digeni Street, Agios Dimitrios, Athens 17342, Greece. [4]Department of Otorhinolaryngology, University Hospital of Ioannina, Medical School of Ioannina University, 51 Napoleontos Zerva Street, Ioannina 45332, Greece.

References
1. Koufman JA, Aviv JE, Casiano RR, Shaw YG. Laryngopharyngeal reflux: position statement of the Committee on Speech, Voice, and Swallowing Disorders of the American Academy of Otolaryngology-Head and Neck Surgery. Otolaryngol Head Neck Surg. 2002;127:32–5.
2. Cheung TK, Lam PK, Wei WI, Wong WM, Ng ML, Gu Q, et al. Quality of life in patients with laryngopharyngeal reflux. Digestion. 2009;79:52–7.
3. Belafsky PC, Postma GN, Koufman JA. Validity and reliability of the reflux symptom index (RSI). J Voice. 2002;16:274–7.
4. Lin CC, Wang YY, Wang KL, Lien HC, Liang MT, Yen TT, et al. Association of heartburn and laryngopharyngeal symptoms with endoscopic reflux esophagitis, smoking, and drinking. Otolaryngol Head Neck Surg. 2009;141(2):264–71.
5. Sanghoon P, Hoon JC, Bora K, Chang-Sub U, Seung-Kuk B, Kwang-Yoon J, et al. An electron microscopic study—Correlation of gastroesophageal reflux disease and laryngopharyngeal reflux. Laryngoscope. 2010;120:1303–8.

6. Habermann W, Schmid C, Neumann K, DeVaney T, Hammer H. Reflux symptom index and reflux finding score in otolaryngologic practice. J Voice. 2012;26(3):e123–7.

7. Feng GJ, Zhang LH, Zhao LL, Liu YL. A pilot study on diagnosing laryngopharyngeal reflux disease by pH monitoring in laryngopharynx. Zhonghua Yi Xue Za Zhi. 2008;88(12):805–8.

8. Gupta R, Sataloff RT. Laryngopharyngeal reflux: current concepts and questions. Curr Opin Otolaryngol Head Neck Surg. 2009;17(3):143–8.

9. Reulbach TR, Belafsky PC, Blalock PD, Koufman JA, Postma GN. Occult laryngeal pathology in a community-based cohort. Otolaryngol Head Neck Surg. 2001;124:448–50.

10. Koufman JA. The Otolaryngologic manifestations of gastroesophageal reflux disease (GERD): A clinical investigation of 225 patients using ambulatory 24 h pH monitoring and an experimental investigation of the role of acid and pepsin in the development of laryngeal injury. Laryngoscope. 1991;101 Suppl 52:1–78.

11. Hopkins C, Yousaf U, Pedersen M. Acid reflux treatment for hoarseness. The Cochrane Database of Systematic Reviews 2006, Issue 1. Art. No.: CD005054. doi:10.1002/14651858.CD005054.pub2.

12. Vincent DA, Garrett JD, Radionoff SL, Reussner LA, Stasney CR. The proximal probe in esophageal pH monitoring: development of a normative database. J Voice. 2000;14(2):247–54.

13. Ozturk O, Oz F, Karakullukcu B, Oghan F, Guclu E, Ada M. Hoarseness and laryngopharyngeal reflux: a cause and effect relationship or coincidence? Eur Arch Otorhinolaryngol. 2006;263:935–9.

14. Sone M, Katayama N, Kato T, Izawa K, Wada M, Hamajima N, et al. Prevalence of laryngopharyngeal reflux symptoms: comparison between health checkup examinees and patients with otitis media. Otolaryng Head Neck Surg. 2012;146:562–6.

15. Reavis KM, Morris CD, Gopal DV, Hunter JG, Jobe BA. Laryngopharyngeal reflux symptoms better predict the presence of esophageal adenocarcinoma than typical gastroesophageal reflux symptoms. Ann Surg. 2004;239:849–56.

16. Galli J, Cammarota G, Volante M, De Corso E, Almadori G, Paludetti G. Laryngeal carcinoma and laryngo-pharyngeal reflux disease. Acta Otorhinolaryng Ital. 2006;26:260–3.

17. Lowden M, McGlashan JA, Steel A, Strugala V, Dettmar P. Prevalence of symptoms suggestive of extra-oesophageal reflux in a general practice population in UK. Logoped Phoniatr Vocol. 2009;34:32–5.

18. Kamani T, Penney S, Midra I, Pothula V. The prevalence of laryngopharyngeal reflux in the English population. Eur Arch Otorhinolaryngol. 2012. doi:10.1007/S00405-012-2028-1.

19. Printza A, Kyrgidis A, Oikonomidou E, Triaridis S. Assessing laryngopharyngeal reflux symptoms with the reflux symptom index: validation and prevalence in the Greek population. Otolaryngol Head Neck Surg. 2011;145:974–80.

20. Gasiorowska A, Poh CH, Fass R. Gastroesophageal reflux disease (GERD) and irritable bowel syndrome (IBS)–is it one disease or an overlap of two disorders? Dig Dis Sci. 2009;54(9):1829–34.

21. Ruigomez A, Rodriguez LA, Wallander MA, Johansson S, Graffner H, Dent J. Natural history of gastro-oesophageal reflux in a general practice population in the UK. Aliment Pharmacol Ther. 2004;20:751–60.

22. Lai YC, Wang PC, Lin JC. Laryngopharyngeal reflux in patients with reflux esophagitis. World J Gastroenterol. 2008;14(28):4523–8.

23. Saruç M, Aksoy EA, Vardereli E, Karaaslan M, Çiçek B, İnce Ü, et al. Risk factors for laryngopharyngeal reflux. Eur Arch Otorhinolaryngol. 2012;269:1189–94.

24. Thompson WG, Heaton KW. Heart burn and globus in apparently healthy people. Can Med Assoc J. 1982;126:46–8.

25. Martinucci I, de Bortoli N, Savarino E, Nacci A, Romeo SO, Bellini M, et al. Optimal treatment of laryngopharyngeal reflux disease. Ther Adv Chronic Dis. 2013;4:287–301.

18

Frequency of mitochondrial m.1555A > G mutation in Syrian patients with non-syndromic hearing impairment

Hazem Kaheel[1], Andreas Breß[1], Mohamed A. Hassan[1,2,6], Aftab Ali Shah[3], Mutaz Amin[4*], Yousuf H. Y. Bakhit[5] and Marlies Kniper[1]

Abstract

Background: Mitochondrial maternally inherited hearing impairment (HI) appears to be increasing in frequency. The incidence of mitochondrial defects causing HI is estimated to be between 6 and 33% of all hearing deficiencies. Mitochondrial m.1555A > G mutation is the first mtDNA mutation associated with non-syndromic sensorineural deafness and also with aminoglycoside induced HI. Its prevalence varied geographically between different populations.

Methods: We carried out PCR, restriction enzyme based screening, and sequencing of 337 subjects (including 132 patients diagnosed clinically with hereditary deafness) from 54 families from Syria for m.1555A > G mitochondrial mutation.

Results: Mitochondrial m.1555A > G mutation was detected in one of fifty-four families (1.85%), six out of the 132 (4.5%) of all patients with NSHI and one propositus of the 205 individuals with normal hearing (0.48%).

Conclusion: This is the first study to report prelingual deafness causative gene mutations identified by sequencing technology in Syrian families. It is obvious from the results that the testing for the m.1555A > G mutation is useful for diagnosis of hearing loss in Syrian patients and should also be considered prior to treatment with aminoglycosides in predisposed individuals.

Keywords: m.1555A > G, Non-syndromic, Hearing impairment, Syria, mtDNA

Background

Hearing impairments (HI) is as one of the most disabling disorders in the world, limiting a person's ability to communicate with others [1]. It is caused by genetic and/or environmental factors. Genetically caused HI is 70% non-syndromic and 30% syndromic [2], with each form related to specific genes. Non-syndromic hearing impairment (NSHI) is isolated hearing deficit without other medical derangements [3]. It affects about 0.1% of live newborns and 4% of all people below 45 years of age [4]. This number increases dramatically in countries and regions where consanguineous marriages are common, like Syria and other Middle Eastern countries [5–7]. Up to 75–80% of cases of non-syndromic hearing impairment have an autosomal recessive cause, 10–15% inherited as autosomal dominant, and few are X-linked or mitochondrial [8].

Mitochondria are intracellular organelles that contain their own DNA (mtDNA). A substitution of A- > G nitrogenous bases in position 1555 of the mitochondrial *12S rRNA* gene is the most prevalent mutation in the mitochondrial genome, associated with both late onset and congenital NSHI. It is of particular interest being a key cause of antibiotic-induced HI [9]. This mutation occurs in a highly conserved region of the *12S rRNA* gene, where aminoglycosides are known to bind and result in defective ATP production in cochlear cells [10].

The m.1555A > G mutation has been identified in more than 120 families throughout the world with frequencies differing according to the population's ethnic group [11–14]. So far, no report exists regarding the involvement of the mtDNA mutations in pathogenesis of deafness in Syria. Syria is a country in the Middle East,

* Correspondence: mtz88@hotmail.co.uk
[4]Department of Biochemistry, Faculty of Medicine, University of Khartoum, P. O. Box 102, Khartoum, Sudan
Full list of author information is available at the end of the article

along the eastern shore of the Mediterranean Sea. The purpose of this study was to determine the prevalence of m.1555A > G mitochondrial mutation among patients with NSHI from Syria.

Methods

All subjects were recruited from Aleppo, which lies in the northwestern region of Syria, with the help of deafness related schools and institutes. The examined group consisted of 337 subjects including 132 affected patients from 54 Syrian families with 2 or more affected subjects (up to 6) with prelingual, profound, sensorineural, bilateral, non-syndromic hearing loss and 205 unrelated healthy controls.

Patients

In this study 175 females and 162 males were participated, with an age range between two and 72 years (mean age 18.2 years). Detailed family pedigrees were drawn. Information on consanguinity, age at onset of HL, detailed prenatal and perinatal history, use of ototoxic drugs (aminoglycosides), etc. was obtained through a detailed questionnaire. Physical examination was performed to exclude syndromic forms of hearing impairment at Alrazi Hospital (Aleppo), ENT examination such as Tympanometry, and BERA (Brainstem Electric Response Audiometry) were also applied at ENT department of the hospital Alrazi.

Mutation Screening

10 ml of peripheral venous blood was obtained from each affected and healthy family members. Genomic DNA was extracted using Qiagen FlexiGene kits in accordance with the manufacturer's instructions. Mitochondrial DNA m.1555A > G mutation was detected using PCR-RFLP strategy (m.1555A > G, F: AGAAAT GGGCTACATTTTCTACCC; m.1555A > G, R: GTTCG TCCAAGTGCACCTTCCA) as mentioned in [15] followed by BsmAI-digest (site: GTC TCN/) (New England Bio Labs®). Products with m.1555A > G mutation showed one band with 248 bp and wild individual displayed two bands (192 bp and 56 bp) after polyacrylamide gel electrophoresis (6%)(Fig. 1a).

The presence of the m.1555A > G mutation was verified using standard Sanger sequencing. Detected mutation was confirmed at least two times and compared with the reference sequence (NC_012920).

Results

The m.1555A > G mutation was found in only one out of 54 families with NSHI(Fig. 1a). The family consisted of four generations. The m.1555A > G mutation was detected in six out of the 132 NSHI patients and in one of the 205 individuals with normal hearing. This result was confirmed by direct sequencing of the corresponding PCR product (Fig. 1b).

The family pedigree of patients with m.1555A > G mutation is shown in Fig. 2. Proposita (I: 2, Fig. 2.) is a 72 year old female with age related hearing impairment (presbycusis). She had eight offspring (4 males and 4 females) all with congenital, profound, bilateral and sensorineural deafness since childhood in accordance with mitochondrial inheritance (Fig. 2). Unfortunately drug history of aminoglycoside usage in this family was

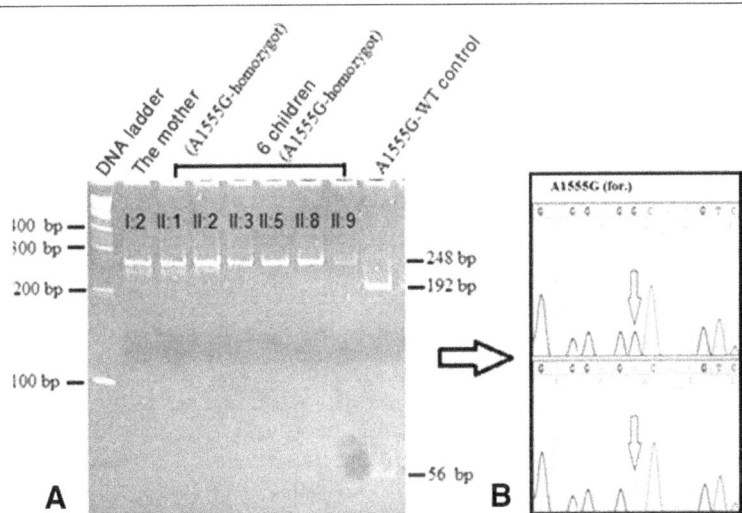

Fig. 1 (a): PCR-RFLP analysis of the only Syrian family found with m.1555A > G mutation: a 248 bp PCR fragment is digested with BsmAI. DNA ladder (the first panel). The wild-type mtDNA is cleaved in to tow fragments, 192 and 56 bp in length (the last panel). PCR product containing the m.1555A > G mutation is not cleaved (the other left panels). **(b):** Partial Sequence chromatograms from a normal hearing individual (down) and affected proband with the m.1555A > G mutation in the mitochondrial *12S rRNA* gene (top) with the forward and reverse primers. The small arrows indicate the localization of the change of an Adenine to Guanine nucleotide at position 1555 of the *12S rRNA* gene

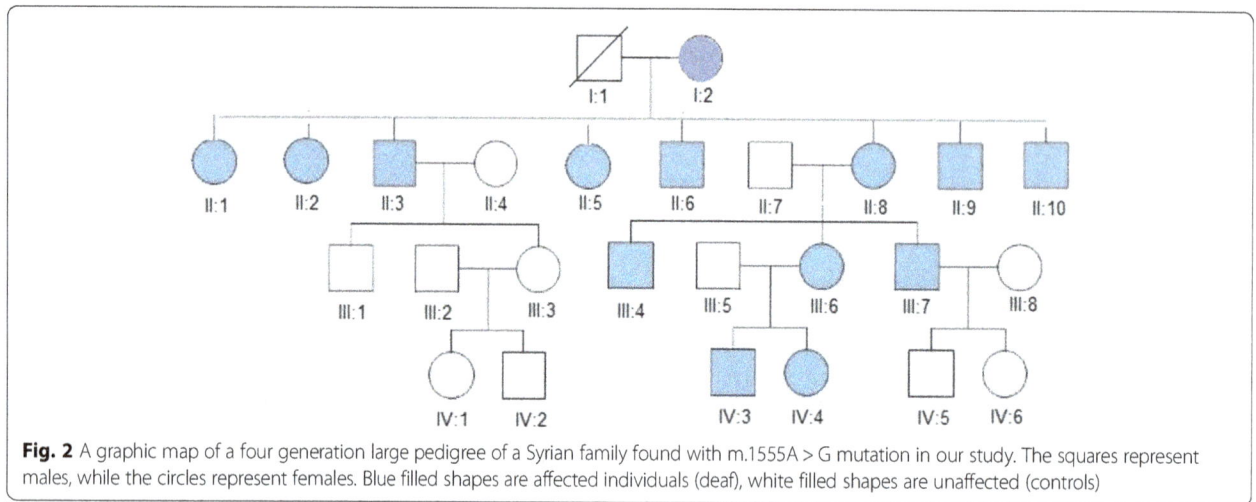

Fig. 2 A graphic map of a four generation large pedigree of a Syrian family found with m.1555A > G mutation in our study. The squares represent males, while the circles represent females. Blue filled shapes are affected individuals (deaf), white filled shapes are unaffected (controls)

unavailable. The m.1555A > G mutation in the mitochondrial *12S rRNA* gene was found in this mother and all her investigated offspring (Fig. 2).

Discussion

The mtDNA m.1555A > G mutation is the most prevalent mutation of mitochondrial genome, associated with both late onset and congenital NSHI, with aminoglycoside-induced hearing loss, in people with different ethnic backgrounds [16]. This is the first study to report the prevalence of m.1555A > G mitochondrial mutation in Syria, one of the Middle East countries. We found the m.1555A > G mutation in one out fifty-four families (1.85%), six out of the 132 NSHI patients (4.5%) and one proposita of the 205 individuals with a normal hearing (0.48%). It shows that the average frequency of the m.1555A > G mutation is 1.85% in the Syrian deaf population. Similar results were previously found in Egypt [17] and reports from other Caucasian populations [7, 12, 18], but not other Middle Eastern countries like Qatar [19], and Iran [20] probably due to the ethnic differences between these populations and the population under study.

Even though it has now been clearly shown that the Prevalence this mutation (1.85%) is not so high in familial cases in Syria, it has nevertheless a very important role. Detection of this mutation would delay the onset of the disease or even prevent it through a lifelong strict avoidance of taking aminoglycosides. When indicated, such a genetic analysis prior to the administration of aminoglycosides would be very valuable, since even a single, small parenteral administration may cause bilateral deafness as a serious side effect.. These findings will help the establishment of effective diagnosis for nonsyndromic hearing loss, improve genetic counselling, and serve as a potential therapeutic platform in the future for the affected patients in Syria.

Conclusion

This is the first study to report prelingual deafness causative gene mutations identified by sequencing technology in Syrian families. It is obvious from the results that the testing for the m.1555A > G mutation is useful for diagnosis of hearing loss in Syrian patients and should also be considered prior to treatment with aminoglycosides in predisposed individuals.

Abbreviations
ATP: Adenosine Tri Phosphate; ENT: Ear Nose Throat; HI: Hearing Impairement; mDNA: mitochondrial Deoxy-ribonucleic Acid; NSHI: Non-syndromic Hearing Impairment; PCR: Polymerase Chain Reaction

Acknowledgements
This study was supported by the *Jürgen ManchotStiftung*, we thank all the families, patients and control individuals for their cooperation in this study.

Authors' contributions
HK designed the study, AB, MH and AS collected and analysed the data, MA and YB wrote the manuscript, MK revised and critically appraised it. All authors read and approved the final manuscript.

Competing interests
The authors declare that they have no competing interests.

Author details
[1]University, HNO –universities Klink-Tubingen, Tubingen, Germany.
[2]Department of Bioinformatics, Africa city of technology, Khartoum, Sudan.
[3]Faculty of Biotechnology, University of Malakand, Khyber Pakhtunkhwa, Pakistan. [4]Department of Biochemistry, Faculty of Medicine, University of Khartoum, P. O. Box 102, Khartoum, Sudan. [5]Department of Basic Medical Sciences, Faculty of Dentistry-University of Khartoum, Khartoum, Sudan.
[6]Division of Molecular Genetics, Institute of Human Genetics, University of Tübingen, Tübingen, Germany, African city of Technology, Khartoum, Sudan.

References
1. Newborn Hearing Screening: Overview, Prevalence of Hearing Loss, The High-Risk Register [Internet]. [cited 2017 Apr 16]. Available from: http://emedicine.medscape.com/article/836646-overview
2. Smith RJ, Shearer AE, Hildebrand MS, Van Camp G. Deafness and Hereditary Hearing Loss Overview [Internet]. GeneReviews(®). University of Washington, Seattle; 1993 [cited 2017 Apr 16]. Available from: http://www.ncbi.nlm.nih.gov/pubmed/20301607

3. Schrijver I. Hereditary non-syndromic sensorineural hearing loss: transforming silence to sound. J Mol Diagn [Internet]. 2004 Nov [cited 2017 Apr 16];6(4):275–84. Available from: http://www.ncbi.nlm.nih.gov/pubmed/15507665.

4. Smith RJ, Jones M-KN. Nonsyndromic Hearing Loss and Deafness, DFNB1 [Internet]. GeneReviews(®). University of Washington, Seattle; 1993 [cited 2017 Apr 18]. Available from: http://www.ncbi.nlm.nih.gov/pubmed/20301449

5. Othman H, Saadat M. Prevalence of consanguineous marriages in syria. J Biosoc Sci [Internet]. 2009 Sep 12 [cited 2017 Apr 18];41(5):685. Available from: http://www.ncbi.nlm.nih.gov/pubmed/19433003

6. Essammak BF, Ashour MJ, Sharif FA. Non-Syndromic autosomal recessive deafness in Gaza strip: A study of five GJB2 Gene mutations. Int J Genet Genomics [Internet]. 2014 [cited 2017 Apr 18];2(5):92–96. Available from: http://www.sciencepublishinggroup.com/j/ijgg

7. Bener A, Mohammad RR. Global distribution of consanguinity and their impact on complex diseases: Genetic disorders from an endogamous population. Egypt J Med Hum Genet [Internet]. 2017 [cited 2017 Apr 18]; Available from: http://www.sciencedirect.com/science/article/pii/S1110863017300174

8. Bitner-Glindzicz M. Hereditary deafness and phenotyping in humans. Br Med Bull [Internet]. 2002 Oct 1 [cited 2017 Apr 18];63(1):73–94. Available from: https://academic.oup.com/bmb/article-lookup/doi/10.1093/bmb/63.1.73

9. Perez-Fernandez D, Shcherbakov D, Matt T, Leong NC, Kudyba I, Duscha S, et al. 4'-O-substitutions determine selectivity of aminoglycoside antibiotics. Nat Commun [Internet]. 2014 Jan 28 [cited 2017 Apr 18];5:486–501. Available from: http://www.nature.com/doifinder/10.1038/ncomms4112

10. Min-Xin G. Mitochondrial DNA Mutations Associated with Aminoglycoside Ototoxicity. J Otol [Internet]. 2006 [cited 2017 Apr 18];1(2):65–75. Available from: http://www.sciencedirect.com/science/article/pii/S1672293006500169

11. Ouyang XM, Yan D, Yuan HJ, Pu D, Du LL, Han DY, et al. The genetic bases for non-syndromic hearing loss among Chinese. J Hum Genet [Internet]. 2009 Mar [cited 2017 Apr 18];54(3):131–140. Available from: http://www.ncbi.nlm.nih.gov/pubmed/19197336

12. Bae JW, Kim D-B, Choi JY, Park H-J, Lee JD, Hur DG, et al. Molecular and Clinical Characterization of the Variable Phenotype in Korean Families with Hearing Loss Associated with the Mitochondrial A1555G Mutation. Moran M, editor. PLoS One [Internet]. 2012 Aug 6 [cited 2017 Apr 18];7(8):e42463. Available from: http://dx.plos.org/10.1371/journal.pone.0042463

13. Estivill X, Govea N, Barceló A, Perelló E, Badenas C, Romero E, et al. Familial Progressive Sensorineural Deafness Is Mainly Due to the mtDNA A1555G Mutation and Is Enhanced by Treatment with Aminoglycosides. Am J Hum Genet. 1998;62(1):27–35.

14. Giordano C, Pallotti F, Walker WF, Checcarelli N, Musumeci O, Santorelli F, et al. Pathogenesis of the deafness-associated A1555G mitochondrial DNA mutation. Biochem Biophys Res Commun. 2002;293(1):521–9.

15. Kupka S, Tóth T, Wróbel M, Zeißler U, Szyfter W, Szyfter K, et al. Mutation A1555G in the 12S rRNA gene and its epidemiological importance in German, Hungarian, and Polish patients. Hum Mutat [Internet]. 2002 Mar 1 [cited 2017 Aug 21];19(3):308–309. Available from: http://doi.wiley.com/10.1002/humu.9017

16. Liu XZ, Angeli S, Ouyang XM, Liu W, Ke XM, Liu YH, et al. Audiological and genetic features of the mtDNA mutations. Acta Otolaryngol [Internet]. 2008 Jul [cited 2017 Apr 18];128(7):732–738. Available from: http://www.ncbi.nlm.nih.gov/pubmed/18568513

17. Fassad MR, Desouky LM, Asal S, Abdalla EM. Screening for the mitochondrial A1555G mutation among Egyptian patients with non-syndromic, sensorineural hearing loss. Int J Mol Epidemiol Genet [Internet]. 2014 [cited 2017 Aug 21];5(4):200–204. Available from: http://www.ncbi.nlm.nih.gov/pubmed/25755848

18. Berthomieu B, Menasche M. An enumerative approach for analyzing time Petri nets [Internet]. Proceedings IFIP. 1983:41–6. Available from: http://citeseerx.ist.psu.edu/viewdoc/summary?doi=10.1.1.11.4063

19. Khalifa Alkowari M, Girotto G, Abdulhadi K, Dipresa S, Siam R, Najjar N, et al. GJB2 and GJB6 genes and the A1555G mitochondrial mutation are only minor causes of nonsyndromic hearing loss in the Qatari population. Int J Audiol [Internet]. 2012 Mar 21 [cited 2017 Aug 21];51(3):181–185. Available from: http://www.ncbi.nlm.nih.gov/pubmed/22103400

20. Zohour MM, Tabatabaiefar MA, Dehkordi FA, Farrokhi E, Akbari MT, Chaleshtori MH. Large-Scale Screening of Mitochondrial DNA Mutations Among Iranian Patients with Prelingual Nonsyndromic Hearing Impairment. Genet Test Mol Biomarkers [Internet]. 2012 Apr [cited 2017 Aug 21];16(4):271–278. Available from: http://www.ncbi.nlm.nih.gov/pubmed/22077646

19

Knowledge and care seeking practices for ear infections among parents of under five children in Kigali, Rwanda

Kaitesi Batamuliza Mukara[1*], Peter Waiswa[2], Richard Lilford[3] and Debara Lyn Tucci[4]

Abstract

Background: Infections affecting the middle ear are a common childhood occurrence. Some cases may present with ear discharge through a tympanic membrane perforation which may heal spontaneously. However, up to 5% or more cases of those affected have persistent ear discharge. A number of barriers contribute towards delayed presentation at health facilities for treatment of ear infections. We conducted a study to evaluate parents' and caregivers' knowledge and care seeking practices for ear infections in children under five in Gasabo district in Kigali, Rwanda.

Methods: Parents/guardians ($n = 810$) were interviewed using a structured questionnaire to elicit their knowledge of ear infections in children under five and their attitude to seeking care for their children.

Results: The mean age of the respondents was 31.27 years (SD = 7.88, range 17–83). Considering an average of knowledge parameters which included causes, symptoms, prevention, treatment and consequences of ear infections, we found that 76.6% (622) of respondents were knowledgeable about ear infections. We defined a positive practice as seeking medical treatment (community health workers or health facility) and this was found in 89.1% (722) respondents. Correlating knowledge with choice of seeking treatment, respondents were 33% less likely to practice medical pluralism (OR = 0.33, CI 0.11–0.97, $P = 0.043$) if they were familiar with infections. Moreover, urban dweller were 1.7 times more likely to know ear infections compared to rural dwellers (OR = 1.70, CI 1.22–2.38, $P = 0.002$).

Conclusion: The majority of respondents had good knowledge and positive attitudes and practices about ear infection. However, medical pluralism was common. There is need to improve the community's awareness and access to primary health care facilities for the care of ear infections especially in rural areas of Rwanda.

Keywords: Ear infections, Parents, Knowledge, Care seeking, Under five

Background

Infections affecting the middle ear are a diverse entity and a common childhood occurrence [1–4]. Acute otitis media (AOM) is an inflammation of the middle ear mucosa presenting acutely with symptoms of otalgia and fever [4]. These infections account for the majority

of antibiotic prescriptions in young children [3, 4]. The trend of prescribing antibiotics for acute ear infections continues to grow. Guidelines for treatment of AOM have advocated a 'wait and see' [3], as up to 80% of those affected show spontaneous resolution [4]. By the 3rd birthday, 80% of children have had at least one episode of acute otitis media [5]. Some cases of acute ear infection may present with ear discharge through a tympanic membrane perforation. The perforation may heal spontaneously in 2–14 days [4]. However, up to 41% of cases have persistent ear discharge; chronic

* Correspondence: kaibat@hotmail.com
[1]ENT department, College of medicine and health Sciences, University of Rwanda, and Health Policy, Planning and Management, Makerere University School of Public Health, Kampala, Uganda
Full list of author information is available at the end of the article

suppurative otitis media (CSOM) [6]. This disease entity also presents with symptoms of tinnitus, hearing loss and persistent discharge refractive to medical treatment usually implying cholesteatoma. Treatment is by antibiotic ear drops and surgery for repair of the persistent tympanic membrane perforation and treatment of complications. Complications are dire and include neck abscesses, mastoiditis, facial nerve paralysis, labyrinthitis, lateral sinus thrombosis, meningitis and brain abscess [4, 7].

It is estimated that 330 million people have CSOM of which 60% have hearing loss; the majority of those affected are children [5]. Hearing loss adversely affects speech and language development and school performance in children [1, 8–10] and may eventually diminish prospects for gainful employment in adulthood. Moreover, 28,000 deaths are attributed to complications due to CSOM [7]. Data on ear infections in sub-Saharan Africa is limited. Published studies estimate CSOM among school going children at 1.6% reported in Tanzania [11] and 2.4% in Kenya [12]. Babigambe (2005) reported a prevalence of 13.2% of CSOM among children aged 6–60 months living in a slum in Uganda [13].

Compelling evidence shows that the painless nature of CSOM renders it an overlooked condition [14–17]. For instance, in their study on prevalence of CSOM among children living in two slums of Dhaka City in Bangladesh, Kamal and Joarder (2014) found that a third of mothers of children examined and found to have CSOM were not aware that their child had this condition, and neither were they aware of the possible sequelae of untreated disease. Moreover, 60% of mothers were not familiar with CSOM nor its treatment and 47% of those who had CSOM, did not seek treatment for it [18].

Risky health seeking practices have been shown to significantly contribute towards an increase in otitis media [19]. In this paper, risky health seeking behaviour is defined as seeking curative services from a source other than that recognised by the Rwandan Health system to treat ear infections. This includes self-medicating with the use of herbs or any other alternative treatment. This definition is modified from the World Health Organisation's (WHO) working definition [20].

Optimal health seeking behaviour often depends on accessibility of health facilities coupled with knowledge and understanding of the benefit of modern medical treatment as opposed to local customs and beliefs [21–23]. Regarding use of traditional medicine, the WHO states that *"rampant poverty is the prime cause for use, misuse and abuse of traditional medicine"* [20]. Cultural beliefs could supersede education even among people with high literacy levels living in regions with strong cultural beliefs and practices, thus resulting in unhealthy care seeking practices [24].

Unpublished clinical data in Rwanda shows a high prevalence of ear infections in 2013. Up to 21% of patients seen in the ENT department at a referral hospital were diagnosed with ear infections, among whom were young adults who report having infections since childhood. Not only have clinicians noticed delays in presentation for those seeking treatment, but also noted reports of patients using traditional medicine for ear infections regardless of high access to medical insurance. Against this background, we conducted this study to determine the extent of knowledge and care seeking practices of parents and care givers for ear infections in children under 5.

Methods
Study design, setting and population
This was a community based study conducted in Gasabo district, one of the 3 districts of Kigali City with a population of 530,907 inhabitants (national census, 2012) and a population density of 1237 persons per square kilometre. It has both rural and urban settlements with 486 villages, 229 of which are rural while 257 are urban [25]. This district is home to one Private referral hospital which offers ENT services among others as well as 3 district hospitals, 17 health centres and 20 functional health posts. According to Integrated Household Living Conditions Survey (EICV3) of 2010/11, the mean transit time by foot to a health facility in Gasabo district is 43.6 min [26]. Each village has 100–150 households and is supervised by 2 Community Health Workers (CHW) called cell coordinators, assisted by 1 assistant cell coordinator.

Data collection
Using random tables, we sampled 30 villages. CHWs provided a list of households with children aged below 5 years in the sampled villages from which 27 households within each village and an extra 3 households for replacement were sampled. One child from an eligible household was selected using Kish table.

The set exclusion criteria was parents who refused to consent to participate in the study or who refused to give consent for their children to participate. However, no respondent was excluded. A total of 810 parents or guardians were interviewed and 810 children of these parents examined.

We collected data in March 2016. Experienced research assistants carried out data collection while two trained medical students in their ENT clerkship examined the children. We collected data regarding demographics, household characteristics and assets, knowledge, perceptions and care practices of the parents or guardians regarding ear infections. Additional file 1 shows the questionnaire used for data collection.

Quality control and ethics

Before starting data collection, we held a 1 day training of research assistants where they were familiarised with the study, the questionnaire and data collection procedure. A pre-test session was conducted in a different district of Rwanda and changes incorporated into the pre-designed questionnaire. Our study proposal was submitted and approved by both the College of Medicine and Health Sciences Research Ethics Committee of the University of Rwanda (approval notice: No. 355/CMHS IRB/2015) and the Makerere University School of Public Health Higher Degree Research and Ethics Committee (approval date: 07th December 2015). Parents or guardians with children under 5 in their household provided written consent availed to them both in Kinyarwanda and English to participate in the study.

Data analysis

We entered data using CSpro 6.2 software after which we performed data cleaning aided by the same software. We used STATA 13.0 for statistical analysis. Given the wide range in the age of respondents, we classified the age into groups with 15 years class interval as follows ≤30, 31–45, 46–60 and >60. Although this last group includes respondents aged 61–83 years, there were only 7 respondents and this was considered a single group.

Knowledge about ear infections and care seeking practices were derived as frequencies and proportions of the responses obtained. Knowledge was subdivided into causes, symptoms, prevention, treatment and consequences of ear infections. The following responses were considered causes of ear infections: poor hygiene, wetting the ears, wax, foreign body and/or microbes. Ear discharge, hearing loss and pain are the cardinal symptoms of ear infections. Respondents who knew 2 of the 3 or any other symptoms were considered knowledgeable of symptoms. Prevention and treatment parameters were rated as 'yes' or 'no' and respondents who reported 'yes' were considered knowledgeable. Respondents who reported hearing loss, persistence of disease, extension into adjacent structures and death as consequences of hearing loss were considered knowledgeable.

We defined a positive practice as seeking medical treatment (CHW or health facility) while positive attitude was derived from responses for choice for treatment seeking and the reason for seeking alternative treatment. Respondents who reported 'not being worried', 'no need for treatment', and 'incurable' were categorised as negative attitude. Moreover choice for information seeking (CHW, health professional) was categorised as positive attitude. To build a knowledge, attitude and practices model, a sum average of each of the responses for each parameter was computed. Additional file 1 gives details of positive and negative ratings for knowledge, attitude and practices.

Socioeconomic status (SES) was derived using Principal Component analysis computed using STATA. We weighted variables of household size and occupancy, source of water supply, types of flooring materials, sanitation facilities and assets. The mean SES was computed and categorised in to Low, Middle and High.

Chi square test and logistic regression analysis were used to derive associations between knowledge of the parents or guardians, SES, residence (urban or rural) and their care seeking practices. The level of significance was set at $p < 0.05$.

Results

We obtained data for 810 respondents whose results we present. Results from the examination of children will be presented in a subsequent paper.

Parents'/guardians' characteristics

The majority of respondents were female; 96% (777). The mean age was 31.27 years (SD = 7.88, range 17–83). A higher proportion of eligible parents took part in the study in urban areas compared to rural areas, accounting for 53% (432) of the study sample. Forty-seven percent (383) of respondents fell in the low SES while 12% (95) were in the high SES category. Fifty eight percent (465) had completed primary school education. More details are shown in Table 1 below.

Knowledge and perceptions of ear infections

Sixty-nine percent (561) said they were aware of ear infections, 88.4% (716) said they could be treated while 67.4% (546) said they could actually be prevented. Ear

Table 1 Socio-demographic characteristics of the respondents

Characteristic		Frequency (n = 810)	Percent
Gender	Males	33	4
	Females	777	96
Age group	≤30	429	52.9
	31–45	346	42.7
	46–60	28	3.5
	>60	7	0.9
Average age	31.27 years		
Residence	Rural	378	46.7
	Urban	432	53.3
Level of education	None	50	6.2
	Primary	465	57.5
	Secondary	220	27.2
	Vocational	74	9.1
Socioeconomic status	Low	383	47.3
	Middle	332	41
	High	95	11.7

infections were perceived to be caused by poor hygiene in 50.4% (408) of respondents and water entering the ear in 27% (219).

Hearing loss was the most common consequence of ear infections. This was reported by 94% (764) of respondents. Other consequences included poor performance in school reported by 26% (212), persistence of the disease, 14% (115), extension of disease to other organs, 13% (106) and death 7% (70). In contrast, 3% (25) respondents said that ear infections have no consequences.

Table 2 above gives details on knowledge among respondents. We computed the average knowledge of respondents considering all knowledge parameters and found that 76.6% (622) of respondents were knowledgeable about ear infections. Moreover, 47% (381) and 8.5% (69) respondents knew two symptoms or three or more symptoms of ear infections respectively.

Using bivariate and multivariate analysis, there was no statistically significant difference in knowledge when we compared age groups, level of education or socioeconomic status. However, rural dwellers were 1.7 times more likely to have knowledge about ear infections compared to urban dwellers both on bivariate and multivariate analysis as shown in Table 3 below. While respondents were a third of times less likely to practice medical pluralism if they knew about ear infections on bivariate analysis, this was not significant at multivariate analysis.

Attitudes towards ear infections

A positive attitude was found in 79.6% (645) respondents. This entailed averaged evaluation of the reasons for their reported choice of treatment seeking, their rating of services provided by the health system as well as the source of information.

Respondents in the 31–45 age range were 50% less likely to have negative attitudes compared to other age groups. Similarly, respondents with secondary education or higher and respondents from middle socioeconomic status were less likely to have a negative attitude towards ear infections. Respondents with a positive attitude were 1 in 5 times less likely to seek treatment at both modern and traditional healers compared to those with a negative attitude. These results were significant both on bivariate and multivariate analysis as shown in Table 4 below.

Care seeking practices with regards to ear infections

Practices were established considering where parents sought information and treatment. Positive practices was found in 89.1% (722) of respondents.

While as 96% (780) of respondents would seek treatment from a health facility, 19% (153) would seek help from a traditional healer. The main reason for seeking traditional treatment was poverty (low affordability) 66% (538), ignorance and lack of knowledge in 62% (504) and lack of a health insurance 41% (333). Community health workers and health professionals were the preferred source of health information for 77% (621) and 60% (452) respondents respectively. Table 5 gives further detail.

Urban dwellers were almost 2 times more likely than rural dwellers to have health enhancing practices for ear infections (OR = 1.85, CI 1.18–2.90, P = 0.008). Comparing education with practices, we found that while respondents with secondary and higher education were twice likely to have positive practices, (OR = 2.08, CI 0.89–4.87, P = 0.091), respondents with vocational education were almost 8 times more likely to have positive practices (OR = 7.90, CI 1.62–38.34, P = 0.010). Table 6 below elaborates these findings further.

Discussion

In this study which assessed knowledge and care seeking practices of parents of under-five children with ear infections, we found that the majority (76.6%) of respondents were knowledgeable about ear infections while 89.1% had positive care seeking practices. We found no relationship between age group of parent and knowledge of ear infections nor care seeking practices. However, parents in the age range of 31–45 years were less likely to have negative attitudes to healthy care seeking compared to other age groups. We found no study looking at the influence of parental age on care seeking practices to compare with our results. Those who practiced medical pluralism or sought traditional treatment attributed it to poverty (low affordability) in 66% while 62% and 41% cited ignorance (lack of knowledge) and lack of a health insurance respectively. These findings are similar to

Table 2 Knowledge of respondents on ear infections

		Frequency	Percent
Knowledge of symptoms of ear infections	None	61	7.5
	1 symptom	299	36.9
	2 symptoms	381	47.0
	≥3 symptoms	69	8.5
Knowledge about prevention	Yes	546	67.4
	No	264	32.6
Knowledge about treatment	Yes	716	88.4
	No	94	11.6
Knowledge of causes of ear infections	Yes	525	64.8
	No	285	35.2
Knowledge about consequences of infections	Yes	789	97.4
	No	21	2.6

Table 3 Knowledge of ear infections

| | Knowledge of ear infections | | | |
	Crude OR (CI)	P-value	Adjusted OR (CI)	P- value
Age group				
≤ 30	1		1	
31–45	0.8 (0.57–1.12)	0.192	0.89(0.62–1.26)	0.511
46–60	2(0.91–4.40)	0.086	2.26(0.10–5.12)	0.064
> 60	0.51(0.61–4.32)	0.54	0.57(0.06–4.92)	0.638
Residence				
Rural	1		1	
Urban	1.7(1.22–2.38)	0.002*	1.69(1.17–2.44)	0.003**
Level of education				
None	1		1	
Primary education	1.48(0.67–3.24)	0.333	1.55(0.68–3.53)	0.228
Secondary & higher	1.92(0.85–4.34)	0.116	1.61(0.67–3.84)	0.24
Vocational education	1.69(0.67–4.25)	0.267	1.31(.48–3.60)	0.483
Socioeconomic status				
Low	1		1	
Middle	1.35(0.95–1.91)	0.095	1.25(0.87–1.80)	0.254
High	1.23(0.72–2.09)	0.446	1.13(0.63–2.01)	0.783
Where they would seek treatment				
None	1		1	
Modern treatment	0.47(0.18–1.24)	0.126	0.45(0.17–1.24)	0.123
Traditional medicine	0.62(0.22–1.77)	0.371	0.71 (0.24–2.10)	0.533
Medical pluralism	0.33(0.11–0.97)	0.043*	0.35(0.11–1.04)	0.06

*significant at bivariate analysis, **significant at multivariate analysis

those of Srikanth in their study on knowledge, attitudes and practices with respect to OM in a rural community in India [22], and also Adeyemo [27] in Nigeria where they found low overall knowledge of otitis media. Only 47% of respondents could identify 2 symptoms of ear infections. Ear discharge, hearing loss and pain were the most common symptoms of ear infections reported, while awareness of other symptoms was low. Pain is a key symptom in acute otitis media [2, 28] while ear discharge is an integral pointer to CSOM [2, 29]. This study looked at ear infections globally and the wide range of symptoms is explained by the nature of ear infections. However, responses given depict more knowledge and awareness of CSOM as compared to acute otitis media.

We found a significant difference in knowledge of ear infections among parents living in rural areas compared to urban areas. Parents in rural areas were more likely to seek traditional treatment for ear infections. Our respondents were more likely to seek modern treatment if they were familiar with ear infections, if they had attained secondary education and beyond and if they lived in an urban setting. Consequently, children from rural areas are at a higher risk of delayed presentation or practicing medical pluralism and developing complications. This is alluded to by Shaheen and colleagues who found treatment seeking in favour of traditional medicine [14]. To overcome this, factors found to result in risky health-seeking behaviour in this study like those found in other studies, which include unaffordable health cost, poor point of care service delivery, distance barriers [22, 30], shortage of medicine in health facilities, and lack of involvement of male parents in child care [30] should be addressed. Findings from a study in Nigeria showed that strong traditional beliefs and practices were more important than level of education in making choices on health. Therefore, health promotion activities can go a long way to foster good health seeking practices.

Respondents who sought traditional treatment attributed this to poverty, lack of awareness and lack of insurance. This finding underscores that CSOM is a disease of poverty [31, 32]. Poverty was associated with inability to pay for services as well as failing to meet transport costs even if the child had medical insurance. Currently,

Table 4 Attitude towards ear infections

	Attitudes to ear infections			
	OR (CI)	P-value	Adjusted OR (CI)	P- value
Age group				
≤ 30	1		1	
31–45	0.59(0.41–0.84)	0.004*	0.54 (0.37–.79)	0.001**
46–60	1.27(0.54–2.96)	0.586	1.19(0.49–2.87)	0.704
> 60	1		1	
Residence				
Rural	1		1	
Urban	0.91(0.65–1.28)	0.6	1.07(0.73–1.61)	0.677
Level of education				
None	1		1	
Primary education	1.02(0.51–2.01)	0.962	0.10(0.49–2.09)	0.965
Secondary & higher	0.44(0.21–0.95)	0.037*	0.41(0.18–0.94)	0.034**
Vocational education	0.67(0.28–1.63)	0.383	0.72(0.27–1.94)	0.516
Socioeconomic status				
Low	1		1	
Middle	0.56(0.38–0.81)	0.002*	0.59(0.39–0.87)	0.009**
High	0.65(0.37–1.16)	0.143	0.80(0.42–1.51)	0.487
Where they would seek treatment				
None	1			
Modern treatment	0.58(0.21–1.58)	0.286	0.39(0.14–1.13)	0.082
Traditional medicine	0.45(0.15–1.38)	0.163	0.12(0.09–0.89)	0.031**
Medical pluralism	0.18(0.05–0.59)	0.005*	0.12(0.04–0.43)	0.001**

*significant at bivariate analysis, **significant at multivariate analysis

adherence to the Community Based Health Insurance is 91% having increased steadily since being rolled out in 2000 [33]. Consequently more people are able to visit health facilities resulting in long queues that may be a discouragement to patients especially farmers. Holding a Community Based Health Insurance did not therefore preclude traditional medicine as an option for care seeking among our respondents. Health communication and education drives are necessary to help parents understand the nature of ear infections and their treatment to enhance care seeking practices.

The varying attitude and willingness to seek medical treatment seen among our respondents might be due to low level of knowledge, poverty, unsatisfactory service provision at point of first contact and delays in referral health system factors such as long queues. This finding is reported in other studies [30, 34]. Markedly, up to 85% of patients with CSOM in a study in Bangladesh preferred to seek over the counter treatment from untrained local village drug vendors instead of seeking help from qualified staff [14]. Overall, the social context may have the upper hand in determining care seeking behaviour. Participatory planning and provision of services

involving beneficiaries as well as improvement of services could help increase utilisation of services thus increase awareness, prevention and treatment of ear infections.

The policy and practice implications of these findings include re-thinking inclusion of ear and hearing care among the attributes of CHWs. The WHO has outlined primary ear and hearing care manuals which can be tailored to a local context [35]. The manuals can help to address the lack of awareness and offer guidance to the scope of practice of era and hearing care at the different levels. This will increase awareness among CHWs which will in turn modify care seeking practices among parents. There is need to improve available ear care services at the primary health care facilities to make them the preferred choice of source of care.

Study limitations

This study has several strengths but also some limitations. It is the first of its kind to be conducted in Rwanda. In addition, it was a large study that included both a rural and urban context meaning that the findings could be representative of Rwanda and similar

Table 5 Care seeking practices

		Frequency	Percent
Where they seek treatment	Health facility[a]	780	96
	Traditional medicine[a]	153	19
	Community health worker	68	8
	Self-medication	17	2
	I would not seek treatment	8	1
Why they seek alternative therapy	Poverty[a]	538	66
	Ignorance[a]	504	62
	No health insurance[a]	333	41
	Not worried about it	23	3
	No need, its incurable	17	2
	Others[a]	86	11
Source of information	Community Health worker[a]	621	77
	Health professional[a]	452	60
	Family or neighbours	44	5
	Others	28	4
	I don't need it	8	1
Consequences of infections	Hearing loss[a]	764	94
	Persistence of the disease[a]	115	14
	Extension to other organs[a]	106	13
	Death	70	7
	None	25	3
	Others	16	2

[a]Outcomes with multiple responses

settings elsewhere. The limitations include the fact that the questionnaire was formulated in English then translated into Kinyarwanda and back. However, Kinyarwanda lack terminologies equivalent to those in English causing some responses to be missed or generalized. For instance, ear discharge is synonymous with CSOM in Kinyarwanda yet that is not the case in English nor in this study. In addition, dichotomising knowledge maybe crude since this could have multiple connotations.

Conclusions

The majority of respondents had good knowledge and positive attitudes and practices about ear infection. The preferred point for care seeking is heavily dependent upon knowledge of ear infections and less on age of the parent, gender and SES. Parents in rural settings are more likely to practice medical pluralism. While consequences of ear infections are known, parents still cling to risky health seeking practices for their children. More effort should be put in improving health service accessibility and delivery since this is a barrier to health care seeking practices. Medical professionals and CHW should be educated on ear infection since this is the preferred source of information. More research is required to assess the impact of training and health promotion on knowledge of parents and care seeking practices for ear infections.

Table 6 Practices for ear infections

	Practices of ear infections			
	OR (CI)	P value	Adjusted OR (CI)	P- value
Age group				
≤ 30	1		1	
31–45	0.74(0.47–1.17)	0.202	0.80(0.42–1.56)	0.519
46–60	0.63(0.21–1.92)	0.42	0.17(0.22–6.25)	0.855
> 60	Not computed			
Residence				
Rural	1		1	
Urban	1.85(1.18–2.90)	0.008*		
Level of education				
None	1		1	
Primary education	1.6(0.74–3.48)	0.232	0.98(0.29–3.25)	0.972
Secondary & higher	2.08(0.89–4.87)	0.091	1.65(0.43–6.41)	0.468
Vocational education	7.9(1.62–38.34)	0.01*	2.57(0.34–19.24)	0.359
Socioeconomic status				
Low	1		1	
Middle	1.48(0.91–2.39)	0.112	1.74(0.87–3.48)	0.121
High	1.4(0.67–2.97)	0.377	1.70(0.50–5.77)	0.394

*significant at bivariate analysis

Abbreviations

AOM: Acute otitis media; CHW: Community Health Worker; CSOM: Chronic suppurative otitis media; ENT: Ear, Nose and Throat department; SES: Socioeconomic status; WHO: World Health Organisation

Acknowledgements

Thanks to Mr. Ntambara Juvenal for his insight patience and guidance in data collection and data entry and Drs Kosuke, Hinda and Ndahindwa for guidance in data analysis. Many thanks to CARTA and all facilitators who in one way or another contributed to this work.

Funding

"This research was supported by the Consortium for Advanced Research Training in Africa (CARTA). CARTA is jointly led by the African Population and Health Research Center and the University of the Witwatersrand and funded by the Wellcome Trust (UK) (Grant No: 087547/Z/08/Z), the Department for International Development (DfID) under the Development Partnerships in Higher Education (DelPHE), the Carnegie Corporation of New York (Grant No: B 8606), the Ford Foundation (Grant No: 1100-0399), Google.Org (Grant No: 191994), Sida (Grant No: 54100029) and MacArthur Foundation Grant No: 10-95915-000-INP".

Authors' contributions

All authors were involved in developing the study design and implementation. KBM collected and analysed data while PW, RL and DT provided overall supervision. KBM wrote the draft. PW, RL and DT reviewed the draft and approved the final manuscript. All authors read and approved the final manuscript.

Competing interests

The authors declare that they have no competing interests.

Author details

[1]ENT department, College of medicine and health Sciences, University of Rwanda, and Health Policy, Planning and Management, Makerere University School of Public Health, Kampala, Uganda. [2]Department of Health Policy, Planning and Management, Makerere University School of Public Health, Uganda and Global Health Division, Karolinska Institutet, Stockholm, Sweden. [3]Warwick Medical School, University of Warwick, Coventry, UK. [4]Head and Neck Surgery & Communication Sciences, Duke University, Durham, USA.

References

1. Yiengprugsawan V, Hogan A, Strazdins L. Longitudinal analysis of ear infection and hearing impairment: findings from 6-year prospective cohorts of Australian children. BMC Pediatr. 2013;13:28.
2. Todberg T, et al. Incidence of otitis media in a contemporary Danish National Birth Cohort. PLoS One. 2014;9(12):e111732.
3. Barber C, et al. Acute otitis media in young children - what do parents say? Int J Pediatr Otorhinolaryngol. 2014;78(2):300–6.
4. Qureishi A, et al. Update on otitis media – prevention and treatment. Infect Drug Resist. 2014;7:15–24.
5. Monasta L, et al. Burden of disease caused by otitis media: systematic review and global estimates. PLoS One. 2012;7(4):e36226.
6. Macfadyen C, et al. Topical quinolone vs. antiseptic for treating chronic suppurative otitis media: a randomized controlled trial. Tropical Med Int Health. 2005;10(2):190–7.
7. Acuin J, Chronic suppurative otitis media: burden of illness and management options. 2004.
8. Smith AW. WHO activities for prevention of deafness and hearing impairment in children. Scand Audiol Suppl. 2001;53:93–100.
9. Sanders M, et al. Estimated prevalence of hearing loss and provision of hearing services in Pacific Island nations. J Prim Health Care. 2015;7(1):5–15.
10. Baltussen R, Smith A. Cost-effectiveness of selected interventions for hearing impairment in Africa and Asia: a mathematical modelling approach. Int J Audiol. 2009;48(3):144–58.
11. Bastos I, et al. Middle ear disease and hearing impairment in northern Tanzania. A prevalence study of schoolchildren in the Moshi and Monduli districts. Int J Pediatr Otorhinolaryngol. 1995;32(1):1–12.
12. Smith AW, et al. Randomised controlled trial of treatment of chronic suppurative otitis media in Kenyan schoolchildren. Lancet. 1996;348(9035):1128–33.
13. Babigamba TE, Prevalence and types of chronic suppurative otitis media among children aged six months to five years in slum dwelling of Kamwokya-Kifumbira, Kampala district, in ENT department. 2005, Makerere University.
14. Shaheen MM, Raquib A, Ahmad SM. Chronic suppurative otitis media and its association with socio-econonic factors among rural primary school children of Bangladesh. Indian J Otolaryngol Head Neck Surg. 2012;64(1):36–41.
15. Orji F. A survey of the burden of management of chronic suppurative otitis media in a developing country. Ann Med Health Sci Res. 2013;3(3):598–612.
16. Ologe FE, Nwawolo CC. Prevalence of chronic suppurative otitis media (CSOM) among school children in a rural community in Nigeria. Niger Postgrad Med J. 2002;9(2):63–6.
17. Morris P. Chronic suppurative otitis media. BMJ Clin Evid. 2012;2012. p. 0507.
18. Kamal N, Joarder AH. Prevalence of chronic suppurative otitis media among the children living in two selected slums of Dhaka City. Bangladesh Med Res Counc Bull. 2004;30:95–104.
19. Rupa V, Jacob A, Joseph A. Chronic suppurative otitis media: prevalence and practices among rural South Indian children. Int J Pediatr Otorhinolaryngol. 1999;48:217–24.
20. World Health Organization, WHO traditional medicine strategy 2002-2005. Geneva: 2002.
21. Lasisi AO, Ajuwon JA. Beliefs and Perceptions of Ear, Nose and Throat-Related Conditions among Residents of a Traditional community in Ibadan, Nigeria. Afr J Med Med Sci. 2001;31(1):49–52.
22. Srikanth S, et al. Knowledge, attitudes and practices with respect to risk factors for otitis media in a rural South Indian community. Int J Pediatr Otorhinolaryngol. 2009;73(10):1394–8.
23. Poole N, et al. Knowledge, attitudes, beliefs and practices related to chronic suppurative otitis media and hearing impairment in Pokhara, Nepal. J Laryngol Otol. 2016;130(01):56–65.
24. Njoroge GN, Bussmann RW. Traditional management of ear, nose and throat (ENT) diseases in Central Kenya. J Ethnobiol Ethnomed. 2006;2(1):1.
25. National Institute of Statistics of Rwanda (NISR) and Ministry of Finance and Economic Planning (MINECOFIN), Fourth Population and Housing Census, Rwanda, 2012. Thematic report: Characteristics of households and housing. 2014.
26. National Institute of Statistics of Rwanda. The Third Integrated Household Living Conditions Survey (EICV 3) Main indicators report. Kigali: Ministry of Finance and Economic Planning; 2012.
27. Adeyemo AA. Knowledge of caregivers on the risk factors of otitis media. Indian J Otol. 2012;18(4):184.
28. Curry MD, et al. Beliefs about and responses to childhood ear infections: a study of parents in eastern North Carolina. Soc Sci Med. 2002;54(8):1153–65.
29. Acuin J. Chronic suppurative otitis media. BMJ Clin Evid. 2007;2007. p. 0507.
30. Mbonye AK. Prevalence of Childhood Illnesses and Care-Seeking Practices in Rural Uganda. Sci World J. 2003;3:721–30.
31. Clarke S, et al. A study protocol for a cluster randomised trial for the prevention of chronic suppurative otitis media in children in Jumla, Nepal. BMC Ear Nose Throat Disord. 2015;15(1):4.
32. Li MG, et al. Is chronic suppurative otitis media a neglected tropical disease? PLoS Negl Trop Dis. 2015;9(3):e0003485.
33. Ministry of Health Rwanda. Third Health Sector Strategic Plan July 2012–June 2018. Kigali: Ministry of Health; 2012.
34. Lasisi AO. Otolaryngological Practice in Developing Country: A Profile of Met and Unmet Needs. East Central Afr J Surg. 2008;13(2):101–4.
35. World Health Organization. Primary ear and hearing care training manuals. Geneva: World Health Organization; 2006.

20

Hibernoma: a rare case of adipocytic tumor in head and neck

Alexandra Rodriguez Ruiz[1], Sven Saussez[1,2], Thibaut Demaesschalck[1] and Jérôme R. Lechien[1,2*]

Abstract

Background: Hibernoma is a rare soft tissue tumor stem from persistent fetal brown fat tissue. This benign tumor may occasionally occur in head and neck area and, in most cases, is characterized by an asymptomatic slow growth.

Case presentation: We presented an uncommon case of hibernoma of the posterior cervical triangle occurring in a 30-year-old man referred to the department of otolaryngology. The patient suffered from a right, very painful, and rapidly growing mass since 3 months. MRI examination reported both an infiltrating mass and a homogenous enhancement of an underlying vascularization after the injection of intravenous contrast. According to the risk of sarcoma, a surgical procedure was made to completely excise the mass that was a hibernoma.

Conclusions: Hibernoma may occur with an uncommon clinical presentation imitating malignancy. MRI plays a key role in the differential diagnosis and surgery remains the better therapeutic approach.

Keywords.: hibernoma,, head,, neck,, tumor,, lipoma

Background

Hibernoma is a rare benign tumor originating from persistent fetal brown fat tissue [1]. The brown fat has a thermogenesis function, especially in the first years of a child's life, but it regresses with age [1]. In adults, the most common residual areas of brown fat are usually located in the inter-scapular region, mediastinum, retroperitoneum, back, thigh and, sometimes, in head and neck [2–4]. Widely, the remaining of brown fat still remains asymptomatic and has no impact on the homeostasis. In rare cases, the remaining tissue can slowly grow, leading to the occurrence of a soft-tissue tumor. Thus, some cases of hibernoma are well described in the current literature and they are commonly found in chest, abdominal cavity and head and neck [3, 4]. In this paper, we reported an unusual case of hibernoma in a patient with a painless mass at the base of the neck. The current literature was reviewed about epidemiology, clinical course, diagnosis and treatment.

---

* Correspondence: Jerome.Lechien@umons.ac.be
[1]Department of Otolaryngology - Head and Neck Surgery, CHU Saint Pierre, Free University of Brussels, rue Haute 322, B1000 Brussels, Belgium
[2]Laboratory of Anatomy and Cell Biology, Faculty of Medicine, UMONS Research Institute for Health Sciences and Technology, University of Mons (UMons), Mons, Belgium

Case presentation

A 30-year-old man was referred to the Department of Otolaryngology and Head and Neck Surgery for mass located in the right posterior cervical triangle of the neck. The patient had this mass since several months but it recently started to grow in a context of substantial neck pain. The patient had no difficulty to breathe and swallow. Clinical examination exhibited a relatively mobile, soft mass located in the supraclavicular area. No cervical node was found. Both clinical and ultrasound examinations led to suspect a soft tissue mass, and the magnetic resonance imaging (MRI) revealed a 38 mm along the axis tumor (Fig. 1) between the elevator scapulae and the right scalene muscles. The tumor infiltrated the scalene muscles and the injection of intravenous contrast (gadolinium) reported a homogenous enhancement of an important underlying vascularization, a nodular structure of the tissue, and the presence of septa > 2 mm. According to the clinical features and the MRI characteristics (especially T1 sequence), we highly suspected liposarcoma of the neck. The fine needle aspiration biopsy was made but non-contributory. Thus, a surgical procedure was made to completely excise the mass and the macroscopic examination revealed an

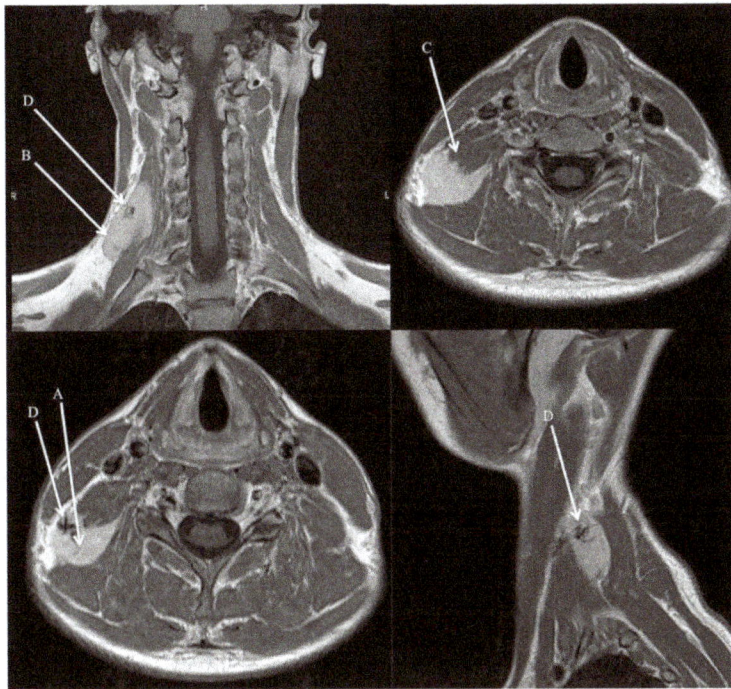

Fig. 1 MRI of the hibernoma. The MRI (T1) revealed a 38 mm along the axis mass of the posterior cervical triangle with septa > 2 mm (**a**), nodular structures (**b**), muscular invasion (**c**), and a high vascularization (**d**).

encapsulated taned-brown polylobulated tumor. The immediate post-operative follow-up was unremarkable. The definitive histopathological examination retained the diagnosis of a hibernoma, which was characterized by mature fat cells, abundant eosinophilic cells with small cytoplasmic vacuoles and regular, small, round cell nuclei (Fig. 2). The 4-years follow-up was unremarkable and the patient had no recurrence.

Discussion

Since the first case described in 1906 [5], approximately ten cases of cervical hibernoma have been reported [6].

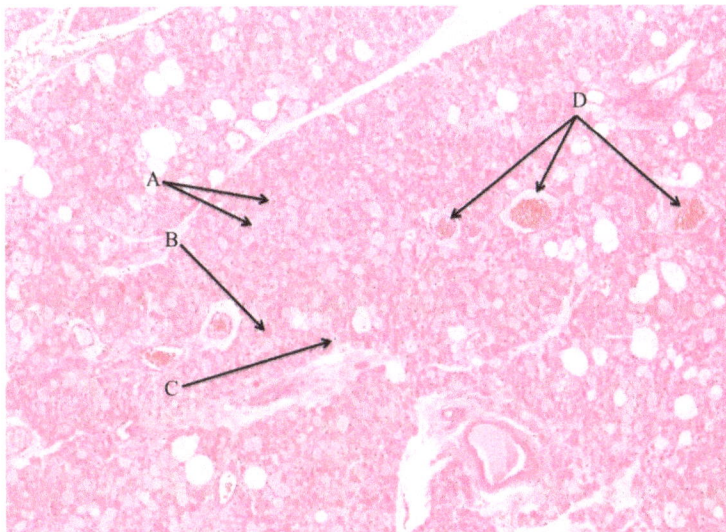

Fig. 2 Histopathological findings. The histopathological findings (10×, hematoxylin & eosin) showed mature fat cells (**a**), abundant eosinophilic cells (**b**) with small cytoplasmic vacuoles and regular, small, round nuclei (**c**). The tissue was characterized by a high vascularization (**d**).

Among these, only three patients had hibernoma in the posterior cervical triangle but it seems highly probable that the diagnosis is widely underestimated [7, 8]. Indeed, with the contribution of modern technological advancements in positron emission tomography, some recent research supports the theory that the true prevalence of brown fat in adult is between 30 and 100%, suggesting an increased possibility to develop hibernoma, though often misdiagnosed or confused with lipoma [9]. Yet, it is important to make the difference between lipoma and hibernoma since, to date, no case of malignant transformation of hibernoma has been reported, which is not the case of lipoma. From an epidemiological standpoint, hibernoma is mostly seen in the third, fourth and fifth decades of life with a slightly higher female prevalence [6, 10].

Clinically, most patients with neck hibernoma are usually asymptomatic over time even if the slow growth of the tumor may, at some point, compress the adjacent structures [7, 8]. In our patient, the rapid growth and the related pain are uncommon manifestations and prompted us to quickly carry out additional examinations to exclude malignancy. To the best of our knowledge, only one reported case was characterized by similar clinical findings [6]. Among the complementary examinations, computed tomography (CT), MRI, and angiography can provide additional usefulness informations. So, hibernomas are usually depicted as well-circumscribed and variably homogeneous tumors with marked contrast enhancement. The differentiation with lipoma is possible with MR imaging because hibernoma still remains more vascularized, with large septa (>2 mm; easily seen with contrast agent), and, unlike to lipoma, the hibernoma tissue can be differentiated to the fat with MRI STIR or T2 Fat Sar sequences [11,

12]. Table 1 summarizes the clinical and imaging characteristics of lipoma, liposarcoma and hibernoma.

In our patient, the MRI examination showed a 38 mm along the axis, relatively well circumscribed tumor with intermediate signal intensity between subcutaneous fat and muscle. Moreover, the observed tumor was homogenous, relatively well circumscribed, with septa > 2 mm and some nodular areas. All of these features led us to exclude lipoma but the critical point concerned the differential diagnosis with liposarcoma. Indeed, the high vascularization, the large septa, and the fast arteriovenous contrast enhancement may mislead to liposarcoma diagnosis. Thus, as reported in the current literature, even with imaging, the characteristics of this tumor remain difficult to differentiate from malignant fat tumors and some very rare tumors such as angiolipoma and malignant fibrous histocytoma [6, 13, 14].

The final diagnosis is made after a fine needle aspiration procedure or after the surgical excision [6]. As showed in our patient, the histopathological findings include small, round, brown fat-like cells, variable numbers of mature fat cells with i) uniform, small eosinophilic cytoplasmic vacuoles, ii) regular, small, and round cell nuclei; and iii) delicate branching capillaries. Hypervascularization combined with abundant mitochondria give hibernomas their color. Concerning the histopathological differential diagnosis with liposarcoma, some cytology features (i.e. admixture of multivacuolated and univacuolated fat cells; a rich, delicate, capillary-like vasculature) are known to lead to a misdiagnosis of liposarcoma and the pathologists must take into consideration these similar characteristics. To date, hibernoma can be classified by morphologic or histological characteristics such as the presence of multivacuolated or univacuolated cells found in brown fat or normal fat

Table 1 Clinical and imaging characteristics of lipoma, liposarcoma and hibernoma.

Clinical features	Lipoma	Liposarcoma	Hibernoma
Size	<5 cm (80% cases)	>5 cm	>5 cm
Growth	Slow	Slow/moderate/high	Slow/moderate/high
Age	25-65y	>50y	30-50y
Clinic	Asymptomatic +++	Asymptomatic ++	Asymptomatic ++
Sexe ratio	M = F	M > F	F > M
MR Imaging	Well-homogeneous	Variably homogeneous	Variably homogeneous
Characteristics	Well-circumscribed	Well-circumscribed	Well-circumscribed
	Less vascularized	Variably vascularized (C+)	Variably vascularized (C+)
	No nodular lesion	Possible nodular lesion	Possible nodular lesion
	T1: Hyper (as fat)	T1: Hyper (less than fat/lipoma)	T1: Hyper (less than fat/lipoma)
	T2: Hyper (as fat)	T2: Hyper	T2: Hyper
	STIR/T2 Fat Sat: removing signal	STIR/T2 Fat Sat: no removing signal	STIR/T2 Fat Sat: no removing signal
	Septa:<2 mm (C+)	Septa:>2 mm (C+)	Septa:>2 mm (C+)

C + = contrast +; F = female; M = male; y = year. Many case presentations allowed the realization of this Table [2, 3, 6–8, 12, 13].

[6]. Morphological, four variants of hibernoma are described: typical, myxoid, spindle cell, and lipoma-like [15]. Typical hibernoma included eosinophilic, pale, and mixed cell types. The myxoid variant contained a loose basophilic matrix while the spindle cell hibernoma had features of spindle cell lipoma. The lipoma-like variant only contained scattered cells. The present histopathological case corresponds to the typical variant. The 4-years follow-up of our patient did not report recurrence that seems to be in line with the other cases reported in the literature [6].

Conclusion

Hibernoma is a rare benign tumor that can mimic malignant lesion of the soft tissue such as liposarcoma. In this paper, we report an unusual presentation of hibernoma of the posterior cervical triangle characterized by both severe pain and rapid growth. MRI plays a key role in the differential diagnosis, especially with other benign tumors but still remains limited for the differential diagnosis with malignancy. The biopsy and the surgery procedure correspond to the gold standard approaches for the final diagnosis, the exclusion of liposarcoma, and to select the appropriate treatment. To date, there is no described case of recurrence or malignant transformation.

Abbreviations.
CT : Computed tomography; MRI: Magnetic resonance imaging.

Acknowledgments
Dr. Sarah Saxena, MD, native English speaker for the collaboration in proofreading of the article. Dr. Stelianos Kampouridis for the MRI pictures.

Competing Interests.
The authors declare that they have no competing interests.

Funding
None.

Authors contributions.
AR wrote the paper et realized the surgical approach with TD. SS and JRL reviewed and corrected the paper. All authors read and approved the final manuscript.

References.
1. Cannon B, Nedergaard J. Brown Adipose Tissue: Function and Physiological. Significance. Physiol Rev. 2004;84:277–359.
2. Chen CL, Chen WC, Chiang JH, Ho CF. Intercapsular hibernoma-Case report and literature review. Kaohsiung J Med Sci. 2011;27:348–52.
3. Della Volpe C, Salazard B, Casanova D, Vacheret H, Bartoli JF, Magalon G. Hibernoma of the antero-lateral thigh. Br J Plast Surg. 2005;58:859–61.
4. Hertoghs M, Van Schil P, Rutsaert R, Van Marck E, Vallaeys J. Intrathoracic hibernoma: Report of two cases. Lung Cancer. 2009;367–70.
5. Merkel H. Über ein Pseudolipon der Mamma. Beitr Path Anat Allge Path. 1906; 39:152–157. [article in German].
6. Trujillo O, Cui IH, Malone M, Suurna M. An unusual presentation of a rare benign tumor in the head and neck: A review of hibernomas. Laryngoscope. 2015;125(7):1656–9.
7. Florio G, Cicia S, Del Papa M, Carnì D. Neck hibernoma: case report and literature review. G Chir. 2000;21(8–9):339–41.
8. Arsa J. Minié. Hibernoma: unusual location in the submental space. J Craniomaxillofac Surg. 1992;20:264–5.
9. Nedergaard J, Bengtsson T, Cannon B. Three years with adult human brown adipose tissue. Ann N Y. Acad Sci. 2010;1212:E20–36.
10. Khattala K, Elmadi A, Bouamama H, Rami M, Bouabdallah Y. Cervical hibernoma in a two year old boy. Pan Afr Med J. 2013;16:27.
11. Papathanassiou ZG, Alberghini M, Taieb S, Errani C, Picci P, Vanel D. Imaging of hibernomas: A retrospective study on twelve cases. Clin Sarcoma Res. 2011;1(1):3.
12. DeRosa DC, Lim RB, Lin-Hurtubise K, Johnson EA. Symptomatic hibernoma: a rare soft tissue tumor. Hawaii J Med Public Health. 2012;71(12):342–5.
13. Jaroszewski DE, Petris GD. Giant hibernoma of the thoracic pleura and chest wall. World J Clin Cases. 2013;1(4):143–5.
14. Salim B, Belkacem C. Hibernoma of the thigh: a report of four cases. J Orthop Surg. 2014;22(1):118–21.
15. Furlong MA, Fanburg-Smith JC, Miettinen M. The morphologic spectrum of hibernoma: a clinicopathologic study of 170 cases. Am J Surg Pathol. 2001; 25(6):809–14.

21

Generic quality of life in persons with hearing loss

Øyvind Nordvik[3*] (iD), Peder O. Laugen Heggdal[1,2], Jonas Brännström[4], Flemming Vassbotn[1,2], Anne Kari Aarstad[1,5] and Hans Jørgen Aarstad[1,2]

Abstract

Background: To the best of our knowledge, no empirically based consensus has been reached as to if, and to what extent, persons with hearing loss (HL) have reduced generic Quality of life (QoL). There seems to be limited knowledge regarding to what extent a hearing aid (HA) would improve QoL. The main aim of the present study was to review studies about the relationship between HL and QoL. A supporting aim was to study the association between distress and HL.

Methods: Literature databases (Cinahl, Pub Med and Web of Science) were searched to identify relevant journal articles published in the period from January 2000 to March 17, 2016. We performed a primary search pertaining to the relationship between HL, HA and QoL (search number one) followed by a supporting search pertaining to the relationship between distress/mood/anxiety and HL (search number two). After checking for duplications and screening the titles of the papers, we read the abstracts of the remaining papers. The most relevant papers were read thoroughly, leaving us with the journal articles that met the inclusion criteria.

Results: Twenty journal articles were included in the present review: 13 were found in the primary search (HL and QoL), and seven in the supporting search (HL and distress). The literature yields equivocal findings regarding the association between generic QoL and HL. A strong association between distress and HL was shown, where distressed persons tend to have a lowered generic QoL. It is suggested that QoL is lowered among HL patients. Some studies suggest an increased generic QoL following the use of HA, especially during the first few months after initiation of treatment. Other studies suggest that HA use is one of several possible factors that contribute to improve generic QoL.

Conclusions: The majority of the studies suggest that HL is associated with reduced generic QoL. Using hearing aids seem to improve general QoL at follow-up within the first year. HL is a risk factor for distress. Further research is needed to explore the relationship between HL and generic QoL, in addition to the importance of influencing variables on this relationship.

Keywords: Quality of life, Hearing loss, Impairment, Distress, Depression, Anxiety, Hearing aid

Background

In 2012, the World Health Organization (WHO) estimated that 360 million people, i.e. 5.3% of the world's population, were living with disabling hearing loss (HL), while around 15% of the world's adult population had some degree of HL [1]. Furthermore, sensory diseases have been estimated to be the world's second most common group of chronic disability when measured by years lived with disability [2]. HL increases with age, mostly because of age-related HL, generally referred to as presbyacusis. This term represents the sum of the environmental, sensory, metabolic and neural causes that to various extents are suggested to contribute to age-related physiological hearing loss [3, 4]. Presbyacusis cause reduced speech understanding in noisy environments, declined processing of acoustic information and impaired localization of sound sources [4]. Hearing loss is present in nearly two thirds of adults

* Correspondence: oyvind.nordvik@hvl.no
[3]Faculty of Health and Social Sciences, Bergen University College, Bergen, Norway
Full list of author information is available at the end of the article

aged 70 years and older in the U.S. population [5]. Even though most people with HL suffer from presbyacusis, other factors such as other ear diseases [6], occupational noise exposure [7] and specific genetic diseases [8] may cause HL. Thus, HL may affect people at all ages and stages in life [9].

HL is often characterized by at which sound pressure level pure tones can be detected employing standard audiometric tests [3]. Presbyacusis typically causes a symmetric bilateral high frequency hearing loss. As human speech is related to relatively high frequencies, even a limited hearing loss at high frequencies may cause impaired speech intelligibility [10]. HL is often not curable, but hearing aids (HA) and other individual sound amplification devices (ISADs) may improve hearing function [11].

Patient reported outcome measures (PROMs), such as Quality of life (QoL) questionnaires, should ideally be systematically implemented in health care practices [12] as there seems to be a need for a more "holistic" approach within a modern view of health care. This calls for the inclusion of both disease-specific and generic QoL outcome measures [13]. QoL measures constitute important outcome- and state measures [14, 15], as well as an area of focus for research in its own right [14, 15]. However, there is no universally accepted definition for the concept of QoL [16, 17]. Even so, we all have a notion about what QoL is, and most people seem to have an intuitive understanding of their own QoL by referring to their own perception [16]. Thus, the concept QoL will hold different contents among different people [16].

WHO defines QoL as "An individual's perception of their position on life in the context of the culture and value systems in which they live and in relation to their goals, expectations, standards and concerns." This is a broad-ranging concept related to a person's physical health, psychological state, level of independence, social relationships, personal beliefs and their relationship to salient features of their own environment. The WHO QoL definition is closely related to the WHO's definition of health from 1948, which describes health as "physical, mental and social well-being, and not merely the absence of disease or infirmity" [16]. This is also a wide definition, in which in addition to a physical dimension, the WHO also includes well- being, environmental and psychological factors as part of health. Hence, both generic and disease-specific QoL become relevant as to disease and health [18].

Many different questionnaires have been developed with the intent of directly measuring the functional consequences of a disease; these may be termed "disease-specific" QoL questionnaires. Thus, QoL instruments intended to study the specific consequences of

HL may be considered examples of such instruments [19]. The effect of HL on hearing function can usually be measured by hearing-specific questionnaires [20], but to what extent HL affects generic QoL is not well agreed upon and constitutes the main aim of this study.

The most commonly used generic QoL questionnaire is the SF- 36, with more than 13,000 "hits" on Pubmed as of 2016. The SF-36 measures functional status and wellbeing [21]. This questionnaire was first used in a provisional edition in 1988 and in a standard form in 1990 [22]. Shortened questionnaires have been developed from this original, i.e. the 12-item questionnaire SF-12 [23]. Another commonly used generic questionnaire is the Euro-QoL instrument (EQ-5D). This is a standardized questionnaire intended to measure generic QoL [24], and it may be utilized within a wide range of health conditions. The EQ-5D describes five dimensions: mobility, self-care, usual activities, pain/discomfort and anxiety/depression. An index value is calculated for each individual, ranging from 1, which indicates no problems in all five dimensions, to 15, which indicate severe problems in all five dimensions. Other generic questionnaires that may be used are the Health Utility Index (HUI) and the Sickness Impact Profile (SIP) [25, 26]. General parts of disease-related questionnaires, such as the European Organization for the Research and Treatment of Cancer (EORTC) Quality of Life Questionnaire (QLQ) may also be considered generic QoL instruments [27]. Disease specific questionnaires may also include some questions about generic QoL. However, generic QoL instruments measure many aspects of QoL, and are often intended for use over a wide range of diseases. Such questionnaires are often also applicable to healthy people. Thus, generic QoL questionnaires allow comparing QoL between patient groups, as well as to data from general populations [16, 28]. The specific main aim of the present study is to review the existing literature on generic QoL obtained by generic instruments among hearing-impaired patients.

In order to assess generic QoL within a disease context, important modulating factors known to contribute to QoL may be assessed alongside the QoL measure. This may include psychosocial factors [29], personality [30, 31] and factors related to activities of daily living [32]. To study potential modulating conditions in the relationship between HL and QoL has therefore been a supporting aim when reviewing the literature in the present study.

QoL as a construct seems to be closely associated with distress, anxiety, and mood, when measured primarily in generic, but also to some extent in disease-specific QoL questionnaires [20, 33–35]. Hence, it should be of interest to study the impact of HL on distress, mood and depression. Anxiety and depression can be defined using standardized classification manuals such as the ICD-10 [36] or DSM-5 [37], while distress seems to have no such clear and universal definition. However, one may understand psychological distress as a unique discomforting, emotional state experienced by an individual that results in harm to the person, either temporarily or permanently [38]. In psychological research, distress is often quantified as the sum of anxiety and lowered mood [39]. Distress may also be utilized as an indicator of mental disease [39]. Thus, as QoL, distress, mood and anxiety are closely related concepts [40], we have conducted a search for the major publications on associations between HL and distress, anxiety and mood in order to present a more complete picture of the associations between HL and generic QoL.

Aim of this paper

So far, no empirically based consensus about if, and in case to what extent, HL patients have reduced generic QoL has been reached. The main aim of this study was to review studies on the relationship between HL and generic QoL published in the period 2000 to present day. As a supporting aim we have also determined noted psychological explaining factors reported in the above-identified publications. As an additional investigational tool, we have reviewed papers from the same period that study HL and distress, anxiety and mood. This was done because level of distress, anxiety and mood seems closely associated to generic QoL.

Method
Design

Data were collected using a systematized literature review design. We performed two separate searches for relevant papers. Search number one targeted HL, HA and QoL, whereas search number two targeted HL and distress, anxiety and depression. The Prisma 2009 checklist [41] was applied during the process of writing this paper, and is available as Additional file 1.

Searches

We suggest that literature produced over the past 15–16 years would contain most of the significant findings and results from prior studies [42]. Based on this, we set the time frame from the year 2000 up to the search date to obtain relevant literature. Moreover, we only included studies based on empirical data with an available abstract. To help narrow down the two searches in order to meet the specific aims of this study, we excluded studies concerning the hearing impaired peers or family or other caregivers. Other exclusion criteria were studies

on deafness, persons with cochlea implants, dual or multi-sensorial loss, tinnitus, stigma and HL, assistive listening devices, bone-anchored hearing aids, HL and psychiatric disease, HA usage, sudden sensorineural HL, conductive HL and surgical interventions on HL. We also excluded qualitative studies as well as studies on psychiatric diseases and depression or anxiety prior to the HL.

Search number one - HL, HA and QoL

In the primary search, we included peer reviewed original papers in English published in the period from January 2000 to March 17, 2016 (search date). Studies on QoL or health-related QoL in adult persons with sensorineural hearing loss or presbyacusis were included.

To identify relevant studies, we performed a search in the databases Cinahl, Pub Med and Web of Science. We used combinations (AND) of the following keywords:

1. *Hearing disorders OR deafness OR hearing loss/partial + OR hearing loss/sensorineural + OR Tinnitus AND hearing aid OR Hearing aid fitting AND hearing loss OR hard of hearing OR loss of hearing OR hearing impair* OR hearing disorder* OR deaf* OR hearing aid* OR hearing assistive technology.*
2. *Quality of life + OR Quality of Life OR health-related Quality of life OR HRQoL OR qol.*

A total of 3280 papers were found in the introductory search. After checking for duplications and screening the titles of the papers, 151 papers remained; Cinahl ($n = 17$), Pub Med ($n = 43$) and Web of Science ($n = 91$). After reading the abstracts, the remaining 35 papers were retained and thoroughly read. This left us with 13 journal articles that met the inclusion criteria (Fig. 1).

Search number two - HL and distress, anxiety and depression

From the supporting search we included peer-reviewed original papers in English published in the period from January 2000 to October 26, 2016 (search date). This search was aimed at studies on distress, depression and/or anxiety caused by the hearing impairment, in adults with sensorineural HL.

To identify relevant studies, we performed a search on October 26, 2016, using the databases Cinahl, Pub Med and the Web of Science.

A total of 1157 papers were found in the introductory search: Cinahl ($n = 238$), Pub Med ($n = 325$), Web of Science ($n = 594$). After checking for duplications, 908 papers remained. Screening the titles of the papers, reading abstracts and then thoroughly reading the most

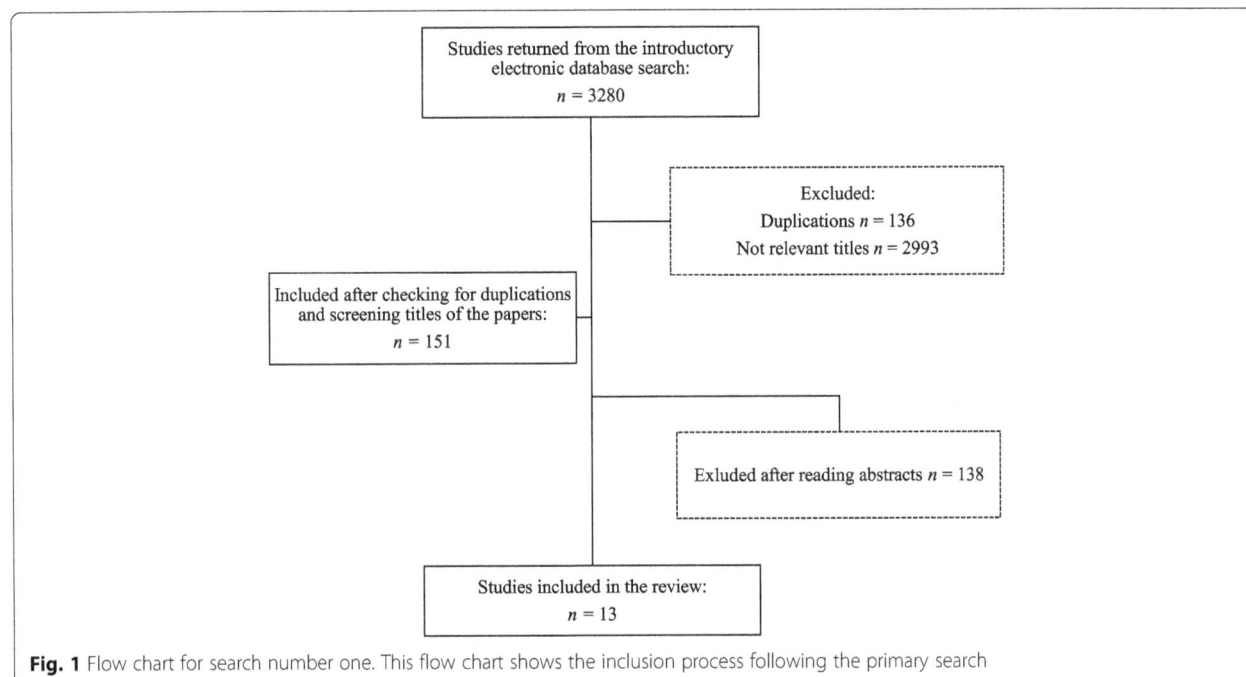

Fig. 1 Flow chart for search number one. This flow chart shows the inclusion process following the primary search

relevant papers left us with seven journal articles to be included in this review (Fig. 2).

Quality according to the Crowe critical appraisal tool (CCAT)

To assess the quality of the papers that met the inclusion criteria and thus were included in this review, we used the Crowe Critical appraisal tool (CCAT). The tool consists of a CCAT form and a CCAT user guide [43]. The CCAT form consists of nine category items. The first eight categories are scored from 0 to 5. The 9th item states the total sum score calculated from scores at categories 1 to 8. Thus, sum scores may range from 0 to 40 points. By using this tool, we had the opportunity to systematically assess the quality of the included papers. The sum score of the CCAT for each study is presented in Tables 1 and 2.

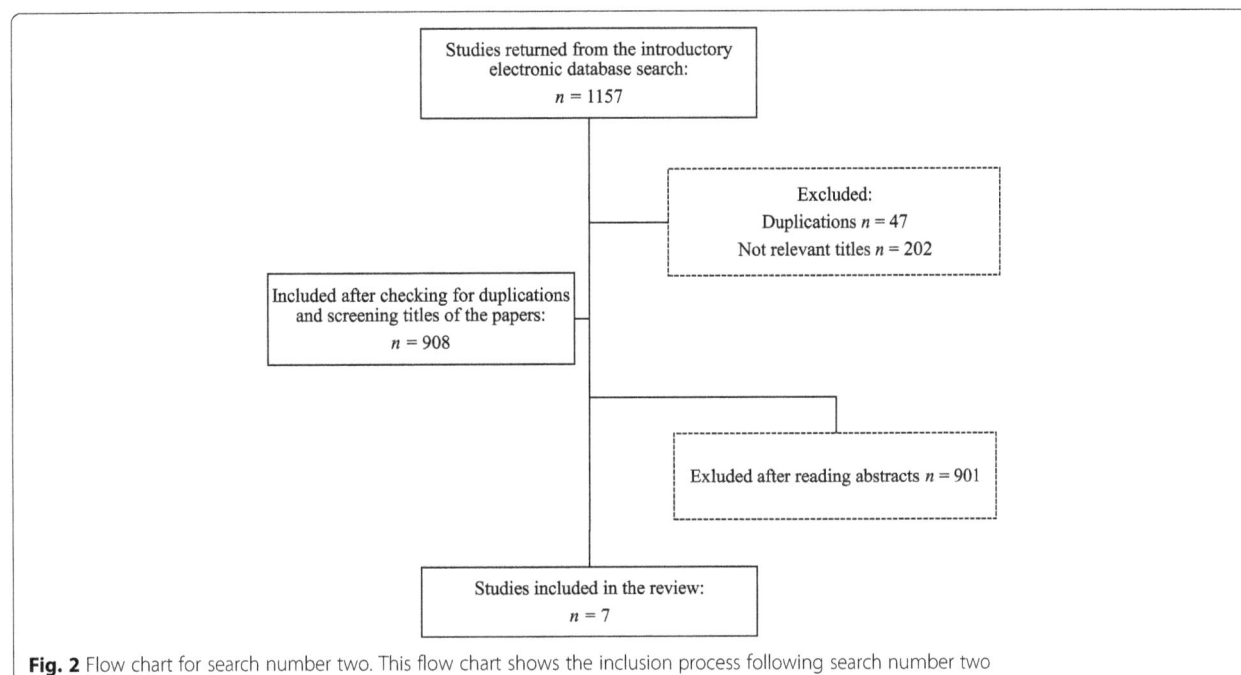

Fig. 2 Flow chart for search number two. This flow chart shows the inclusion process following search number two

Table 1 Included studies from the primary search

Study	Type of study	QoL Questionnaire used in study	First time/ experienced users?	Number of participants in study	Age	Unilateral or Bilateral HL	Range and character - HL	HA fitting	Results	CCAT score
Capoani Garcia Mondelli, M. F. and P. J. Soalheiro de Souza, 2012 [46]	Cross sectional/ Longitudinal	Generic WHOQOL - bref	First time	30 (57% male)	Range: 60–90 years, mean age 76.8 years	bilateral	Moderate hearing loss. No further definition.	Before HA fitting (ISAD) and after 3 months.	Using HA (ISAD) improved the overall QoL	25
Chew, H. S. and S. Yeak, 2010 [49]	Cross sectional	Generic: SF 36	First time	80 (41% male)	Range: 50 years and over. Median age 69 years	bilateral	>25 dB PTA in the better ear.	Not specified	SF-36 lacked specificity and sensitivity in assesing the impact on HL on QoL	21
Chia, E.-M., et al., 2007 [50]	Cross sectional	Generic: SF 36	Not specified	2431	Mean age: 67 years	Unilateral and bilateral	Unilateral HI defined as HI in one ear and no HI in the other ear. Bilateral HI defined as HI in both ears. HI defined as >25 dB PTA	Not specified	Unilateral HL: No significant difference in QoL than those whitout HL. Bilateral HL: Poorer QoL than those whitout HL.	27
Dalton, D. S., et al., 2003 [44]	5- year follow-up Longitudinal	SF-36 (Generic)	Not specified	2688, (42% male)	53–97 years, mean age 69 years	Not specified	Mild: 26–440 dB PTA HL in eighter ear. Moderate to severe: >40 dB PTA in eighter ear	Not specified	HL was associated with reduced QoL.	36
Espmark, A. K. K., et al., 2002 [47]	Cross sectional	HMS (26 questions, where 4 of 20 items where related to QoL)	First time	154 (38% male)	Born 1920 or earlier	Not specified	Three groups: Normal to slight HL: <30 dB PTA. Mild HL: 30–39 dB PTA. Moderate to severe HL: ≥ 40 dB PTA	Not specified	HL was significantly associated with reduced QoL in all four dimensions in females and in two of four in males.	27
Hallberg, L. R., et al., 2008 [51]	Cross sectional	PGWB	Mixed	79 (39% male)	48–92 years, mean age 68.7 years	Bilateral	PTA low at Freq. 0.5, 1 and 2 kHz was 39.6 dB. PTA high at Freq. 2,3,4 and 6 kHz was 55.5 dB	Not specified	HL was significantly associated with reduced QoL. Psychsocial consequenses of HI, such as lowered QoL, cannot be predicted from audiometric data alone.	33
Helvik, A. S., et al., 2006 [52]	Cross sectional	PGWB	Mixed, mean duration of the HI was 15.1 years	343 (55% male)	21–94 years, mean age 69 years	Not specified	Mean threshold of hearing for the total sample was 43.0 dB	Not specified	Psychological well-being was associated with activity limitation and participation restriction, but not with the degree of HL	28

Table 1 Included studies from the primary search *(Continued)*

Study	Type of study	QoL Questionnaire used in study	First time/ experienced users?	Number of participants in study	Age	Unilateral or Bilateral HL	Range and character - HL	HA fitting	Results	CCAT score
									and use of communication strategies	
Lotfi, Y., et al., 2009 [48]	Cross sectional/ Longitudinal	HHIE	First time users	207 (71% male)	'60 years, mean age 73.01 years	Not specified	Moderate HL: 56– 70 dB Profound HL: 71– 90 dB	Before HA fitting and after 3 months	Significant improvement in QoL after HA fitting	19
Meyer, J. M. and S. Kashubeck-West, 2013 [55]	Cross sectional	HHIA and The meassure of psychological well-being (generic)	Not specified	277 (25% male)	18–65 years Mean age 49 years	Not specified	Not specified	Not specified	Relationship between perceived severity and perceived disability acted as direct predictors to well-being and as a indirect predictors through their relationship with coping. No significant association between QoL and HL	30
Miyakita, T., et al., 2002 [54]	Cross sectional	Generic, LISZ, 13 questions about QoL	Not specified	210 retired workers, gender not specified	56–65 years, mean age 60.6 years	Not specified	Not specified	Not specified	Hearing disabillities was associated with deterioration in QoL. No significant association between QoL and HL	23
Niemensivu, R., et al., 2015 [45]	Prospective study Including control group	Generic 15D	First time HA	949 with HI (42% male), Control group 4685 persons	Mean age: 73.8 years	Not specified	Frequencies 0.5,1,2 and 4 kHz. Four categories of HL. Mild: 25–40 dB, moderate: 41–70 dB, Severe 71–95 dB and very severe: >95 dB.	Before HA fitting (in the better ear) and after six monthts	Significant improvement in QoL after unilateral HA fitting	29
Stark, P. and L. Hickson, 2004 [53]	Cross sectional/ Longitudinal	Generic SF- 36	First time HA	131 (67% male)	47–90 years, mean age 71.7 years	Not specified	Not devided in groups. PTA at 0.5, 1 and 2 kHz in the better ear.	Before HA fitting and after 3 months	No significant improvements in HRQoL after HA fitting.	30

Table 1 Included studies from the primary search *(Continued)*

Study	Type of study	QoL Questionnaire used in study	First time/ experienced users?	Number of participants in study	Age	Unilateral or Bilateral HL	Range and character - HL	HA fitting	Results	CCAT score
							25 dB or less: $n = 18$			
							26–35 dB: $n = 44$			
							36–46 dB: $n = 23$			
							46–55 dB: $n = 8$			
Vuorialho, A., et al., 2006 [56]	Cross sectional/ Longitudinal	Generic EQ-5D in combination with HHIE-S	First time HA	98 (50% male)	61–87 years (median 77 years)	Not specified	Not specified	Before HA fitting and after 6 months	No s ignificant QoL i mprovement after HA- fitting	30

EQ-5D EuroQol Group- 5 Dimensions
SF- 36 Medical Outcome Study (MOS) Short Form- 36 Health Survey Scale
15D 15 Dimension (a standardized self-administered measure of Health related Quality of Life)
LISZ Life Satisfaction Index, version Z
HMS Hearing Measurement Scale
PGWB Psychological General Well Being index
WHOQOL – bref Abbreviated version of the WHO QoL- 100 Quality of Life assessment
HHIE/HHIA Hearing Handicap Inventory for the Elderly/Adults
HHI-S HHIE - Screening version

Results

HL and generic QoL

The range of HL was presented differently in the included studies. Five studies presented HL in groups from mild to severe HL [44–48] and five presented the number of participants over different hearing range groups [49–53]. Three studies gave no information on this [54–56]. Still, it seems that in most of the included studies, the lower limit of hearing loss was defined by a mean hearing loss exceeding 25 dB HL in the better ear at the octave frequencies from 0.5 to 4 kHz [57] (Table 1).

The included studies have used self-report questionnaires concerning QoL in adult persons with HL. The number of participants varied from 30 to 2688 (Table 1). Of the 13 studies included, 11 studies were cross-sectional, one was longitudinal [44] and one was prospective [45]. Seven studies used a generic QoL questionnaire [45, 46, 49–52, 54]. Two used a disease-specific QoL questionnaire only [47, 48], while the remaining four studies used a combination of generic and disease-specific questionnaires (Table 1). Four studies used the SF-36 in order to measure generic QoL, of which three employed the SF-36 alone [44, 49, 50]. One study combined SF-36 and a disease-specific questionnaire, the Hearing Handicap Inventory for Elderly (HHIE) [53].

In general, two of the included papers concluded that HL is substantially associated with a reduced QoL [44, 54], whereas six claimed there is a weak correlation [47,

50–53, 56] and five no [45, 46, 48, 49, 55] significant correlation between HL and generic QoL.

One study investigated both unilateral and bilateral hearing loss (HL) [50], three studies reported bilateral HL only [46, 49, 51] while the remaining nine studies provided no information on this matter. In the study that reported both unilateral and bilateral HL, persons with unilateral HL did not report significantly lower generic QoL than persons without HL. In one study, worse hearing at the high frequencies in male patients than in female patients was reported [51]. Despite this, the males had significantly better scores on generic QoL compared to the females. Furthermore, non-verbal behavior that alleviates the consequences of HL on generic QoL, such as pretending to hear, guessing what was said and avoiding interactions, was reported less used by men than by women [51].

In one study, the disease-specific questionnaire (HHIE) and the SF-36 questionnaire were employed [49]. These authors suggests that the SF-36 form lacks sensitivity and specificity in assessing the impact of HL on QoL, and suggests that untreated HL results in a significant decline in QoL, as measured with the HHIE questionnaire.

A study based on a relatively small population of 30 individuals, suggested that Individual Sound Amplification Devices (ISADs) improved the overall QoL of the individuals assessed [50]. At the same time, poor social relationships and coping skills were risk factors for

Table 2 Studies included from search number two

Authors	Type of study	Hearing loss and Distress OR anxiety OR depression	Sample size and gender	Age	Results	CCAT score
Gopinath, B., et al. (2012) [62]	Survey	Distress	811 (control group = 687) No data on gender	≥ 55 years	Older patients with HL are significantly more likely to experience emotional distress directly due to their HL.	31
Nachtegaal, J., et al. (2009) [61]	Cross-sectional	Distress, depression	1511 No data on gender	18–70 years. Divided into 5 age strata (18–29, 30–39, 40–49, 50–59 and 60–70 years)	HL is negatively associated with higher distress, depression, somatization and lonliness in young and middle- aged groups.	33
Tseng, C. C., et al. (2016) [58]	Longitudinal	Depression	1717 (control group = 6868) 55% male	39–63 years. Median = 51 years	Patients with sudden sensorineural hearing loss (SSHNL) are 2.17 times more at risk for depressive disorders, compared to those without SSNHL. Especially in age groups ˂ 60 years.	29
Li et al. (2014)	Survey	Depression	18,318 Male = 48%	Adults 18 years or older. 18–44 years: 49.4% 45–69 years: 39.1% ≥ 70 years: 11.5%	HL is significantly associated with depression, particulary in women and those younger than 70 years.	25
Kramer, S. E., et al. (2002) [63]	Longitudinal (part of the LASA- study)	Depression and other chronic diseases	1506 (in the LASA- study)	55–85 years	Elderly with HL report significantly more depressive symptoms, in addition to negative association to other psychosocial variables.	20
Cetin, B., et al. (2010) [60]	Prospective	Depression and anxiety	90 (contol group = 90). All participants were male, military personel	21–30 years Mean age = 21.72 years	Higher level of depression and anxiety in the patient group, compared to the control group in the study. The duration of the HL was positevely correlated with anxiety and depression.	20
Carlsson, P.-I., et al. (2015) [24]	Retrospective	Depression and anxiety	1247 mean age = 67 years. Male = 51%	19–101 years, mean age 68 years	This study indicate greater levels of anxiety and depression among patients with severe or profound HL, than in the general population.	32

reduced QoL. The study suggested that HL is one of several reasons why the elderly have depression, anxiety or other noxious emotions.

The authors of a study that investigated the effect of age at HL onset suggested that late onset HL seem to be negatively correlated to QoL [24]. That is, people who are born with HL or acquire HL in younger years seem to adapt to their HL better, without the HL affecting their QoL in adult life. This study also found that the education level was lower in persons with HL, as only 14% of the participants had university-level education [24].

One study found that there probably is an indirect connection between HL and lower QoL. The authors explain this with a decline in general health that may occur with increased age [50]. This is supported by a study that included subjects with an average age of 71.7 years that found that older people have more health problems in general. Moreover, this study suggests that QoL has many modulating factors, with HL being one of those factors [53]. Furthermore, this study suggests that it is important to understand the synergetic effect of present co-morbidities. This latter point is also addressed by a study that suggests that a varying perception of HL may be influenced by general life circumstances, and that one should not ignore the synergetic effect of multiple co-morbidities on the generic QoL scores [49].

HA use and generic QoL

Five studies measured QoL before the HA fitting, as well as after three [46, 48, 53] or six [45, 56] months following HA fitting. Four of these studies used generic questionnaires to measure QoL, while one used a disease-specific questionnaire [48]. There seems to be evidence that using HA alleviates HL and improves the quality of social relationships. The study conducted by Stark and Hickson [53] showed that the degree of HL, and extent of HA use, seems to be important for improved hearing-specific QoL. However, no significant improvement in generic QoL was reported in this study. The two other studies where QoL was measured after 3 months [46, 48], showed an improved QoL after using HA. In the two studies where QoL was measured after 6 months, one study reported that generic QoL measures yielded equivocal results [56], perhaps due to the sensitivity of the questionnaire being used. The other study [45] suggests a marginal improvement in generic QoL in adults with HL after using HA.

HL and distress, anxiety and/or depression

In the included studies, self-report questionnaires concerning distress, anxiety or depression were collected from participants who were adult persons over 18 years with HL. The number of participants in the studies varied from 90 to 18,318 (Table 2). The gender distribution reported varied from 48 to 55% male participants [24, 58, 59]. One of the studies only had male participants [60] (see Table 2). Three studies [59, 61, 62] used data collected from large population surveys, in which data on the correlation of HL and anxiety, depression and/or distress were available. Two of the studies were based on data collected from a national health register [24] or a database [58]. The remaining two studies had data collected from a prospective study [60] and a longitudinal study [63]. The study conducted by Nachtegaal et al. [61] presented results on both distress and depression, whereas Gopinath et al. [62] presented results from distress. The rest of the included studies presented results on anxiety and depression [24, 58–60, 63]. In these studies, associations between HL and distress, anxiety or depression were only part of the results and conclusions about factors negatively associated with HL.

Of the two included studies on distress, one study suggested that hearing loss is associated with higher distress and present depression. For every decibel increase in signal to noise ratio (SNR), the distress score increased by 2%, while the odds for developing moderate or severe depression increased by 5% [61]. The other study suggested that older HL adult patients are significantly more likely to experience emotional distress [62].

In a study conducted by Hallberg et al. [51], the authors suggest that the psychosocial consequences of the HL cannot be predicted from audiometric data alone, but must be seen in the context of coping strategies, such as communication strategies. In one of these studies, two of the exclusion criteria were dementia and psychiatric disease [49], while one study used limited psychiatric disease as an exclusion criterion [46].

In general, there seems to be significantly higher levels of both anxiety and depression in patients with severe or profound HL compared to a reference population. This seems to be the case even when taking into consideration that some of the patients may have developed anxiety or depression prior to the onset of HL [24]. The duration of HL seems to be positively correlated with anxiety and depression levels, thereby suggesting that the longer the amount of time with HL, the higher the levels of anxiety and depression [60]. However, many of the studies conclude that this conclusion is best supported among females and younger individuals [58, 61].

In conclusion, there seems to be a strong association between HL and depression [58, 59, 63], particularly in women and those younger than 70 years [58, 61]. Anxiety [24, 60] and distress [61, 62] also seem more prevalent among patients with HL. Thus, there is highly likely an association between distress and HL.

Discussion

The literature included in this review yield equivocal findings regarding the association between generic QoL and HL. Some authors argue that there are strong associations [44, 54], while others find less strong [47, 50–53, 56] or no relationships at all [45, 46, 48, 49, 55]. All the included studies on associations between distress and HL give firmly support to such a conclusion, in particular concerning depression among younger individuals [58, 59, 61].

One of the two studies with the highest number of subjects, supported an association between generic QoL and HL and focused on older adults [44]. These subjects showed more severe HL the older they were. The association between increased age and severity of the HL in this study makes it difficult to conclude whether the age or the HL caused the change in generic QoL. Furthermore, when studying older adults by the use of self-reported questionnaires like a QoL questionnaire, it is important to ensure that the informants have the cognitive capacity needed to understand and complete the questionnaire. We have found no report concerning this matter in any of the published studies included in this survey. This should be a matter of future improvement of the investigational design.

Age is an example of a demographic variable that may influence generic QoL [32]. Therefore, such variables should be reported, and analyses carried out in order to estimate the relative importance of these variables. Furthermore, one should preferably adjust the QoL scores by these variables as additional analyses. This has to some extent been reported within the included papers, but no exhaustive study on this matter has been presented. Most of the included studies, however, do not lend any substantial support to the claim that demographic variables are of high importance concerning generic QoL and HL.

HL may be unilateral or bilateral. Standard procedure would be to report hearing levels from the least affected ear [64]. Nevertheless, to differentiate between the two conditions should be of importance and this was done in one investigation [50]. It should be of interest to study subjects with unilateral HL more extensively in order to acquire knowledge of any impaired QoL in this group.

Many of the studies yielding the highest CCAT-scores employed SF-36 as QoL measure, which only to some extent represents a generic HRQoL instrument. The SF-36 does not cover the full range of QoL. General symptoms are not covered [49]. More specifically health related QoL generic questionnaires could additionally be utilized in order to study whether HL affects a broader array of symptoms in persons with HL [44, 49, 53].

The associations between HL and distress, anxiety and depression are better documented than the general relationship between QoL and HL. Many factors may explain this relationship. HL may be the causative factor secondary to the social isolation caused by HL. Furthermore present comorbidity may explain both. This needs to be studied further. Distressed persons are expected to have lowered generic QoL [40]. Therefore, solely based on this association, generic QoL is suggested to be lowered among HL patients.

Regarding justifying HL treatment, improvements in both generic and disease-specific QoLs are important outcome measures, both clinically and for researchers [20]. To what extent individuals with untreated HL have lower generic QoL [49] is therefore interesting to study. A low generic QoL baseline subsequently improved after treatment constitutes an excellent HA treatment argument. A low baseline QoL among HL patients would also lend support to offering a larger range of treatments to this group beyond fitting a hearing aid [65]. The studies where generic QoL were measured following HA fitting after 3 months [46, 48, 53] or 6 months [45, 56]

show equivocal findings. Some of these studies suggest increased generic QoL caused by the use of a HA, while other studies explain HA use as one of several possible factors that leads to better generic QoL. In conclusion, future generic QoL studies should be encouraged since a firm conclusion about HL and generic QoL has not yet been reached.

Despite the fact that HL may cause poorer generic QoL, and that using a HA may improve generic QoL, some studies suggest that many who are fitted with HAs, used their HA only to a limited degree [66]. This may be caused by the patients not receiving sufficient help and follow-up to master the HA [67]. Other studies on treatment show that HAs are an important contributor to increased QoL in HL patients [65]. Some studies suggest that using HAs over time seems to reverse the adverse effects of HL on QoL [62]. The process of HA fitting may also carry a placebo- effect. If so, this could also indicate that, as previously suggested [33, 68–70] concerning other diseases, generic QoL to a large extent mainly originates from the personality and thus stays more or less stable, regardless of the severity of HL.

We suggest a need for including both PROMs and physical measures in all hearing assessments [50]. Many modern HAs have the capability to log the actual use of the HAs in addition to the patient's self-reported use. By collecting both physical and QoL data repeatedly, more robust data would be available to evaluate the strength of the relationship between the actual use of HAs and eventual improvements in QoL. By including control groups within research, one could in addition obtain more conclusive answers as to whether an improved QoL following HA fitting may be considered a Hawthorne effect [71], i.e. if the QoL improvement during HA fitting is due to the attention in this period.

For researchers, it also seems reasonable to measure additional potentially explaining variables, at several time points, when trying to determine what affects the QoL in persons with HL. Such screening would provide the opportunity to unravel why and to what extent patients with HL has lowered QoL, or even psychiatric disease. This could provide important clues on how to better help these patients. Systematic studies of HL treatment, with this perspective included, could likely provide evidence on how to better the health care services for patients with HL.

Data were collected using a literature review design with the aim to identify relevant literature published from the timespan 2000–2016 concerning patients with HL and the evaluation of their generic QoL. When using a limited time span there will always be a risk of missing important publications. This represents a possible weakness in our study that could have been overcome by extending the timespan to include previous years.

Furthermore, we did not systematically search the reference list of the included papers for additional papers. This may have provided additional relevant papers and this represents a weakness in our design. Also, differences in sample sizes, age of subjects, hearing loss configurations and methodological presentations between studies complicated the comparison of results between studies.

Conclusions

The main aim of this study was to review studies about the relationship between HL and QoL. Results of our review show that the majority of such studies suggest that HL reduces QoL. Those studies that also measured QoL after fitting of HAs suggest that HA fitting to some degree improves generic QoL at follow-up within the first year. A supporting aim was to review studies on the relationship between HL and distress, anxiety and mood. Results of our review show that HL is a risk factor for distress. We suggest that systematic studies of HL treatment, with a QoL perspective included, could provide evidence on how to better the health care services for patients with HL. As a consequence of our findings we suggest a need for including both PROMs and physical measures in persons with hearing loss, both at baseline and as outcome measures. Further research is needed to explore the relationship between HL and generic QoL, as well as the importance of various influencing variables on this relationship.

Abbreviations

HA: Hearing aids; HL: Hearing loss; ISAD: Individual sound amplification device; PROM: Patient reported outcome measure; QoL: Quality of life

Acknowledgements

Not applicable.

Funding

This research received no specific grant from any funding agency in the public, commercial or not-for-profit sector.

Authors' contributions

ØN performed the literature search and read all abstracts. ØN and PH read relevant papers to identify those that met the inclusion criteria. ØN wrote the initial results section. ØN and PH wrote an initial manuscript based on these results. JB, FV, AKA and HJA contributed substantially to the revision of all parts of the initial manuscript. All authors read and approved the final manuscript.

Competing interests

The authors declare that they have no competing interests.

Author details

[1]Department of Otolaryngology/Head and Neck Surgery, Haukeland University Hospital, Bergen, Norway. [2]Department of Clinical Medicine, Faculty of Medicine and Dentistry, University of Bergen, Bergen, Norway. [3]Faculty of Health and Social Sciences, Bergen University College, Bergen, Norway. [4]Department of Clinical Science, Section of Logopedics, Phoniatrics and Audiology, Lund University, Lund, Sweden. [5]Department of Health Science, Faculty of Health Sciences, University of Stavanger, Stavanger, Norway.

References

1. Olusanya BO, Neumann KJ, Saunders JE. The global burden of disabling hearing impairment: a call to action. Bull World Health Organ. 2014;92(5): 367–73.
2. Vos T, Allen C, Arora M, Barber RM, Bhutta ZA, Brown A, Carter A, Casey DC, Charlson FJ, Chen AZ. Global, regional, and national incidence, prevalence, and years lived with disability for 310 diseases and injuries, 1990-2015: a systematic analysis for the global burden of disease study 2015. Lancet. 2016;388(10053):1545.
3. Pacala JT, Yueh B. Hearing deficits in the older patient:"I didn't notice anything". JAMA. 2012;307(11):1185–94.
4. Gates GA, Mills JH. Presbycusis. Lancet. 2005;366(9491):1111–20.
5. Lin FR, Thorpe R, Gordon-Salant S, Ferrucci L. Hearing loss prevalence and risk factors among older adults in the United States. J Gerontol A Biol Sci Med Sci. 2011;66(5):582–90.
6. Vila PM, Thomas T, Liu C, Poe D, Shin JJ. The burden and epidemiology of eustachian tube dysfunction in adults. Otolaryngol Head Neck Surg. 2017; 156(2):278–84.
7. Masterson EA, Deddens JA, Themann CL, Bertke S, Calvert GM. Trends in worker hearing loss by industry sector, 1981–2010. Am J Ind Med. 2015; 58(4):392–401.
8. Naz S, Imtiaz A, Mujtaba G, Maqsood A, Bashir R, Bukhari I, Khan MR, Ramzan M, Fatima A, Rehman AU. Genetic causes of moderate to severe hearing loss point to modifiers. Clin Genet. 2017;91(4):589–98.
9. Shargorodsky J, Curhan SG, Curhan GC, Eavey R. Change in prevalence of hearing loss in US adolescents. JAMA. 2010;304(7):772–8.
10. Sprinzl G, Riechelmann H. Current trends in treating hearing loss in elderly people: a review of the technology and treatment options–a mini-review. Gerontology. 2010;56(3):351–8.
11. Laplante-Lévesque A, Hickson L, Worrall L. Rehabilitation of older adults with hearing impairment: a critical review. J Aging Health. 2010;22(2): 143–53.
12. Wehrlen L, Krumlauf M, Ness E, Maloof D, Bevans M. Systematic collection of patient reported outcome research data: a checklist for clinical research professionals. Contemp Clin Trials. 2016;48:21–9.
13. Cocks K, King MT, Velikova G, Martyn St-James M, Fayers PM, Brown JM. Evidence-based guidelines for determination of sample size and interpretation of the European Organisation for the Research and Treatment of Cancer Quality of Life Questionnaire Core 30. J Clin Oncol. 2010;29(1):89–96.
14. Reeve BB, Wyrwich KW, Wu AW, Velikova G, Terwee CB, Snyder CF, Schwartz C, Revicki DA, Moinpour CM, McLeod LD. ISOQOL recommends minimum standards for patient-reported outcome measures used in patient-centered outcomes and comparative effectiveness research. Qual Life Res. 2013;22(8): 1889–905.
15. Terwee C, Prinsen C, Garotti MR, Suman A, De Vet H, Mokkink L. The quality of systematic reviews of health-related outcome measurement instruments. Qual Life Res. 2016;25(4):767–79.

16. Fayers PM, Machin D. Quality of life: the assessment, analysis and interpretation of patient-reported outcomes. John Wiley & Sons, Wiley Online Library; 2013.

17. Fayed N, De Camargo OK, Kerr E, Rosenbaum P, Dubey A, Bostan C, Faulhaber M, Raina P, Cieza A. Generic patient-reported outcomes in child health research: a review of conceptual content using World Health Organization definitions. Dev Med Child Neurol. 2012;54(12):1085–95.

18. Cieza A, Oberhauser C, Bickenbach J, Chatterji S, Stucki G. Towards a minimal generic set of domains of functioning and health. BMC Public Health. 2014;14(1):218.

19. Heggdal L. Clinical application and psychometric properties of a Norwegian questionnaire for the self-assessment of communication in quiet and adverse conditions using two revised APHAB subscales. J Am Acad Audiol. 2018;29(1):25–34.

20. Ciorba A, Bianchini C, Pelucchi S, Pastore A. The impact of hearing loss on the quality of life of elderly adults. Clin Interv Aging. 2012;7:159.

21. Sirgy MJ, Michalos AC, Ferriss AL, Easterlin RA, Patrick D, Pavot W. The qualityity-of-life (QOL) research movement: past, present, and future. Soc Indic Res. 2006;76(3):343–466.

22. Ware JE Jr, Sherbourne CD. The MOS 36-item short-form health survey (SF-36): I. Conceptual framework and item selection. Med Care. 1992; 30(6):473–83.

23. Ware JE Jr. SF-36 health survey update. Spine. 2000;25(24):3130–9.

24. Carlsson P-I, Hjaldahl J, Magnuson A, Ternevall E, Edén M, Skagerstrand Å, Jönsson R. Severe to profound hearing impairment: quality of life, psychosocial consequences and audiological rehabilitation. Disabil Rehabil. 2015;37(20): 1849–56.

25. Coons SJ, Rao S, Keininger DL, Hays RD. A comparative review of generic quality-of-life instruments. PharmacoEconomics. 2000;17(1):13–35.

26. Németh G. Health related quality of life outcome instruments. Eur Spine J. 2006;15(1):S44–51.

27. Fayers P, Bottomley A, Group EQoL. Quality of life research within the EORTC—the EORTC QLQ-C30. Eur J Cancer. 2002;38:125–33.

28. Ludwig K, Schulenburg J-MG, Greiner W. Valuation of the EQ-5D-5L with composite time trade-off for the German population–an exploratory study. Health Qual Life Outcomes. 2017;15(1):39.

29. Larsen FB, Pedersen MH, Friis K, Glümer C, Lasgaard M. A latent class analysis of multimorbidity and the relationship to socio-demographic factors and health-related quality of life. A national population-based study of 162,283 Danish adults. PLoS One. 2017;12(1):e0169426.

30. Monzani D, Galeazzi G, Genovese E, Marrara A, Martini A. Psychological profile and social behaviour of working adults with mild or moderate hearing loss. Acta Otorhinolaryngol Ital. 2008;28(2):61.

31. Wahl H-W, Heyl V, Schilling O. Robustness of personality and affect relations under chronic conditions: the case of age-related vision and hearing impairment. J Gerontol B Psychol Sci Soc Sci. 2012;67(6):687–96.

32. Montejo P, Montenegro M, Fernández MA, Maestú F. Memory complaints in the elderly: quality of life and daily living activities. A population based study. Arch Gerontol Geriatr. 2012;54(2):298–304.

33. Dunne S, Mooney O, Coffey L, Sharp L, Desmond D, Timon C, O'Sullivan E, Gallagher P. Psychological variables associated with quality of life following primary treatment for head and neck cancer: a systematic review of the literature from 2004 to 2015. Psycho-Oncology. 2017;26(2):149–60.

34. Aarstad AK, Beisland E, Osthus AA, Aarstad HJ. Distress, quality of life, neuroticism and psychological coping are related in head and neck cancer patients during follow-up. Acta Oncol. 2011;50(3):390–8.

35. Beisland E: Health-related quality of life, distress and psychosocial factors in head and neck and renal cancer patients. Quality of life in HNSCC and RCC patients. 2015.

36. World Health Organization. ICD-10 Version: 2016. http://apps.who.int/classifications/icd10/browse/2016/en. Accessed 16 Dec 2016.

37. Association AP. Diagnostic and statistical manual of mental disorders. (DSM-5). Washington, DC: American Psychiatric Association; 2013.

38. Ridner SH. Psychological distress: concept analysis. J Adv Nurs. 2004;45(5): 536–45.

39. Keyes KM, Nicholson R, Kinley J, Raposo S, Stein MB, Goldner EM, Sareen J. Age, period, and cohort effects in psychological distress in the United States and Canada. Am J Epidemiol. 2014;179(10):1216–27.

40. Faller H, Schuler M, Richard M, Heckl U, Weis J, Küffner R. Effects of psycho-oncologic interventions on emotional distress and quality of life in adult patients with cancer: systematic review and meta-analysis. J Clin Oncol. 2013;31(6):782–93.

41. Liberati A, Altman DG, Tetzlaff J, Mulrow C, Gøtzsche PC, Ioannidis JP, Clarke M, Devereaux PJ, Kleijnen J, Moher D. The PRISMA statement for reporting systematic reviews and meta-analyses of studies that evaluate health care interventions: explanation and elaboration. PLoS Med. 2009;6(7):e1000100.

42. Cronin P, Ryan F, Coughlan M. Undertaking a literature review: a step-by-step approach. Br J Nurs. 2008;17(1):38–43.

43. Crowe M. Crowe critical appraisal tool (CCAT) user guide. Scotland: Conchra House; 2013.

44. Dalton DS, Cruickshanks KJ, Klein BE, Klein R, Wiley TL, Nondahl DM. The impact of hearing loss on quality of life in older adults. The Gerontologist. 2003;43(5):661–8.

45. Niemensivu R, Manchaiah V, Roine RP, Kentala E, Sintonen H. Health-related quality of life in adults with hearing impairment before and after hearing-aid rehabilitation in Finland. Int J Audiol. 2015;54(12):967–75.

46. Mondelli MFCG, de Souza PJS. Quality of life in elderly adults before and after hearing aid fitting. Braz J Otorhinolaryngol. 2012;78(3):49–56.

47. Espmark A-KK, Rosenhall U, Erlandsson S, Steen B. The two faces of presbyacusis: hearing impairment and psychosocial consequences: Los dos rostros de la presbiacusia: Impedimento auditivo y consecuencias psicosociales. Int J Audiol. 2002;41(2):125–35.

48. Lotfi Y, Mehrkian S, Moossavi A, Faghih-Zadeh S. Quality of life improvement in hearing-impaired elderly people after wearing a hearing aid. Arch Iran Med. 2009;12(4):365–70.

49. Chew H, Yeak S. Quality of life in patients with untreated age-related hearing loss. J Laryngol Otol. 2010;124(8):835–41.

50. Chia E-M, Wang JJ, Rochtchina E, Cumming RR, Newall P, Mitchell P. Hearing impairment and health-related quality of life: the Blue Mountains hearing study. Ear Hear. 2007;28(2):187–95.

51. Hallberg LR-M, Hallberg U, Kramer SE. Self-reported hearing difficulties, communication strategies and psychological general well-being (quality of life) in patients with acquired hearing impairment. Disabil Rehabil. 2008; 30(3):203–12.

52. Helvik A-S, Jacobsen G, Hallberg LR. Psychological well-being of adults with acquired hearing impairment. Disabil Rehabil. 2006;28(9):535–45.

53. Stark P, Hickson L. Outcomes of hearing aid fitting for older people with hearing impairment and their significant others. Int J Audiol. 2004;43(7):390–8.

54. Miyakita T, Ueda A, Zusho H, Kudoh Y. Self-evaluation scores of hearing difficulties and quality of life components among retired workers with noise-related hearing loss. J Sound Vib. 2002;250(1):119–28.

55. Meyer JM, Kashubeck-West S. Well-being of individuals with late-deafness. Rehabil Psychol. 2013;58(2):124.

56. Vuorialho A, Karinen P, Sorri M. Effect of hearing aids on hearing disability and quality of life in the elderly: Efecto de los auxiliares auditivos (AA) en la discapacidad auditiva y la calidad de vida de los ancianos. Int J Audiol. 2006;45(7):400–5.

57. Agrawal Y, Platz EA, Niparko JK. Prevalence of hearing loss and differences by demographic characteristics among US adults: data from the National Health and Nutrition Examination Survey, 1999-2004. Arch Intern Med. 2008; 168(14):1522–30.

58. Tseng C-C, Hu L-Y, Liu M-E, Yang AC, Shen C-C, Tsai S-J. Risk of depressive disorders following sudden sensorineural hearing loss: a nationwide population-based retrospective cohort study. J Affect Disord. 2016;197:94–9.

59. Li C-M, Zhang X, Hoffman HJ, Cotch MF, Themann CL, Wilson MR. Hearing impairment associated with depression in US adults, National Health and nutrition examination survey 2005-2010. JAMA Otolaryngol Head Neck Surg. 2014;140(4):293–302.

60. Cetin B, Uguz F, Erdem M, Yildirim A. Relationship between quality of life, anxiety and depression in unilateral hearing loss. J Int Adv Otol. 2010;6(2):252-7.

61. Nachtegaal J, Smit JH, Smits C, Bezemer PD, Van Beek JH, Festen JM, Kramer SE. The association between hearing status and psychosocial health before the age of 70 years: results from an internet-based national survey on hearing. Ear Hear. 2009;30(3):302–12.

62. Gopinath B, Schneider J, Hickson L, McMahon CM, Burlutsky G, Leeder SR, Mitchell P. Hearing handicap, rather than measured hearing impairment, predicts poorer quality of life over 10 years in older adults. Maturitas. 2012;72(2):146–51.

63. Kramer SE, Kapteyn TS, Kuik DJ, Deeg DJ. The association of hearing impairment and chronic diseases with psychosocial health status in older age. J Aging Health. 2002;14(1):122–37.

64. Gurgel RK, Jackler RK, Dobie RA, Popelka GR. A new standardized format for reporting hearing outcome in clinical trials. Otolaryngol Head Neck Surg. 2012;147(5):803–7.

65. Chisolm TH, Johnson CE, Danhauer JL, Portz LJ, Abrams HB, Lesner S, McCarthy PA, Newman CW. A systematic review of health-related quality of life and hearing aids: final report of the American Academy of Audiology task force on the health-related quality of life benefits of amplification in adults. J Am Acad Audiol. 2007;18(2):151–83.

66. McCormack A, Fortnum H. Why do people fitted with hearing aids not wear them? Int J Audiol. 2013;52(5):360–8.

67. Lupsakko TA, Kautiainen HJ, Sulkava R. The non-use of hearing aids in people aged 75 years and over in the city of Kuopio in Finland. Eur Arch Otorhinolaryngol Head Neck. 2005;262(3):165–9.

68. Aarstad AK, Aarstad HJ, Olofsson J. Personality and choice of coping predict quality of life in head and neck cancer patients during follow-up. Acta Oncol. 2008;47(5):879–90.

69. Aarstad H, Aarstad A, Birkhaug E, Bru E, Olofsson J. The personality and quality of life in HNSCC patients following treatment. Eur J Cancer. 2003; 39(13):1852–60.

70. Beisland E, Aarstad AKH, Osthus AA, Aarstad HJ. Stability of distress and health-related quality of life as well as relation to neuroticism, coping and TNM stage in head and neck cancer patients during follow-up. Acta Otolaryngol. 2013;133(2):209–17.

71. Wickström G, Bendix T. The "Hawthorne effect"—what did the original Hawthorne studies actually show? Scand J Work Environ Health. 2000;26(4): 363–7.

22

Three year experience with the cochlear BAHA attract implant: a systematic review of the literature

Panagiotis A. Dimitriadis[1*], Matthew R. Farr[1], Ahmed Allam[1,2] and Jaydip Ray[1]

Abstract

Background: Bone conduction devices are widely used and indicated in cases of conductive, mixed or single sided deafness where conventional hearing aids are not indicated or tolerated. Percutaneous bone-conduction devices gave satisfactory hearing outcomes but were frequently complicated by soft tissue reactions. Transcutaneous bone conduction devices were developed in order to address some of the issues related to the skin-penetrating abutment. The aim of this article is to present a systematic review of the indications, surgical technique and audiological, clinical and functional outcomes of the BAHA Attract device reported so far.

Methods: A systematic computer-based literature search was performed on the PubMed database as well as Scopus, Cochrane and Google Scholar. Out of 497 articles, 10 studies and 89 reported cases were finally included in our review.

Results: The vast majority of implanted patients were satisfied with the aesthetics of the device scoring highly at the Abbreviated Profile of Hearing Aid Benefit, Glasgow Benefit Inventory and Client Oriented Scale of Improvement. Overall, hearing outcomes, tested by various means including speech in noise, free field hearing testing and word discrimination scores showed a significant improvement. Complications included seroma or haematoma formation, numbness around the area of the flap, swelling and detachment of the sound processor from the external magnet.

Conclusions: The functional and audiological results presented so far in the literature have been satisfactory and the complication rate is low compared to the skin penetrating Bone Conduction Devices. Further robust trials will be needed to study the long-term outcomes and any adverse effects.

Keywords: BAHA Attract, Transcutaneous bone conduction device, Hearing loss

Background

The notion of bone conduction hearing was mentioned as early as the second century AD by Claudius Galenus [1]. Its principle is that sound can be transferred to the inner ear by skull vibrations, bypassing the external and middle ear. Bone conduction devices (BCD) are commonly used in cases of single-sided deafness or conductive/mixed hearing loss where conventional hearing aids are not indicated or tolerated. Conventional BCD [2] were developed in the early 20th century and included a sound processor attached to spectacles or headbands [3]. Disadvantages of

these devices included problems with the skin and soft tissue under the transducer as well as tension headaches due to a high static pressure of about 2 N [4], sound attenuation due to soft tissue interposition especially in frequencies above 1 kHz and issues with feedback [4]. Implanted BCD transmit sound vibrations directly to skull and were developed to overcome some of the issues mentioned above. They are divided into percutaneous (skin penetrating) and transcutaneous (non-skin penetrating) types.

The Bone Anchored Hearing Aid (BAHA®) was the first available percutaneous BCD. It is a semi-implantable under the skin BCD coupled to the skull via an abutment to a titanium fixture. Presently, there are two companies

* Correspondence: pdimitriadis1@sheffield.ac.uk
[1]Department of Otolaryngology, Sheffield Teaching Hospitals, Sheffield, UK
Full list of author information is available at the end of the article

that manufacture the percutaneous BCD: the Swedish Cochlear Bone Anchored Solutions AB, Mölnlycke, that manufacture the BAHA® and the Danish Oticon, which manufacture the Ponto. Their sound processors continually improve offering higher output capability, improved transduced technology and better fitting procedure. To date, more than 150,000 hard of hearing individuals use BAHA [4–6].

Problems associated with these devices include: wound dehiscence, recurrent soft tissue reactions and infections around the abutment are commonly reported (range 8–59 %) which can be daunting both for the patient and the surgeon and can occasionally lead to revision surgery (range 5-42 %) [2, 7]. Implant loss rate is reported to be 8.3 %; and it is even higher in the paediatric population and individuals with learning disabilities [8]. Aesthetic appearance is also a relative drawback and it is therefore often not widely acceptable people in adolescence or by people from different cultural backgrounds [9].

The Bonebridge from MED-EL, Innsbruck, Austria is a direct-drive BCD that is non-skin penetrating. Its transducer is completely implanted and the external processor is attached to the skin by retention magnets in the implanted unit [10].

The skin-drive or transcutaneous BCD transmit sound vibrations through the skin and were developed in order to address some of the issues related to the presence of the skin-penetrating abutment. Hugh and colleagues developed and implanted the first transcutaneous BCD (Xomed Audiant) and the complication rate dropped significantly [11]. It was soon taken out of the market due to poor clinical and audiological outcomes [12].

Following on from this concept, the Sophono device was developed by Siegert under the name Otomag and has been available since 2006 [13]. It has two magnets implanted to the skull by five titanium screws. It uses a larger contact area, designed to reduce skin pressure, which in turn might lead to flap problems. When the skin flap thickness is more than 6 mm, thinning is recommended [14]. A retrospective study on 20 patients with aural atresia implanted with Sophono, found an average improvement of 28.6 dB HL on Pure Tone Audiometry (PTA) and 61.6 % in speech recognition threshold (SRT) scores compared to the unaided condition [15]. Similar audiometric results were presented in studies by Magliulo et al. [16] and O'Niel et al. [17]. In O'Niel's study, skin problems following fitting were noticed in 36 % of the patients and included swelling, irritation, infection, or pain following prolonged use of the device [17].

The BAHA Attract was launched in 2013 and so far more than 200 patients have been implanted [6].

This device uses a single magnet that is attached to the skull with a single titanium fixture. The sound processor is attached to a corresponding external magnet with a soft pad that is used to distribute pressure over the contact area and decrease skin sensitivity. The innovation in this BCD is that in cases of conversion to Attract, a previously fitted osseointegrated fixture can be used to replace the abutment with an implant magnet. We present here a systematic review of the literature.

Methods

A systematic computer-based literature search was performed on the PubMed database as well as Scopus, Cochrane and Google Scholar. We also searched the grey literature and the manufacturer's leaflets and publications. For each search we used the following free-text search terms: Term A was 'BAHA' or 'transcutaneous' and Term B was 'Attract' or 'hearing'.

Inclusion and exclusion criteria

We have included publications that met the following criteria:

1] Reports on patients that underwent BAHA Attract implantation
2] Published in the English language

We have excluded publications that were:

1] Book chapters, letters to the editor and editorials
2] Publications that were relevant to other transcutaneous devices but BAHA Attract
3] Publications from earlier than 2013 (i.e. before the BAHA Attract was commercially available)

Results
Search results

Our search strategy on PubMed revealed 497 articles. After the eligibility assessment 487 publications were excluded. In total, 10 studies were included in the review. Figure 1 illustrates the paper selection process.

Audiological and otological indications

According to the manufacturer, patients with unilateral or bilateral conductive hearing loss (CHL), especially those with an air-bone gap of more than 30 dB would benefit from an Attract system with good hearing outcomes. In cases of mixed hearing loss, patients with a greater air-bone gap (>30 dB) would benefit more from an Attract system than an air conduction hearing aid. Regarding the sensorineural element of hearing loss, a BAHA Attract could compensate for up to 45 dB HL. Finally patients with singe-sided deafness [and low transcranial attenuation] would be able to hear due to crossing over of vibrations to the healthy cochlea and able to localise sounds better. In cases of large transcranial attenuation or moderate mixed hearing loss the patients would most likely

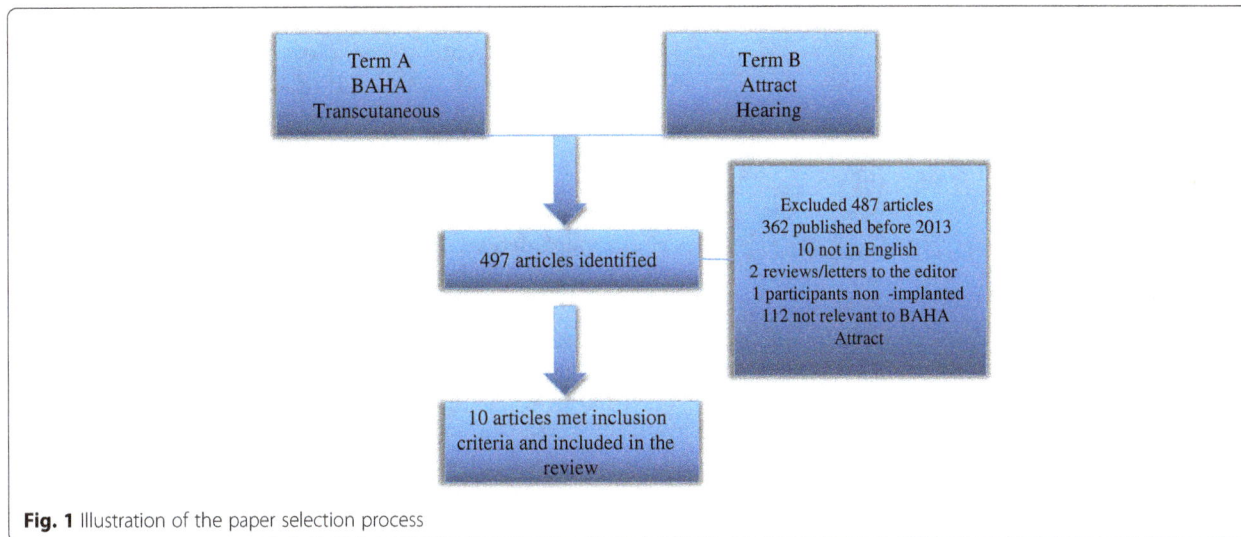

Fig. 1 Illustration of the paper selection process

benefit more from other hearing aid solutions [18]. Patients with the following Ear Nose and Throat (ENT) conditions would benefit from an Attract system: congenital malformations, ear canal stenosis, discharging ears with or without mastoid cavity, previous ear surgery and syndromic hearing loss (such as in Goldenhar or Treacher Collins) [18]. Of course each case should be assessed in its own merits.

Figures 2 and 3 summarize the audiological and otological indications for implantation of BAHA Attract respectively, based on the cases that were found in the published studies. Table 1 includes the demographics of the patients included in the study as well as otological and audiological indications per study.

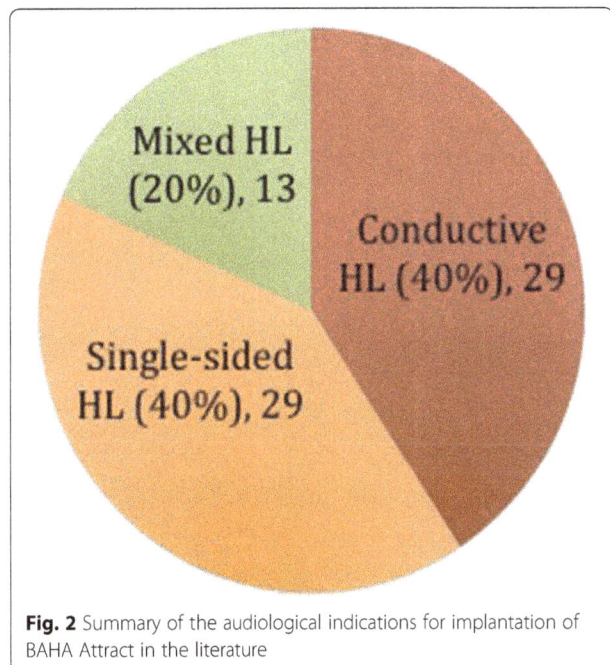

Fig. 2 Summary of the audiological indications for implantation of BAHA Attract in the literature

In particular, out of the 89 patients included in this study, 17 (19.1 %) were children under the age of 16. From the available audiological data in the paediatric population, 5 (55.6 %) had unilateral SNHL and 4 (44.4 %) had CHL (2 had bilateral CHL and 1 contralateral mixed HL). In the adult population, 27 (45 %) had CHL, 22 (36.7 %) had unilateral SNHL and 11 (18.3 %) had mixed hearing loss (bilateral). Otological problems seen in the children included atresia of the external auditory canal (EAC) (36.4 %), COM (27.3 %), EAC stenosis (9.1 %), large vestibular aqueduct and Mondini dysplasia (18.2 %), ossicular abnormality (9.1 %) primary ciliary dyskinesia (9.1 %). In the adults, the majority had COM (53,3 %), followed by otosclerosis (20 %), single sided deafness (8.9 %), atresia (8.9 %), post-viral infection (4.4 %), EAC stenosis (2.2 %) and post-mastoidectomy (2.2 %).

Evaluation of candidates

The air bone gap in the candidate's conductive or mixed hearing loss is a good indicator on whether they would benefit from an Attract system. So, a proper audiological evaluation including PTA, speech audiometry and sound field testing, is essential in the patients' workup. It is also important for the patients to try the Attract in different acoustic environments; this can be done by supplying them with a BAHA on a softband that that they can use for a few weeks. An unnecessary, costly procedure can be prevented that way, if the candidates do not perceive any benefit from the trial.

Surgery

Surgery can be performed under local or general anaesthesia. Gawecki et al. (2016) performed 17 out of 20 cases under local anaesthesia and suggested that it is feasible in most adults [19]. Different implant centres' incision site might differ slightly from that described in the company's

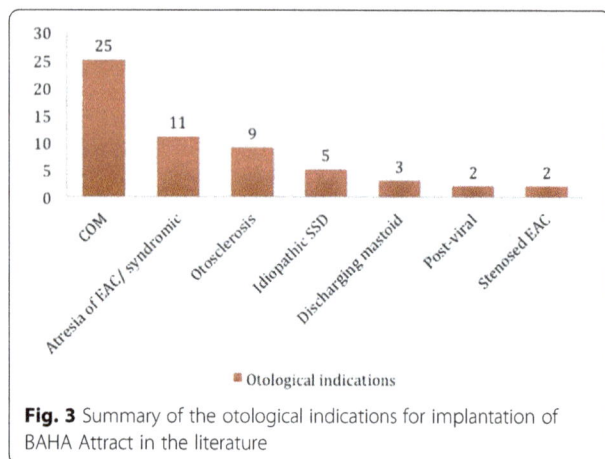

Fig. 3 Summary of the otological indications for implantation of BAHA Attract in the literature

surgery guide [20] but most follow the typical C-shaped incision described in the surgery guide. The incision sites as well as mean surgery time and range per centre are included in Table 2. The site of the implant is marked preoperatively; the superior edge of the processor is 5-7 cm posterior to the ear canal at the level of the temporal line. It is essential that the sound processor does not touch the pinna. A dot of methylene blue dye is injected deep at the centre of the implant site to aid correct placement of the fixture once the flap is raised. Before infiltration of local anaesthesia, skin thickness is measured in several positions of the planned implant site. If the soft tissue is thicker than 6 mm, soft tissue reduction is required to ensure adequate sound transmission [21]. In a study by Briggs et al. [22], 3 out of 5 patients with flap thickness >6 mm, had insufficient magnetic retention, despite flap thinning. A 100^0 to 120^0 C-shaped incision is made 15 mm away from the marked area, down to periosteum and a full-thickness scalp flap is raised. Once adequate dissection is adequate so that the magnet template can be placed in a satisfactory position, a cruciate incision is done in the periosteum, which is raised to expose enough bone for the implant flange. A bone bed indicator can be used to determine whether the surrounding bone requires polishing. Drilling follows at an angle perpendicular to the bone surface, which aims to minimise the need for bone polishing later in the procedure. Once the fixture is in situ, the magnet is screwed into the implant and tightened to 25 Ncm using the torque wrench provided. The wound is closed in layers and a head bandage is applied for 1 to 2 days. A waiting period of 4–6 weeks for osseo-integration to take place is necessary before loading of the sound processor. A BAHA softwear pad is placed in between the skin and the external magnet and provides load distribution over the entire surface of the contact area [2].

Outline of studies and audiological outcomes

Table 3 depicts the study design as well as outcome measures and outcomes per study. Baker et al. (2015) [23], in

Table 1 Patients' demographics, audiological and otological indications for surgery

Study	No of patients	Gender	Mean age (years), age range	Audiological indications	Otological indications
Baker 2015 [23]	6	4 M, 2 F	10.7 (5–15)	5 Unilateral SNHL 1 CHL	N/A
Gawecki 2016 [19]	20	7 M, 13 F	49.8 (25–67)	11 Bilateral Mixed HL 1 Bilateral CHL 8 Unilateral SNHL	8 COM 3 Atresia of EAC 8 otosclerosis 1 post-mumps
Deveze 2015 [6]	1	1 M	65	Unilateral SNHL	Post Ramsey-Hunt
Iseri 2014 [24], Iseri 2015 [9]	16	6 M, 10 F	28 (5–52)	N/A	14 COM 2 Atresia of EAC
Marsella 2015 [25]	3	N/A	25 (8–44)	3 CHL	2 Atresia of EAC 1 post-mastoidectomy
Clamp 2015 [2] Briggs 2015 [22]	27	12 M, 15 F	47.5 (range N/A)	17 CHL 10 Unilateral SNHL	N/A
Powell 2015 [26]	6	N/A	16 (8–46)	2 Bilateral CHL 3 Unilateral CHL, Contralateral Mixed HL 1 Unilateral SNHL	1 SSD 2 LVAS and Mondini 1 Atresia of EAC 1 Meatal stenosis 1 primary ciliary dyskinesia
Carr 2015 [26]	10	5 M, 5 F	45.8 (21–60)	7 CHL 3 Unilateral SNHL	5 COM 1 Otosclerosis 1 Meatal stenosis 3 SSD

CHL: Conductive Hearing Loss, COM: Chronic Otitis Media, EAC: External Auditory Canal, HL: Hearing Loss, N/A: Not available, No: number, M: Male, F: Female, SNHL: Sensorineural Hearing Loss, SSD: Sudden Sensorineural Deafness

Table 2 Surgery time, incision, complications and their management

Study	Mean surgery time in minutes, (range)	Surgical incision	Complications - Management	Outcome
Baker 2015 [23]	N/A	As per manufacturer	1 seroma - Needle aspiration 1 device detaching	1 Resolved 1 Patient not using device
Gawecki 2016 [19]	44 (30–60)	As per manufacturer	2 Haematoma – Compression bandage	Resolved
Deveze 2015 [6]	N/A	Anterior based flap	None	
Iseri 2014 [24], Iseri 2015 [9]	46 (35–65)	Anterior based flap	1 Haematoma – Aspiration 1 Erythema – Reduced magnet strength 3 Erythema and pain – Reduced magnet strength	Resolved
Marsella 2015 [26]	N/A	As per manufacturer	1 swelling soft tissue - Antibiotics	Resolved
Clamp 2015 [2] Briggs 2015 [22]	45 (range N/A)	As per manufacturer	4 Mild erythema 4 Pain – reduced strength of magnet in 1 patient	Resolved
Powell 2015 [26]	N/A	N/A	1 Device detaching despite stronger magnet 1 Sound processor detaching from external magnet plate	N/A
Carr 2015 [27]	57 (40–80)	Inferior based flap	8 Numbness of scalp	None

N/A Not available

their study performed pre-operative audiometry using inset of supra-aural headphones and compared with soundfield post-operatively. Masking was applied to the non-test ear. In average PTA thresholds were improved by 41 dBHL and speech reception thresholds by 56 dBHL. However, measuring hearing thresholds by different means (inset or supra aural headphones vs. soundfield) can affect accuracy of statistical analysis. Post-implantation audiometric data were missing from one child as the magnet was not strong enough to hold the sound processor. Gawecki et al. (2016) [19] reported on their series of 20 adult patients who underwent BAHA Attract implantation.

Table 3 Study design, Outcome measures and results

Study	Study Design	Outcome measures	Results (Mean improvement)
Baker 2015 [23]	Retrospective case series	Soundfield testing: PTA and SRT	PTA: 41 dB HL SRT: 56 dB HL
Gawecki 2016 [19]	Prospective cohort study	QoL questionnaires: GBI, APHAB, BAHU Free field speech in noise audiometry	APHAB: 23.5 % improvement GBI: 29.6 % improvement BAHU: "Good" or "very good" by 85 % of patients Speech in noise: 32.9 %
Deveze 2015 [6]	Case report	N/A	N/A
Iseri 2014 [24], Iseri 2015 [9]	Multicentre retrospective cohort study	Free field PTA and SRT QoL questionnaires: GBI	PTA: 27.3 dB HL SRT: 24 dB HL GBI: 40.5
Marsella 2015 [25]	Prospective case series	Free field PTA and SRT	PTA: 25 dB HL SRT: 63 %
Clamp 2015 [2] Briggs 2015 [22]	Multicentre prospective cohort study	Free field PTA and SRT Speech in noise audiometry QoL questionnaire: APHAB	PTA: 18.4 dB HL SRT: 50 dB HL at 50 dB SPL Speech in noise: 15 dB HL APHAB: significant improvement $p < 0.05$
Powell 2015 [26]	Cross-sectional cohort study	Free field PTA and SRT QoL questionnaires: Bone Anchored Hearing Devices questionnaire	PTA: 30.2 SRT: 72.5 Bone Anchored Hearing Devices Questionnaire: mean score 9.7/10
Carr 2015 [27]	Retrospective cohort study	Free field speech discrimination QoL questionnaires: GBI, COSI	Speech discrimination: 56 % at 50 dBA GBI:82 % and 91 % (for previously aided vs not-previously aided patients) COSI: 86 % of patients could hear in background noise 95 % of the time

APHAB Abbreviated Profile of Hearing Aid Benefit, *BAHU* BAHA Aesthetic, hygiene and Use, *COSI* Client Oriented Scale of Improvement, *GBI* Glasgow Benefit Inventory, *N/A* Not available, *PTA* Pure Tone Audiometry, *QoL:* Quality of Life, *SRT* Speech Reception Thresholds

They divided their patients in two groups, namely Group A: 11 patients with bilateral mixed or CHL and Group B: nine patients with unilateral deafness. The postoperative audiometric evaluation that was performed in 17 (85 %) patients, included speech in noise only and revealed a mean gain of 32.9 %. Iseri et al. (2015) [9] presented the results of a multi-centre study that aimed to compare BAHA Attract with percutaneous bone conduction implants. The BAHA Attract group consisted of 16 patients. Some preliminary results on 12 of them were already published in 2014 [24]. During surgery, bone polishing was required in 5 patients and soft tissue reduction in 4 patients. Post-operatively, the hearing thresholds and SRT were significantly improved (P < 0.05) when the bone conduction implant was on than without it. A between group comparison revealed a significant difference in the SRT results in favour of the percutaneous BCI group. Marsella et al. (2015) [25] reported on their experience of 3 patients implanted with BAHA Attract. The mean gain on PTA was 25 dB. A better gain was seen in the central frequencies and lower gain in the lower (250Hz) and higher frequencies (4 kHz). The SRT post-operatively was 100 % for each patient, with a mean gain of 63 %. Clamp and Briggs (2015) [2] presented some initial results from 8 patients implanted in Melbourne, Australia. This was part of a multicenter study; the other centres were in Santiago, Chile; Haifa, Israel and Hong Kong, China. A subsequent study was published later in 2015 [22] that included another 19 patients. Free field hearing testing showed a mean gain of 18.4 dB HL over the 4 central frequencies. Mean improvement in SRT in quiet was 50 % at 50 dB SPL, 46.4 % at 65 dB SPL and 24.2 % at 80 dB SPL. There was statistically significant improvement in Speech in noise Ratio of 15 dB (SD: 12.8 dB) compared to unaided hearing and 3.8 dB (SD: 7 dB) compared to soft band. For the Australian arm: Mean speech discrimination (monosyllabic words in quiet) score gain with BAHA Attract was 40.7 dB. Speech discrimination in noise was also improved (mean signal to noise difference gain of 10.6 dB). Pure Tone Audiometry results were not available and masking was applied to the contralateral ear at all conditions. Powell et al. (2015) [26] published their results on a study that compared outcomes between 6 patients with BAHA Attract and 6 that were implanted the Sophono Alpha 1. They concluded that both systems improved audiological outcomes and there was no statistically significant difference in aided thresholds or speech discrimination scores between the two devices. Mean unaided PTA was 60.8 dB HL and mean aided PTA 30.6 dB HL. Most gain was noticed at the lower and mid frequencies. At 55 dB, unaided SRT were around 18.5 %, but when aided, they improved to around 87 %. Mean speech perception score gain at 55 dB was 70 %. Carr et al. (2015) [27] reported on 10 patients who

were implanted the BAHA Attract device. They performed word discrimination scores (WDS) in 3 of the patients with CHL using Boothroyd sentences. When aided, there was an increase in WDS of 50 % at 30dBA (from 0 % to 50 %), and 56 % at 50 dBA (32 % to 88 %), which was not statistically significant. Finally, Deveze et al. (2015) [6] reported on one case where a percutaneous bone conduction implant was changed to a BAHA Attract due to recurrent episodes of skin reactions around the abutment (Holgers Grade 3) that failed to improve despite having a longer abutment fitted and local treatment. The initial procedure involved soft tissue reduction. Upon removal of the abutment an interval of 2 months was kept for the skin to heal before re-operating. The authors, concerned about the skin quality and further pressure to skin by the magnet, used a superficial fascia temporalis flap that was stitched around and sheltered the magnet. Audiological results were not presented however the patient reported a decrease in the output compared to the previous percutaneous device. It is commonly accepted that the hearing gain with BAHA Attract is lower than the percutaneous BAHA, therefore they are best used in patients with normal or mildly affected cochlear function. If the hearing deteriorates (e.g. due to aging) conversion to a percutaneous BAHA device should be considered and is a straightforward procedure since there is no need to replace the fixture [2].

The studies from Baker et al. (2015) [23] and Powel et al. (2015) [26] studied predominantly paediatric population and both observed greater improvement in mean aided thresholds (41 dB HL and 30.6 dB HL respectively) compared to other studies with predominantly adult population, such as the one from Briggs et al. (2015) [22] who found improvements of 18.4 dB HL. Similarly, SRT appeared to be better in the paediatric population. This can be explained by the thinner soft tissue and less attenuation of vibration in children.

Functional outcomes

In the study by Gawecki et al. (2016) [19], both groups (Group A: bilateral mixed and conductive hearing loss, Group B: unilateral deafness) reported significant improvement in the Global score of the Abbreviated Profile of Hearing Aid Benefit (APHAB) (mean gain: total 23.5 %, Group A 21.4 %, Group B 26.4 %). Seventeen patients (85 %) reported that the aesthetic effect of the Attract was good or very good. Regarding the Glasgow Benefit Inventory (GBI), the mean total score for both groups was 29.6 (general subscale 40.3, social support 13.3, physical health 3.3). Similarly, in the studies by Iseri et al. (2014,2015) [9, 24], 97 % of patients completed the GBI and the mean score was 40.5 (General subscale 47.6, Social support 28.1, Physical health 23.9). Briggs et al.

(2015) [22] found a significant improvement in the global score of the APHAB (p < 0.05). Powell et al. (2015) [26] designed a new questionnaire (Bone Anchored Hearing Devices Questionnaire) taking into consideration the Entific medical systems questionnaire and the APHAB. Quality of life was improved in all 6 patients and their overall satisfaction on a scale from 0 (very dissatisfied) to 10 (very satisfied) was 9.7. In the study by Carr et al. (2015) [27] the overall satisfaction scores on GBI for those who were aided before implantation was 91 % and for those who were not previously aided was 82 %. Regarding the Client Oriented Scale of Improvement (COSI), 70 % of patients responded that they could hear in noisy environments 75 % to 95 % of the time and all of them agreed that the sound quality was good or very good. Finally, no functional results were presented in the remaining 2 studies [6, 25].

Complications

A pie chart that displays the complication rates is presented in Fig. 4. Table 2 presents the complications per centre along with their management. A common problem reported amongst the studies is linked to the magnet strength; pain and erythema around the implant that resolve by lowering the magnet's strength while weak attachment of the magnet is usually resolved by increasing the magnet strength. There is need to find the ideal balance between the two in each case. Seroma or haematoma formation was reported in 4 patients (4.4 %), which was treated conservatively [9, 19, 23]. Eight patients (8.9 %) reported to have numbness around the area of the flap in a single study [27]. This probably represents a commoner problem that is under-reported. One patient (1.1 %) was treated with antibiotics for a mild swelling that they developed 7 days post-operatively [25]. In another case (1.1 %) the sound processor would detach from the external magnet [26]. No major differences identified in the complications between the paediatric and adult patients. There

have been no reports of persistent adverse reactions of skin due to the magnet up to this intermediate phase. However, it would be important to look out for any long-term complications of its use.

Discussion

Strengths and Limitations of the studies and directions for future studies

A common limitation in the studies described is that they are observational studies (retrospective or prospective cohort studies) or case reports rather than Randomised Controlled Trials; therefore, confounding factors might have influenced reported outcomes. Some of the studies include a small number of patients so caution is needed in generalizing the results. Moreover, the outcome measures (Audiological and Functional) and the timing of testing varied greatly amongst the studies making a direct comparison difficult. Age and gender matching of participants in studies that compared different hearing solutions [9, 26] was not always done although this is hard to achieve in convenience studies. Finally, data on audiological, otological indications or functional outcomes were missing from some of the studies [2, 6, 9, 23, 25]. On the other hand, most studies had a good follow-up rate of their cohort and were able to present data for most of the participants. The manufacturers were not involved in the design, analysis or publication process of most studies. More specifically all but three studies disclosed no conflict of interest. Two studies [6, 23] did not declare any conflict of interest. The study by Briggs et al. (2015) [22] was sponsored by Cochlear Bone Anchored Solutions, Mölnlycke, Sweden.

In the future, more robust, well-designed studies with a higher level of evidence are needed. With rising healthcare costs and a demand for improving technology in an era of rationalization in healthcare, there is an ever-increasing need for hard evidence of the cost benefit ratio of new technology.

Conclusions

This is the first systematic literature review on a new transcutaneous Bone Conduction Hearing Aid device, the BAHA Attract by the Cochlear Bone Anchored Solutions AB Mölnlycke, Sweden that was granted approval in 2013. Once the appropriate candidates have been selected through thorough evaluation the results have been promising. The surgery is relatively simple and quick and can be done under local anaesthesia or general anaesthesia. The functional and audiological results presented in the literature are quite satisfactory and the complication rate is much less compared to the skin penetrating BCD. A multi-centre randomized controlled trial that would test different hearing devices is currently missing from the literature.

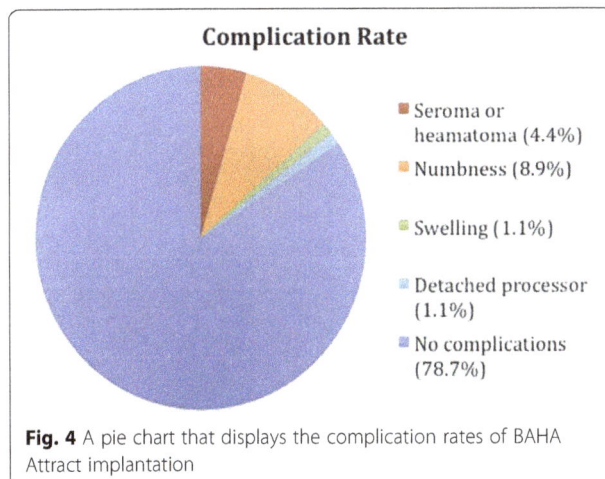

Fig. 4 A pie chart that displays the complication rates of BAHA Attract implantation

Abbreviations

APHAB: Abbreviated Profile of Hearing Aid Benefit; BAHA: Bone Anchored Hearing Aid; BCD: Bone conduction devices; CHL: Conductive hearing loss; COM: Chronic otitis media; COSI: Client Oriented Scale of Improvement; EAC: External auditory canal; ENT: Ear, nose and throat; GBI: Glasgow Benefit Inventory; MeSH: Medical subject headings; MRI: Magnetic resonance imaging; PTA: Pure Tone Audiometry; SRT: Speech recognition thresholds; SSD: Single sided deafness; WDS: Word discrimination scores

Acknowledgements

None.

Funding

No funding was received for this study.

Authors' contributions

PAD: involved in drafting the manuscript, gave final approval of the version to be published, agreed to be accountable for all aspects of the work. MRF: involved in drafting the manuscript, gave final approval of the version to be published, agreed to be accountable for all aspects of the work. AA: involved in revising the manuscript, gave final approval of the version to be published, agreed to be accountable for all aspects of the work. JR: involved in revising the manuscript, gave final approval of the version to be published, agreed to be accountable for all aspects of the work. All authors read and approved the final manuscript.

Author details

[1]Department of Otolaryngology, Sheffield Teaching Hospitals, Sheffield, UK. [2]Department of Otolaryngology, Mansoura University Hospitals, Mansoura, Egypt.

References

1. Berger KW. Early bone conduction hearing aid devices. Arch Otolaryngol. 1976;102:315–8.
2. Clamp PJ, Briggs RJ. The Cochlear Baha 4 Attract System - design concepts, surgical technique and early clinical results. Expert Rev Med Devices. 2015;12:223–30.
3. Mudry A, Tjellström A. Historical background of bone conduction hearing devices and bone conduction hearing aids. Adv Otorhinolaryngol. 2011;71:1–9.
4. Reinfeldt S, Håkansson B, Taghavi H, Eeg-Olofsson M. New developments in bone-conduction hearing implants: a review. Med Devices (Auckl). 2015;8:79–93.
5. Kurz A, Flynn M, Caversaccio M, Kompis M. Speech understanding with a new implant technology: a comparative study with a new nonskin penetrating Baha system. Biomed Res Int. 2014;2014:416205.
6. Devèze A, Rossetto S, Meller R, Sanjuan Puchol M. Switching from a percutaneous to a transcutaneous bone anchored hearing system: the utility of the fascia temporalis superficialis pedicled flap in case of skin intolerance. Eur Arch Otorhinolaryngol. 2015;272:2563–9.
7. Dimitriadis PA, Vlastarakos PV, Nikolopoulos TP. Treatment of sensorineural hearing loss: contemporary rehabilitation and future prospects. In: Dupont JP, editor. Hearing Loss: Classification, Causes and Treatment. New York: NOVA Biomedical Books; 2011. p. 101–37.
8. Dun CA, Faber HT, de Wolf MJ, Mylanus EA, Cremers CW, Hol MK. Assessment of more than 1,000 implanted percutaneous bone conduction devices: skin reactions and implant survival. Otol Neurotol. 2012;33:192–8.
9. Iseri M, Orhan KS, Tuncer U, Kara A, Durgut M, Guldiken Y, et al. Transcutaneous bone-anchored hearing aids versus percutaneous ones: multicenter comparative clinical study. Otol Neurotol. 2015;36:849–53.
10. Sprinzl G, Lenarz T, Ernst A, Hagen R, Wolf-Magele A, Mojallal H, et al. First European multicenter results with a new transcutaneous bone conduction hearing implant system: short-term safety and efficacy. Otol Neurotol. 2013;34:1076–83.
11. Hough J, Himelick T, Johnson B. Implantable bone conduction hearing device: Audiant bone conductor. Update on our experiences. Ann Otol Rhinol Laryngol. 1986;95:498–504.
12. Snik AF, Dreschler WA, Tange RA, Cremers CW. Short- and long-term results with implantable transcutaneous and percutaneous bone-conduction devices. Arch Otolaryngol Head Neck Surg. 1998;124:265–8.
13. Siegert R. Partially implantable bone conduction hearing aids without a percutaneous abutment (Otomag): technique and preliminary clinical results. Adv Otorhinolaryngol. 2011;71:41–6.
14. http://www.sophono.com/professionals/practice-support Accessed 28 Sept 2016.
15. Siegert R, Kanderske J. A new semi-implantable transcutaneous bone conduction device: clinical, surgical, and audiologic outcomes in patients with congenital ear canal atresia. Otol Neurotol. 2013;34:927–34.
16. Magliulo G, Turchetta R, Iannella G, Valperga di Masino R, di Masino RV, de Vincentiis M. Sophono Alpha System and subtotal petrosectomy with external auditory canal blind sac closure. Eur Arch Otorhinolaryngol. 2015;272:2183–90.
17. O'Niel MB, Runge CL, Friedland DR, Kerschner JE. Patient outcomes in magnet-based implantable auditory assist devices. JAMA Otolaryngol Head Neck Surg. 2014;140:513–20.
18. Cochlear™ BAHA 4 Candidate Selection Guide, last accessed 14/08/2016
19. Gawęcki W, Stieler OM, Balcerowiak A, Komar D, Gibasiewicz R, Karlik M, et al. Surgical, functional and audiological evaluation of new Baha(®) Attract system implantations. Eur Arch Otorhinolaryngol. 2016;273(10):3123–30.
20. Cochlear™ Baha® 4 Attract System Surgical Procedure, last accessed 14/08/2016
21. Flynn MC. Design Concept and Technological Considerations for the Cochlear BAHA 4 Attract System. Report E82744. Molnlycke, Sweden: Cochlear Bone Anchored Solutions AB, 2013
22. Briggs R, Van Hasselt A, Luntz M, Goycoolea M, Wigren S, Weber P, et al. Clinical performance of a new magnetic bone conduction hearing implant system: results from a prospective, multicenter, clinical investigation. Otol Neurotol. 2015;36:834–41.
23. Baker S, Centric A, Chennupati SK. Innovation in abutment-free bone-anchored hearing devices in children: Updated results and experience. Int J Pediatr Otorhinolaryngol. 2015;79:1667–72.
24. Işeri M, Orhan KS, Kara A, Durgut M, Oztürk M, Topdağ M, et al. A new transcutaneous bone anchored hearing device - the Baha® Attract System: the first experience in Turkey. Kulak Burun Bogaz Ihtis Derg. 2014;24:59–64.
25. Marsella P, Scorpecci A, Dalmasso G, Pacifico C. First experience in Italy with a new transcutaneous bone conduction implant. Acta Otorhinolaryngol Ital. 2015;35:29–33.
26. Powell HR, Rolfe AM, Birman CS. A comparative study of audiologic outcomes for Two transcutaneous bone-anchored hearing devices. Otol Neurotol. 2015;36:1525–31.
27. Carr SD, Moraleda J, Procter V, Wright K, Ray J. Initial UK experience with a novel magnetic transcutaneous bone conduction device. Otol Neurotol. 2015;36:1399–402.

A questionnaire using vocal symptoms in quality control of phonosurgery: vocal surgical questionnaire

Aleksander Grande Hansen[1]*⊙, Chi Zhang[2], Jens Øyvind Loven[1], Hanne Berdal-Sørensen[1], Magnus TarAngen[1] and Rolf Haye[1,3]

Abstract

Background: Quality control after phonosurgery is important and may be time consuming. Often questionnaires focusing on quality of life are applied. We aimed at investigating the use of organ specific symptoms, such as hoarseness and voice failure with the use of self-reported visual analogue scales (VAS) and Likert-scales.

Methods: A vocal surgical questionnaire using VAS and Likert-scales for hoarseness, voice failure and factors that could influence voice quality was given twice consecutively to a group of healthy volunteers ($n = 57$, 45 female) and a group of voice patients ($n = 34$, 21 females) for a test/re-test study. Secondly, a group of patients undergoing surgery ($n = 90$, 61females) answered the questionnaire preoperatively and postoperatively. The difference between test/retest, healthy volunteers and patients, and between pre- and postoperative results were compared.

Results: There was no significant difference in the test/retest results in healthy volunteers nor in the patient group. There was statistically significant difference between the healthy volunteers and patients, and between the preoperative and postoperative results after phonosurgery.

Conclusion: This short and organ specific questionnaire clearly demonstrates the effect of phonosurgery, making it an easy and relevant tool in quality control and potentially reducing the need of postoperative controls in the outpatient clinic.

Keywords: Laryngology, Questionnaire, Voice assessment, Phonosurgery, Visual analogue scale, Likert scale

Background

Quality control after treatment of vocal disorders is often implemented using mailed questionnaires [1–5]. Most of them focus on quality of life items [6]. Surgeons treating laryngeal lesions are more interested in organ specific vocal symptoms, particularly hoarseness and voice failure, as these symptoms often provide indication for surgery and are considered important in assessing the results of phonosurgery. Hoarseness is a symptom describing a vocal change, e.g. a breathy, creaky or raspy voice. Voice failure describes that the voice "gives out" in the middle of speaking. Surgeons also want to be informed of any change in symptom load, other treatments, occupational as well as social habits that may influence treatment. Ideally, all patients undergoing phonosurgery should be recalled for a postoperative consultation with stroboscopy, but this is challenging in terms of human and financial resources. A clinical postoperative questionnaire would allow to only recall patients with persistent symptoms. Our aim, therefore, was to construct a questionnaire focusing on hoarseness and voice failure, using visual analogue scales (VAS) to compare these symptoms between healthy volunteers and patients, and between preoperative and postoperative symptom load.

Methods

This study was performed at the Department of Oto-Rhino-Laryngology, Head and Neck Surgery of Lovisenberg Diaconal Hospital in Oslo, Norway. The study was approved by the Ethics Committee at the hospital.

* Correspondence: aleksandergrandehansen@gmail.com
[1]Department of Ear, Nose and Throat, Head and Neck Surgery, Lovisenberg Diaconal Hospital, Oslo, Norway
Full list of author information is available at the end of the article

Vocal surgical questionnaire (VSQ)

We constructed a VSQ for a preoperative resume of the patient's symptoms and the relevant clinical data. The preoperative version of the VSQ was twice presented to patients and controls as a test-retest study. In the second presentation we asked if there had been a change in the vocal function since the first response. If there had been a change this test-retest sample was discarded. The preoperative version of the VSQ (Fig. 1) consists of one VAS for hoarseness and another one for voice failure. Both VAS were 10 cm long, marked 0 (= no hoarseness/voice failure) on the left end, and 10 (= complete hoarseness/voice failure) on the right end. The patients were asked to rate their subjective sense of hoarseness and voice failure by putting a mark on the scale. The score was measured in millimetres (mm) from the left end of the scale to this mark.

We also included four point Likert scales for hoarseness and voice failure. The grades were 0 = none/never, 1 = mild/sometimes, 2 = moderate/often and 3 = severe/always. Four point Likert scales were also used in assessing vocal function in different social settings: at home, at work, during leisure, in noisy environment with the options 0 = never, 1 = sometimes, 2 = often, 3 = always. The patients were asked about how often they needed to clear their throat, their smoking habits, hearing

Name

VOCAL SURGICAL QUESTIONNAIRE

Date: ____________

Please mark your opinion of your vocal problem in the appropriate box and on the scale.

	never	sometimes	often	always
Are you bothered by hoarseness? (breathy, creaky or raspy voice)	☐	☐	☐	☐
	none	mild	moderate	severe
Rate your hoarseness:	☐	☐	☐	☐

Mark on the scale below the degree of your hoarseness.

0= none 10= complete

0 I--I 10

	never	sometimes	often	always
Are you bothered by voice failure? ("gives out" in the middle of speaking)	☐	☐	☐	☐

Mark how often you experience voice failure on the 0 to 10 scale below.

0= never 10= always

0 I--I 10

Do you have problems with your voice....

	never	sometimes	often	always
at home?	☐	☐	☐	☐
at work?	☐	☐	☐	☐
at leisure?	☐	☐	☐	☐
in noise?	☐	☐	☐	☐
Do you clear your throat?	☐	☐	☐	☐
Do you smoke?	☐	☐	☐	☐
Do you have problems hearing?	☐	☐	☐	☐
Do you have heartburn (reflux)?	☐	☐	☐	☐

If yes, do you use medication for it?	No ☐	Yes ☐
Do you have asthma?	No ☐	Yes ☐
If yes, do you use inhalers?	No ☐	Yes ☐
Have you had speech therapy?	No ☐	Yes ☐

What kind of work do you do:______________________

Fig. 1 The vocal surgical questionnaire (VSQ) used in the preoperative recording of vocal symptoms

disability, reflux symptoms, asthma and use of related medication. The final items were related to occupation and the use of speech therapy.

The postoperative version of the VSQ contained the same questions as the preoperative one with an additional item about the overall improvement in the voice after surgery. The postoperative version of the VSQ was mailed to the patients 4 months postoperatively together with a cover letter and a pre-paid return envelope.

Subjects

The study population consisted of three groups: controls, i.e. persons without a voice problem, patients included for the test-retest study and an expanded group of patients treated surgically. Persons/patients with an inadequate command of the Norwegian language were excluded.

Healthy volunteers were recruited from different departments at our hospital. They could not complain of voice disorders. The volunteers twice responded to the preoperative version of the VSQ with a minimum time interval of 1 week. To ensure that the two responses evaluated the same vocal function, there should not be any change in vocal function in the time interval between the two responses. They were given a study identification number only known to one of the investigators. The lists with the identification numbers were subsequently destroyed after the responses were obtained.

Patients referred to the department for benign laryngeal diseases were asked to participate in a test-retest study of the preoperative version of the VSQ. The time interval was a minimum of 1 week. Patients with malignant disorders were excluded. To ensure that the two responses evaluated the same vocal function, participants with changes in the vocal function between the two responses were excluded.

Patients with benign laryngeal disorders were asked to respond to the VSQ and also to the postoperative version of the VSQ after 4 months. We included patients with laryngeal papillomatosis, vocal sulcus, atrophic vocal cords, recurrent nerve palsy and spastic dysphonia. Surgery was performed during general anaesthesia. Benign laryngeal lesions were treated microscopically with microsurgical instruments or laser, spastic dysphonia with injections of botulinum toxin and vocal sulcus lesions and atrophic vocal cords with injections of hydroxyapatite.

Statistical analyses

On test-retest studies, the mean and variance of VAS were calculated for both questionnaires. The difference between the answers from the two questionnaires of the same cohort was compared with Wilcoxon signed rank test. Cohen's kappa was computed on test-retest cohorts

to verify the reliability of the questionnaire. Cronbach's alpha was computed on the same cohorts to quantify the internal consistency among questions. We used Spearman's correlation coefficient to quantify the correlation between VAS and Likert scale of hoarseness and voice failure both on pre- and postoperative cohorts. Wilcoxon signed rank test was used to compare the difference between responses to Likert scale questions pre- and postoperatively. All statistics were performed using R, version 3.4.2, with package "psych".

Results

Controls, test-retest

We recruited 57 healthy volunteers (45 females and 12 males) with a mean age of 48.6 years. There was no significant difference in VAS scores of hoarseness and voice failure between their first and second response to the VSQ (Table 1). The ratings between the two responses to vocal function in different social environments, hearing loss, asthma, regurgitation and clearing of the throat were not significantly different (Table 2).

Patients, test-retest

Thirty-four patients (21 females and 13 males) with a mean age of 43.5 years twice responded to the preoperative version of the VSQ. There were six smokers and two patients with asthma. No significant difference was found between the first and second responses to the VAS scores of hoarseness and voice failure (Table 1). Cohen's kappa was computed for Likert scores of vocal function in different social settings, social habits,

Table 1 VAS scores (Standard Deviation) for control group and patient test-retest; comparison between patients and controls and comparison between pre- and postoperative results

Control group

	1. response	2. response	Difference	p-value
Hoarseness	4.83 (12.25)	4.73 (10.57)	0.74	0.63
Voice failure	1.91 (3.84)	2.22 (4.19)	−0.98	0.70

Patient test-retest

	1. response	2. response	Difference	p-value
Hoarseness	70.64 (24.49)	71.74 (19.26)	−0.39	0.89
Voice failure	49.09 (30.06)	54.78 (26.72)	−3.25	0.92

Comparison patients vs. controls using mean of 1. and 2. response

	Patients	Controls	Difference	p-value
Hoarseness	71.19 (22.03)	4.78 (11.44)	66.41	< 0.0001
Voice failure	51.85 (28.44)	2.07 (4.02)	49.78	< 0.0001

Pre and postoperative results compared

	Preoperative	Postoperative	Difference	p-value
Hoarseness	64.25 (23.20)	23.89 (26.78)	41.17	< 0.0001
Voice failure	43.82 (27.53)	17.95 (25.34)	26.08	< 0.0001

Table 2 Comparison between responses of first and second questionnaire in controls (volunteers) and patients

	Controls	Patients
Vocal function		
At home	0.13	0.34
At work	0.10	0.50
In noise	0.47	0.26
At leisure	0.21	0.36
Hawking	0.40	0.40
Smoking	0.55	0.48
Hearing problem	0.58	0.75
Reflux	0.36	0.52
Reflux medication	0.57	0.87
Asthma	0.75	0.65
Asthma spray	0.61	1.00

Cohen's kappa

illnesses and treatments to verify the reliability of the questionnaire and the results were positive (Table 2). The Cronbach's alpha tests for questions of voice function in different social settings showed high values for both the first and second questionnaire (Table 3).

Comparison between controls and patients

VAS scores of hoarseness and voice failure (using the average of the first and second questionnaire) showed significant differences between patients and controls (Table 1).

Results of surgery

We compared the pre and postoperative data of 90 patients (29 males and 61 females) with a mean age of 47.2 years who were surgically treated of benign vocal cord disorders. All patients from the test-retest study were included in the study of the surgical results. We recorded 15 smokers and 11 patients with asthma. The VAS scores for hoarseness and voice failure were significantly different between the pre- and postoperative recordings (Table 1).

We found that the Likert and VAS scores for hoarseness and voice failure were highly correlated both for

Table 3 Reliability of 1. and 2. questionnaire in patients regarding voice failure in different social settings

	1. questionnaire	2. questionnaire
All items	0.89	0.91
At home	0.85	0.85
At work	0.85	0.91
In noise	0.90	0.89
At leisure	0.83	0.85

Chronbach alpha

the pre- and postoperative recordings and the differences between them using Spearman's correlation (Table 4). This is illustrated in Fig. 2.

The Likert scores (using median values) before and after surgery and their differences for vocal function in social settings, hearing problems, smoking, regurgitation, clearing of throat, asthma and treatments are shown in Table 5. Patients reported significant improvement in all items except for smoking, hearing problems, heartburn and asthma.

Discussion

We have assessed the VSQ for use as an instrument in quality control of phonosurgery. The test-retest of controls and of patients did not show any significant change in hoarseness or voice failure when the questionnaire was twice applied to the participants. There was a statistically significant difference in the results between patients and controls for hoarseness, voice failure and vocal function in different social settings. The postoperative results showed a significant improvement in hoarseness, voice failure and vocal function. We therefore believe that our findings could make the VSQ a useful instrument in quality control of phonosurgery.

Studies have shown that short questionnaires give better response rates than longer ones [7]. We, therefore, intended to remove overlapping questions. The scores for hoarseness and voice failure which were recorded both on Likert scales and VAS were comparable. As VAS is a continuous and Likert an interrupted scale we prefer to only use VAS for these items. The VSQ has four different questions about the voice quality in different social settings. As there was no significant difference in improvement after surgery between the different settings, we believe that one item should be sufficient to describe the social aspect of voice function. The voice quality at home was the only one responded to by all patients and therefore best suited for our purpose. Professional voice users could benefit from the evaluation of vocal symptoms in different social settings. Therefore, these questions could remain in the VSQ for professional voice users.

The postoperative responses to hearing problems, asthma, smoking habits, regurgitation and use of medication were only marginally different from the preoperative ones. We, therefore, expect that most of the postoperative responses of these items will remain unchanged. Thus, one open-ended question of any change in smoking habit, hearing, heart burn, asthma, treatments and occupation would be sufficient. The question about speech therapy after surgery should remain. The postoperative questionnaire could thereby be reduced to eight items.

There are several questionnaires in use for assessing the status of the voice before and after treatment [8],

Table 4 Correlation between VAS and Likert scale for pre- and postoperative patients.

	Preoperative	Postoperative	Comparison between pre and post
Hoarseness	0.76	0.91	0.85
Voice failure	0.81	0.87	0.69

Spearman's correlation

and objective measurements often do not correlate with self-assessed voice symptoms [9]. Questionnaires often pose questions on voice impairment (vocal physical symptoms), voice function and the impact of the voice on the patients' emotional wellbeing. Most questionnaires use a

five point Likert scale for each of the questions [10] or VAS [11, 12]. The scores are added for a final result. Each question has equal merit. We wanted to focus on the two main physical aspects of the voice and in addition on the medical conditions and therapies, social habits and

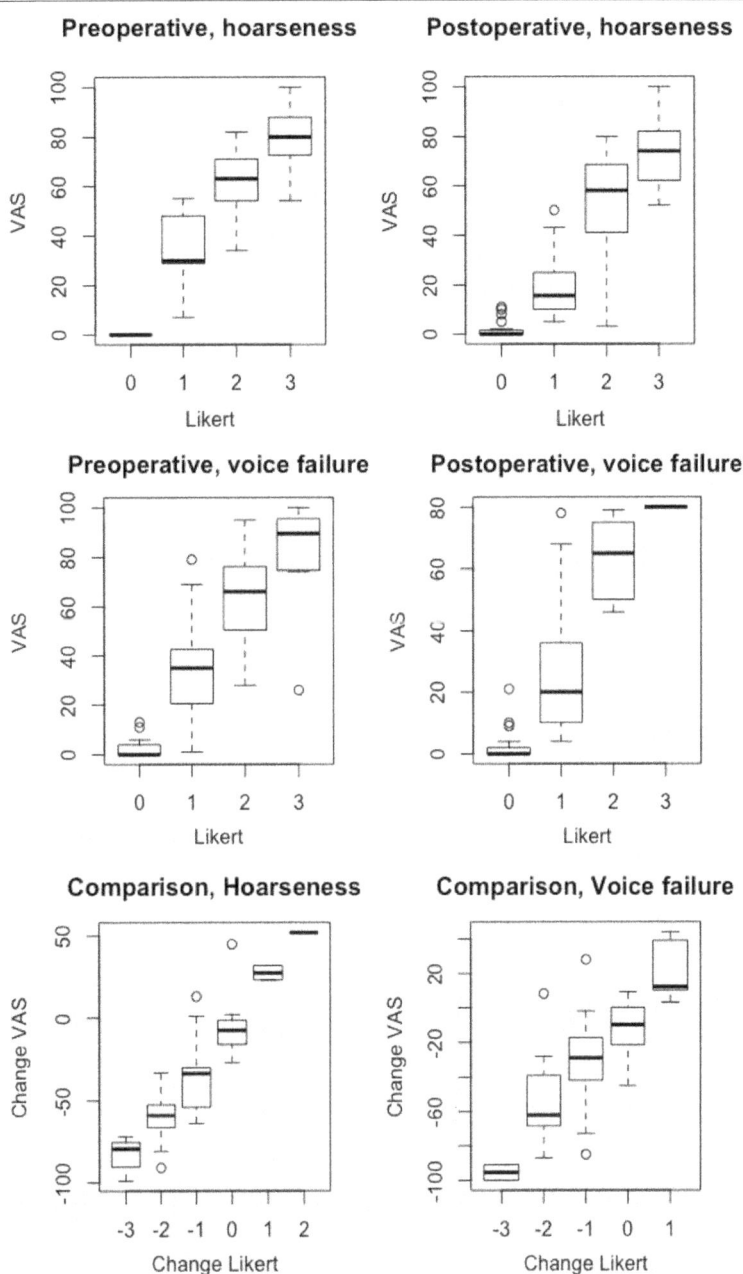

Fig. 2 Comparison between visual analogue scale (VAS) and Likert scores for hoarseness and voice failure, pre-, postoperative and improvement

Table 5 Comparison of Likert scores for vocal symptoms, vocal function, social habits, illness and treatments between pre-, postoperative and change in ratings

	Median pre	Median post	Median change	P-value
Hoarseness	2	1	−1	< 0.0001
Voice failure	1	0	− 1	< 0.0001
Hoarseness at home	2	0	−1	< 0.0001
At work	2	0	−1	< 0.0001
At leisure	2	0	−1	< 0.0001
In noise	2	1	−1	< 0.0001
From others	2	0	−1	< 0.0001
Clear throat	1	1	−1	< 0.0001
Smoking	0	0	0	0.032
Problem hearing	0	0	0	0.937
Heartburn	0	0	0	0.44
Asthma	0	0	0	0.9772

Wilcoxon signed rank test

occupation that may influence the voice. These are important in relation to surgery. Changes in these items may be contributory to improvement or deterioration of the voice, thus they have a natural place in a vocal questionnaire.

The vocal function is important for the patient's emotional well-being, social function and occupation. However, questionnaires do not evaluate the impact of emotions on the vocal function and we acknowledge that changes in the emotions in the time period between the pre- and postoperative questionnaires could have influenced our results.

Conclusions

We believe that this short postoperative questionnaire focusing on hoarseness and voice failure gives a satisfactory assessment of the patient's response to phonosurgery. This will help us decide whether to recall the patient for a new consultation or not. A satisfactory response will obviate the need of a recall and save time for other patients.

Abbreviations
VAS: Visual analogue scale; VSQ: Vocal surgical questionnaire

Acknowledgements
The authors are grateful for the motivation from the clinic management to perform this study.

Funding
Lovisenberg Diaconal Hospital funded the study.

Responsibility
Aleksander Grande Hansen takes responsibility for the integrity of the contents of this study.

Authors' contributions
AGH contributed in conception and design, acquisition and analyses of data, writing, drafting and revising the manuscript critically. CZ contributed in statistical analyses, interpretation of data, constructing figures, writing, drafting and revising the manuscript critically. JØL contributed to design, recruitment and implementation of the study, writing, drafting and revising the manuscript critically. HBS contributed to design, recruitment and implementation of the study, writing, drafting and revising the manuscript critically. MT contributed in data collection, writing, drafting and revising the manuscript critically. RH contributed to design, recruitment of volunteers and patients, interpretation of data, writing, drafting and revising the manuscript critically. All authors read and approved the final manuscript.

Competing interests
The authors declare that they have no competing interests.

Author details
[1]Department of Ear, Nose and Throat, Head and Neck Surgery, Lovisenberg Diaconal Hospital, Oslo, Norway. [2]Institute of Basic Medical Sciences, Faculty of Medicine, University of Oslo, Oslo, Norway. [3]Institute of Clinical Medicine, Faculty of Medicine, University of Oslo, Oslo, Norway.

References
1. Laukkanen AM, Leppanen K, Ilomaki I. Self-evaluation of voice as a treatment outcome measure. Folia Phoniatr Logop. 2009;61(1):57–65.
2. Uloza V. Effects on voice by endolaryngeal microsurgery. Eur Arch Otorhinolaryngol. 1999;256(6):312–5.
3. Aaby C, Heimdal JH. The voice-related quality of life (V-RQOL) measure–a study on validity and reliability of the Norwegian version. J Voice. 2013; 27(2):258 e229–33.
4. Pernambuco L, Silva MP, Almeida MN, Costa EB, Souza LB. Self-perception of swallowing by patients with benign nonsurgical thyroid disease. Codas. 2017;29(1):e20160020.
5. Karlsen T, Grieg AR, Heimdal JH, Aarstad HJ. Cross-cultural adaption and translation of the voice handicap index into Norwegian. Folia Phoniatr Logop. 2012;64(5):234–40.
6. Branski RC, Cukier-Blaj S, Pusic A, Cano SJ, Klassen A, Mener D, Patel S, Kraus DH. Measuring quality of life in dysphonic patients: a systematic review of content development in patient-reported outcomes measures. J Voice. 2010;24(2):193–8.
7. Rosen CA, Lee AS, Osborne J, Zullo T, Murry T. Development and validation of the voice handicap index-10. Laryngoscope. 2004;114(9):1549–56.

8. Birkent H, Sardesai M, Hu A, Merati AL. Prospective study of voice outcomes and patient tolerance of in-office percutaneous injection laryngoplasty. Laryngoscope. 2013;123(7):1759–62.

9. Ma EP, Yiu EM. Voice activity and participation profile: assessing the impact of voice disorders on daily activities. J Speech Lang Hear Res. 2001;44(3):511–24.

10. Deary IJ, Webb A, Mackenzie K, Wilson JA, Carding PN. Short, self-report voice symptom scales: psychometric characteristics of the voice handicap index-10 and the vocal performance questionnaire. Otolaryngol Head Neck Surg. 2004;131(3):232–5.

11. Gillivan-Murphy P, Drinnan MJ, O'Dwyer TP, Ridha H, Carding P. The effectiveness of a voice treatment approach for teachers with self-reported voice problems. J Voice. 2006;20(3):423–31.

12. Rousseau B, Cohen SM, Zeller AS, Scearce L, Tritter AG, Garrett CG. Compliance and quality of life in patients on prescribed voice rest. Otolaryngol Head Neck Surg. 2011;144(1):104–7.

24

The role of tonsillectomy in the Periodic Fever, Aphthous stomatitis, Pharyngitis and cervical Adenitis syndrome

Jostein Førsvoll[1,2]* ⓘ and Knut Øymar[1,2]

Abstract

Background: Tonsillectomy (TE) or adenotonsillectomy (ATE) may have a beneficial effect on the clinical course in children with the Periodic Fever, Aphthous stomatitis, Pharyngitis and cervical Adenitis (PFAPA) syndrome. However, an immunological reason for this effect remains unknown. This literature review summarizes the current knowledge of the effect of TE or ATE in the PFAPA syndrome.

Methods: A search of PubMed, Medline, EMBASE and Cochrane was conducted for papers written in English dated from 1 January 1987 to 31 December 2016. The search included all studies reporting outcomes after TE or ATE from children aged 0 to 18 years with PFAPA.

Results: Two randomized controlled trials reported significantly faster resolution of febrile episodes after TE or ATE in children with PFAPA compared to controls (non-surgery groups). We identified 28 case series including 555 children with PFAPA. The diagnosis was set prospectively before surgery in 440 children and retrospectively after surgery in 115 of the children. TE or ATE had a curative effect in 509 of the 555 children with PFAPA (92%), but few studies were of high quality.

Conclusion: TE or ATE may have a curative effect on children with PFAPA, but the evidence is of moderate quality. Further high-quality randomized controlled studies are still needed.

Keywords: PFAPA, Tonsils, Tonsillectomy, Adenotonsillectomy

Background

The Periodic Fever, Aphthous stomatitis, Pharyngitis and cervical Adenitis (PFAPA) syndrome is the most common paediatric periodic fever syndrome [1, 2], with a cumulative incidence of 2.2 per 10.000 children up to the age of 5 years in a Nordic population [2]. The hallmarks of the disease are short (3–5 days), regularly occurring episodes of high fever accompanied by at least one of the following major symptoms: pharyngitis, cervical adenitis and aphthous stomatitis [3–5]. The febrile episodes are accompanied by a marked inflammatory response with C-reactive protein >100 mg/L with complete

normalization between the episodes [6]. Episodes of PFAPA often start during the first few years of life and often spontaneously resolve during late childhood [2, 7].

PFAPA has not been defined genetically, and the aetiology is unknown. A dysregulated interleukin-1 response may play a part in the aetiology of the disease [8, 9], and PFAPA is currently regarded as an autoinflammatory disease [10]. There is no established international consensus regarding the definition of PFAPA [11]. The clinical entity was first described by Marshall et al. in 1987 [12], and in 1989 they presented the acronym PFAPA and suggested a set of diagnostic criteria for the syndrome [13]. In 1999, Thomas et al. presented a modified set of diagnostic criteria and since then these criteria have been widely used in international studies [4]. The criteria by Marshall and Thomas are principally

---

* Correspondence: jforsvoll@gmail.com
[1]Department of Paediatrics, Stavanger University Hospital, PO BOX 8100, 4068 Stavanger, Norway
[2]Department of Clinical Science, University of Bergen, Bergen, Norway

equivalent, but in addition to excluding cyclic neutropenia, the definition by Marshall et al. also systematically excludes rare hereditary periodic fever syndromes.

As early as in 1989, Abramson et al. reported that in four children with PFAPA, fever episodes ceased after tonsillectomy (TE) [14]. Since then, the outcome after TE or adenotonsillectomy (ATE) has been reported in several case series of children with PFAPA, indicating a beneficial effect of surgery on the clinical course. Based on two randomized controlled studies, a recent Cochrane review concluded that the evidence for the effect of TE in children with PFAPA is of moderate quality [15], but the case series have not been systematically described before.

There is currently no other curative treatment for children with PFAPA, and for those with bothering symptoms highly influencing daily life for the child and family, TE or ATE has become an option to consider [2, 3, 15].

This literature review summarizes the results of all studies reporting the outcome of TE or ATE in children with the PFAPA syndrome.

Methods

A systematic search of the PubMed, Medline, EMBASE and Cochrane databases was performed up to January 31th 2017 using the keywords "Marshall Syndrome", "PFAPA" and "Periodic Fever, Aphthous stomatitis, Pharyngitis and cervical Adenitis". Papers in English language published between 1 January 1987 and 31 December 2016 were checked for relevance, and the references in the relevant papers were also reviewed to identify any articles not found in the systematic search. Papers were included if they reported the outcome after TE or ATE in children aged 0 to 18 years diagnosed with PFAPA. The diagnostic criteria for the diagnosis in each study were noted; according to Marshall [12, 13], Thomas [4] or adapted criteria not clearly based on either of the two.

The outcome after TE or ATE was defined as "curative" if a cessation of febrile episodes occurred; as "partly effective" if the children experienced less frequent, shorter or less severe symptoms during subsequent febrile attacks; and as "not effective" if the disease pattern remained unchanged. The study design was reviewed, and registered if the PFAPA diagnosis was set prospectively before surgery or retrospectively after surgery had been performed. When concurrence of authorship and time, the studies were thoroughly assessed for overlap of patients included.

If a case series included ≥20 patients, a follow-up of ≥24 months and the diagnosis was set prior to surgery, the study was considered as high quality. If two of these criteria were present the study was considered of moderate quality, and with ≤ one criteria of low quality. High quality study

should have included patients according to definitions by Marshall or Thomas. The review was performed according to the Additional file 1: PRISMA guidelines [16].

Results

After omitting duplicates, the search retrieved 558 manuscripts (Fig. 1). After a review of the titles, abstracts, and reference lists of the relevant manuscripts, two randomized controlled trials (RCTs) and 28 case series reporting the outcome after TE or ATE in children with PFAPA were identified. Two Cochrane studies were identified, but no other systematic reviews were found.

The outcome of PFAPA after tonsillectomy with or without adenoidectomy

The first RCT performed by Renko et al. included 26 children with PFAPA (mean age: 4.1 years) [17]. They found that tonsillectomy was curative in all 14 children randomized to the TE group, whereas six of the 12 children in the control group experienced spontaneous resolution of PFAPA episodes within 6 months after inclusion in the study ($p < 0.001$).

In the RCT by Garavello et al., 39 children with PFAPA were randomized to either ATE ($n = 19$) or expectant management ($n = 20$) groups [18]. Twelve of the children in the ATE surgery group had a prompt resolution of symptoms (63%), whereas only one child in the control group experienced spontaneous resolution during the 18 months of follow-up (5%) ($p < 0.001$). The mean number of episodes recorded during the follow-up period was 0.7 (1.2; SD) in the surgery group and 8.1 (3.9) in the control group (p < 0.001). The episodes were further described as less severe in the surgery group.

As summarized in Table 1, the outcome after TE or ATE has been reported in 28 case series, including a total of 555 children with PFAPA. The diagnosis was set prospectively before surgery in 450 children and retrospectively after surgery in 115 of the children. Three studies were categorized as high quality, six as medium quality and 19 as low quality. Surgery was curative in 509 children (92%), partly effective in 14 children and not effective in 32 children. Surgery was curative in 160 of 176 children (91%) in studies with low quality and in 149 of 161 children (93%) in studies with moderate quality. In the high quality studies, surgery was curative in 200 of 218 children (92%). In 16 of the studies, the mean time of observation after surgery was sufficiently given, with a median time of 19 months (11, 26.5) (interquartile range).

Two Cochrane reviews by Burton et al. in 2010 and 2014 studied the clinical effectiveness of TE or ATE compared to nonsurgical treatment in the management of PFAPA [15, 19], both reviews based on the two randomized studies only. They concluded that TE appears to be a

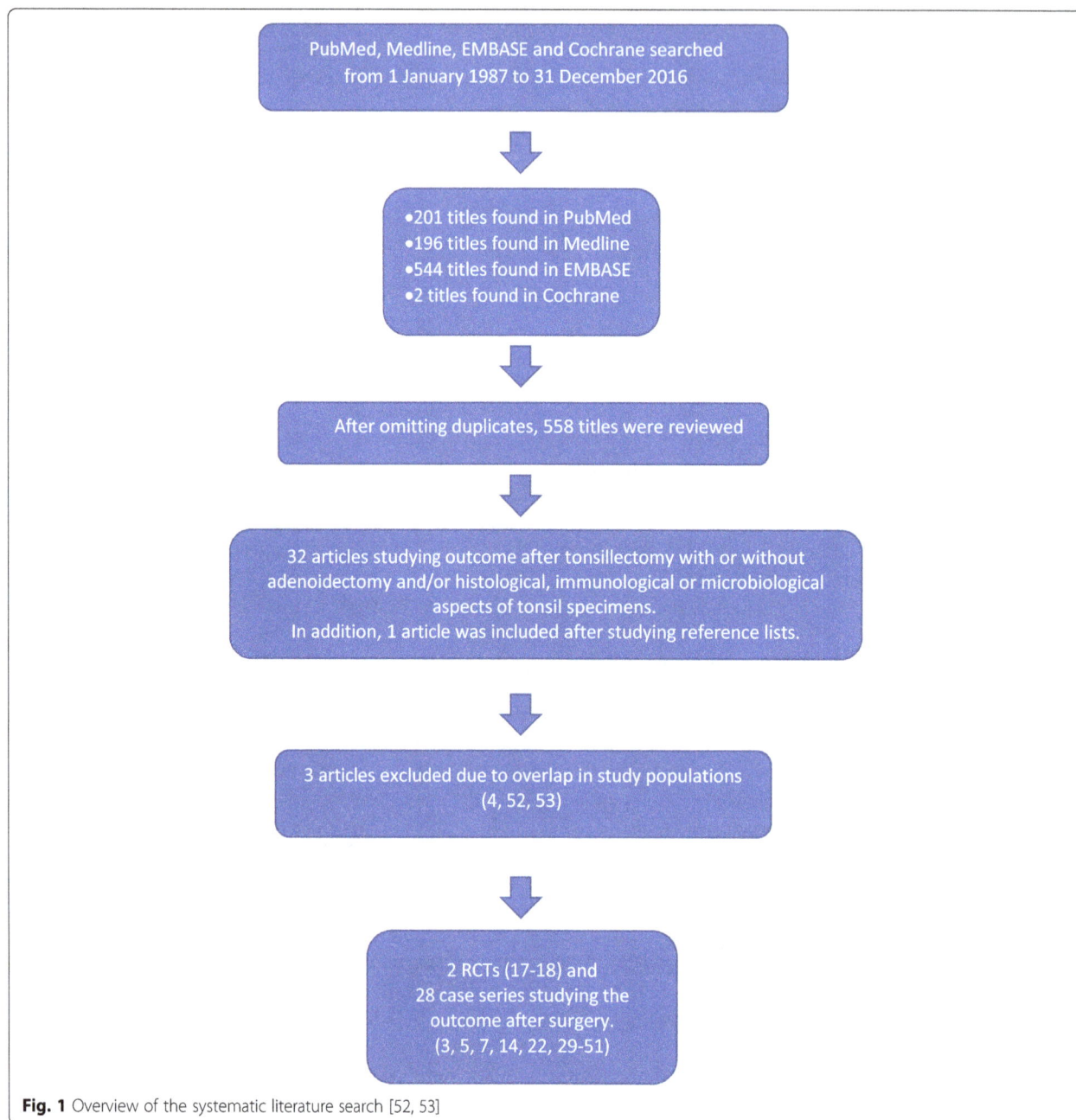

Fig. 1 Overview of the systematic literature search [52, 53]

useful treatment option in the management of children with PFAPA syndrome, with moderate-quality evidence.

Discussion

The two RCTs performed indicate a beneficial effect of TE or ATE in children with PFAPA. The study by Renko et al. had a short time of follow-up, and has also been criticized for vague diagnostic criteria not according to Marshall or Thomas [20, 21]; the large percentage of children described as having PFAPA but with fever as their only symptom may be the reason for the speculation concerning the specificity of the PFAPA diagnosis

in this study. A clear and uniform definition should be applied to compare results from studies and provide generalizability to patient fulfilling these criteria. However, in a recent publication from this study group, they showed that TE may also be effective as a treatment for children with recurring febrile episodes who do not meet the classical diagnostic criteria for PFAPA [22].

Garavello et al. did a thorough diagnostic workup of all children included in their RCT, they applied strict diagnostic criteria for PFAPA, and there was a longer time of follow-up. They performed ATE on all children who underwent surgery and showed favourable

Table 1 Case series reporting the outcome after tonsillectomy and adenotonsillectomy in children with the PFAPA syndrome

	Author/year (reference)	Number of children	Curative	Partly effective	Not effective	Observation post surgery (months, mean)	Adeno-tonsillectomy[a]	Diagnosis set prior to surgery	Criteria for PFAPA diagnosis[b]	Quality
1	Abramson et al. 1989 [14]	4	4	–	–	15	3 (75%)	No	Marshall	Low
2	Padeh et al. 1999 [3]	3	3	–	–	Not clear	0	Yes	Marshall	Low
3	Dahn et al. 2000 [30]	5	5	–	–	3	5 (100%)	No	Adapted	Low
4	Galanakis et al. 2002 [31]	15	15	–	–	Not clear	0	No	Thomas	Low
5	Berlucchi et al. 2003 [32]	5	5	–	–	10	2 (40%)	Yes	Adapted	Low
6	Parikh et al. 2003 [33]	2	0	–	2	Not clear	0	No	Marshall	Low
7	Tasher et al. 2006 [5]	6	6	–	–	19	0	Yes	Thomas	Low
8	Wong et al. 2008 [34]	9	8	1	–	24	0	Yes	Marshall	Medium
9	Pignataro et al. 2009 [35]	9	5	4	–	26	0	Yes	Marshall	Medium
10	Fedrer et al. 2010 [36]	11	11	–	–	18	0	Yes	Thomas	Low
11	Peridis et al. 2010 [37]	9	8	–	1	12	2 (22%)	Yes	Thomas	Low
12	Wurster et al. 2011 [7]	12	6	3	3	Not clear	10 (83%)	Yes	Thomas	Low
13	Licameli et al. 2012 [38] [c]	102	99	–	3	43	102 (100%)	Yes	Marshall	High
14	Førsvoll et al. 2013 [29]	17	17	–	–	Not clear	7 (41%)	Yes	Thomas	Low
15	Krol et al. 2013 [39]	18	18	–	–	Not clear	0	Yes	Thomas	Low
16	Ter Haar et al. 2013 [40]	8	4	3	1	Not clear	Not clear	Yes	Marshall	Low
17	Valenzuela et al. 2013 [41]	9	9	–	–	10	0	Yes	Thomas	Low
18	Kubota et al. 2014 [42]	5	4	–	1	Not clear	0	Yes	Thomas	Low
19	Vigo et al. 2014 [43]	41	27	–	14	69	0	Yes	Marshall	High
20	Dytrych et al. 2015 [44]	10	10	–	–	19	0	Yes	Thomas	Low
21	Førsvoll et al. 2015 [45]	4	4	–	–	27	1 (25%)	Yes	Thomas	Medium
22	Lantto et al. 2015 [46][d]	31	31	–	–	6	11 (35%)	No	Adapted	Low
23	Perko et al. 2015 [47]	28	26	2	–	Not clear	0	Yes	Thomas	Medium
24	Batu et al. 2016 [48][c]	53	50	–	3	Not clear	0	Yes	Thomas	Medium
25	Dusser et al. 2016 [49]	4	3	–	1	Not clear	Not clear	Yes	Thomas	Low
26	Erdogan et al. 2016 [50]	75	74	1	–	24	Not clear	Yes	Thomas	High
27	Lantto et al. 2016 [22][d]	58	56	–	2	107	0	No	Thomas	Medium
28	Rigante et al. 2016 [51]	2	1	–	1	Not clear	0	Yes	Thomas	Low
	Total	555	509	14	32	–	143 (26%)	–		

PFAPA Periodic Fever, Aphthous stomatitis, Pharyngitis and cervical Adenitis
[a]:Adenotonsillectomy performed instead of tonsillectomy alone
[b]:PFAPA diagnosis was set according to criteria by Marshall [13], Thomas [4] or adapted criteria not clearly based on either of the two
[c]and [d]:Possible overlap between study populations

outcomes for these children compared with the control group. Therefore, this study may serve as the best evidence for TE or ATE in children with PFAPA.

Case series have important limitations and provide the lowest level of evidence. A beneficial outcome after TE or ATE in 523 of 555 children is impressive. However, only three studies were considered by us as high quality. In one of these studies, TE was curative in only 66% of patients, but in 92% of patients in all the high quality studies together. Moreover, subgroups of patients may have been selected for the operations, and publication bias may be another important limitation for case series. Several of the case series lack information regarding follow-up or have a brief period of follow-up. Therefore, a firm conclusion on the effect of TE or ATE cannot be drawn based on these studies.

It is not clear if ATE is more effective than TE alone. In the highest-quality study included in this review, the RCT by Garavello et al., ATE was performed in all children. Further studies are needed to confirm these findings and bring clarity to this issue.

Tonsillectomy for PFAPA has also been described in adult patients with PFAPA, but the results are not included in this review. The data are limited, but the procedure seems to be less effective for adults than for children [23–26].

Taken together, a high rate of success of TE or ATE has been shown in two RCTs, of which one with high quality, and in case series with high and moderate quality. In our opinion the current literature therefore supports TE or ATE as a treatment option for children with PFAPA, but with a moderate level of evidence. However, the disease is benign with a high likelihood of spontaneous resolution during childhood [2, 5, 7]. In one study of 59 children with PFAPA, the mean duration of symptoms before resolution was 6.3 years [7], whereas in one study of 46 children, the median age of resolution differed by only 10 months between those who were operated or not [2]. The indication for surgery must therefore be evaluated separately in each child based on the burden of the disease, the impact of recurrent febrile episodes on the family, and signs of impending resolution, such as less-severe and shorter febrile episodes and longer afebrile intervals [2, 5]. The decision must be taken by physicians and parents together based on the degree of symptoms and the best possible knowledge of different outcomes.

Several studies have indicated that a dysregulated immune system may play a part in the aetiology of PFAPA [8, 9, 27–29]. In 2011, Stojanov et al. proposed a model for PFAPA where a microbial trigger initiates a cascade leading to the febrile attacks. They suggested that an immunologically immature host or a host with an inherited or acquired immune abnormality plays a permissive role [8]. However, the observation that removal of the tonsils, which serve as a minor part of the secondary immune system, may be curative for a disease that is possibly caused by a dysregulated immune system remains puzzling.

Conclusion

In conclusion, two RCTs and several case series indicate that TE or ATE has a beneficial effect on the course of PFAPA, but the evidence is of moderate quality. Surgery must be weighed against the chance of spontaneous recovery. More RCTs on the effect of TE with strict diagnostic criteria for PFAPA are needed.

Abbreviations

ATE: Adenotonsillectomy; PFAPA: Periodic fever, aphthous stomatitis, pharyngitis and cervical adenitis; RCT: Randomized controlled trial; TE: Tonsillectomy

Acknowledgements

Not applicable

Funding

The authors received no funding for this work.

Authors' contributions

The authors have contributed equally to the manuscript. KØ wrote the first draft of the manuscript. JF performed the literature search. Both authors revised the manuscript and prepared it for publication. Both authors read and approved the final manuscript.

Competing interests

The authors have no competing interests.

References

1. Masters SL, Simon A, Aksentijevich I, Kastner DL. Horror autoinflammaticus: the molecular pathophysiology of autoinflammatory disease. Annu Rev Immunol. 2009;27:621–68.
2. Forsvoll J, Kristoffersen EK, Oymar K. Incidence, clinical characteristics and outcome in Norwegian children with periodic fever, aphthous stomatitis, pharyngitis and cervical adenitis syndrome; a population-based study. Acta Paediatr. 2013;102:187–92.
3. Padeh S, Brezniak N, Zemer D, Pras E, Livneh A, Langevitz P, et al. Periodic fever, aphthous stomatitis, pharyngitis, and adenopathy syndrome: clinical characteristics and outcome. J Pediatr. 1999;135:98–101.

4. Thomas KT, Feder HM Jr, Lawton AR, Edwards KM. Periodic fever syndrome in children. J Pediatr. 1999;135:15–21.

5. Tasher D, Somekh E, Dalal I. PFAPA syndrome: new clinical aspects disclosed. Arch Dis Child. 2006;91:981–4.

6. Forsvoll JA, Oymar K. C-reactive protein in the periodic fever, aphthous stomatitis, pharyngitis and cervical adenitis (PFAPA) syndrome. Acta Paediatr. 2007;96:1670–3.

7. Wurster VM, Carlucci JG, Feder HM Jr, Edwards KM. Long-term follow-up of children with periodic fever, aphthous stomatitis, pharyngitis, and cervical adenitis syndrome. J Pediatr. 2011;159:958–64.

8. Stojanov S, Lapidus S, Chitkara P, Feder H, Salazar JC, Fleisher TA, et al. Periodic fever, aphthous stomatitis, pharyngitis, and adenitis (PFAPA) is a disorder of innate immunity and Th1 activation responsive to IL-1 blockade. Proc Natl Acad Sci U S A. 2011;108:7148–53.

9. Kolly L, Busso N, von Scheven-Gete A, Bagnoud N, Moix I, Holzinger D, et al. Periodic fever, aphthous stomatitis, pharyngitis, cervical adenitis syndrome is linked to dysregulated monocyte IL-1beta production. J Allergy Clin Immunol. 2013;131:1635–43.

10. Wekell P, Karlsson A, Berg S, Fasth A. Review of autoinflammatory diseases, with a special focus on periodic fever, aphthous stomatitis, pharyngitis and cervical adenitis syndrome. Acta Paediatr. 2016;105:1140–51.

11. Hofer M, Pillet P, Cochard MM, Berg S, Krol P, Kone-Paut I, et al. International periodic fever, aphthous stomatitis, pharyngitis, cervical adenitis syndrome cohort: description of distinct phenotypes in 301 patients. Rheumatology (Oxford). 2014;53:1125–9.

12. Marshall GS, Edwards KM, Butler J, Lawton AR. Syndrome of periodic fever, pharyngitis, and aphthous stomatitis. J Pediatr. 1987;110:43–6.

13. Marshall GS, Edwards KM, Lawton AR. PFAPA syndrome. Pediatr Infect Dis J. 1989;8:658–9.

14. Abramson JS, Givner LB, Thompson JN. Possible role of tonsillectomy and adenoidectomy in children with recurrent fever and tonsillopharyngitis. Pediatr Infect Dis J. 1989;8:119–20.

15. Burton MJ, Pollard AJ, Ramsden JD, Chong LY, Venekamp RP. Tonsillectomy for periodic fever, aphthous stomatitis, pharyngitis and cervical adenitis syndrome (PFAPA). Cochrane Database Syst Rev. 2014;9:CD008669.

16. Liberati A, Altman DG, Tetzlaff J, Mulrow C, Gøtzsche PC, Ioannidis JP, et al. The PRISMA statement for reporting systematic reviews and meta-analyses of studies that evaluate health care interventions: explanation and elaboration. PLoS Med. 2009; https://doi.org/10.1371/journal.pmed.1000100.

17. Renko M, Salo E, Putto-Laurila A, Putto-Laurila A, Saxen H, Mattila PS, et al. A randomized, controlled trial of tonsillectomy in periodic fever, aphthous stomatitis, pharyngitis, and adenitis syndrome. J Pediatr. 2007;151:289–92.

18. Garavello W, Romagnoli M, Gaini RM, Garavello W, Romagnoli M, Gaini RM. Effectiveness of adenotonsillectomy in PFAPA syndrome: a randomized study. J Pediatr. 2009;155:250–3.

19. Burton MJ, Pollard AJ, Ramsden JD. Tonsillectomy for periodic fever, aphthous stomatitis, pharyngitis and cervical adenitis syndrome (PFAPA). Cochrane Database Syst Rev. 2010;9:CD008669.

20. Spalding SJ, Hashkes PJ. The role of tonsillectomy in management of periodic fever, aphthous stomatitis, pharyngitis, and adenopathy: unanswered questions. J Pediatr. 2008;152:742–3.

21. Hofer MF. Cured by tonsillectomy: was it really a PFAPA syndrome? J Pediatr. 2008;153:298.

22. Lantto U, Koivunen P, Tapiainen T, Renko M. Long-term outcome of classic and incomplete PFAPA (periodic fever, Aphthous Stomatitis, Pharyngitis, and adenitis) syndrome after tonsillectomy. J Pediatr. 2016;179:172–7.

23. Padeh S, Stoffman N, Berkun Y, Padeh S, Stoffman N, Berkun Y. Periodic fever accompanied by aphthous stomatitis, pharyngitis and cervical adenitis syndrome (PFAPA syndrome) in adults. Isr Med Assoc J. 2008;10:358–60.

24. Colotto M, Maranghi M, Durante C, Rossetti M, Renzi A, Anatra MG. PFAPA syndrome in a young adult with a history of tonsillectomy. Intern Med. 2011;50:223–5.

25. Cantarini L, Vitale A, Bartolomei B, Galeazzi M, Rigante D. Diagnosis of PFAPA syndrome applied to a cohort of 17 adults with unexplained recurrent fevers. Clin Exp Rheumatol. 2012;30:269–71.

26. Cantarini L, Vitale A, Galeazzi M, Frediani B. A case of resistant adult-onset periodic fever, aphthous stomatitis, pharyngitis and cervical adenitis (PFAPA) syndrome responsive to anakinra. Clin Exp Rheumatol. 2012;30:593.

27. Stojanov S, Hoffmann F, Kery A, Renner ED, Hartl D, Lohse P, et al. Cytokine profile in PFAPA syndrome suggests continuous inflammation and reduced anti-inflammatory response. Eur Cytokine Netw. 2006;17:90–7.

28. Brown KL, Wekell P, Osla V, Sundqvist M, Savman K, Fasth A, et al. Profile of blood cells and inflammatory mediators in periodic fever, aphthous stomatitis, pharyngitis and adenitis (PFAPA) syndrome. BMC Pediatr. 2010;10:65.

29. Forsvoll J, Kristoffersen EK, Oymar K. Elevated levels of CXCL10 in the periodic fever, Aphthous stomatitis, Pharyngitis and cervical adenitis syndrome (PFAPA) during and between febrile episodes; an indication of a persistent activation of the innate immune system. Pediatr Rheumatol Online J. 2013;11:38.

30. Dahn KA, Glode MP, Chan KH. Periodic fever and pharyngitis in young children: a new disease for the otolaryngologist? Arch Otolaryngol Head Neck Surg. 2000;126:1146–9.

31. Galanakis E, Papadakis CE, Giannoussi E, Karatzanis AD, Bitsori M, Helidonis ES. PFAPA syndrome in children evaluated for tonsillectomy. Arch Dis Child. 2002;86:434–5.

32. Berlucchi M, Meini A, Plebani A, Bonvini MG, Lombardi D, Nicolai P. Update on treatment of Marshall's syndrome (PFAPA syndrome): report of five cases with review of the literature. Ann Otol Rhinol Laryngol. 2003;112:365–9.

33. Parikh SR, Reiter ER, Kenna MA, Roberson D. Utility of tonsillectomy in 2 patients with the syndrome of periodic fever, aphthous stomatitis, pharyngitis, and cervical adenitis. Arch Otolaryngol Head Neck Surg. 2003; 129:670–3.

34. Wong KK, Finlay JC, Moxham JP, Wong KK, Finlay JC, Moxham JP. Role of tonsillectomy in PFAPA syndrome. Arch Otolaryngol Head Neck Surg. 2008; 134:16–9.

35. Pignataro L, Torretta S, Pietrograde MC, Dellepiane RM, Pavesi P, Bossi A, et al. Outcome of tonsillectomy in selected patients with PFAPA syndrome. Arch Otolaryngol Head Neck Surg. 2009;135:548–53.

36. Feder HM, Salazar JC. A clinical review of 105 patients with PFAPA (a periodic fever syndrome). Acta Paediatr. 2010;99:178–84.

37. Peridis S, Koudoumnakis E, Theodoridis A, Stefanaki K, Helmis G, Houlakis M. Surgical outcomes and histology findings after tonsillectomy in children with periodic fever, aphthous stomatitis, pharyngitis, and cervical adenitis syndrome. Am J Otolaryngol. 2010;31:472–5.

38. Licameli G, Lawton M, Kenna M, Dedeoglu F. Long-term surgical outcomes of adenotonsillectomy for PFAPA syndrome. Arch Otolaryngol Head Neck Surg. 2012;138:902–6.

39. Krol P, Bohm M, Sula V, Dytrych P, Katra R, Nemcova D, et al. PFAPA syndrome: clinical characteristics and treatment outcomes in a large single-centre cohort. Clin Exp Rheumatol. 2013;31:980–7.

40. Ter Haar N, Lachmann H, Ozen S, Woo P, Uziel Y, Modesto C, et al. Treatment of autoinflammatory diseases: results from the Eurofever registry and a literature review. Ann Rheum Dis. 2013;72:678–85.

41. Valenzuela PM, Araya A, Perez CI, Maul X, Serrano C, Beltran C, et al. Profile of inflammatory mediators in tonsils of patients with periodic fever, aphthous stomatitis, pharyngitis, and cervical adenitis (PFAPA) syndrome. Clin Rheumatol. 2013;32:1743–9.

42. Kubota K, Ohnishi H, Teramoto T, Kawamoto N, Kasahara K, Ohara O, et al. Clinical and genetic characterization of Japanese sporadic cases of periodic fever, aphthous stomatitis, pharyngitis and adenitis syndrome from a single medical center in Japan. J Clin Immunol. 2014;34:584–93.

43. Vigo G, Martini G, Zoppi S, Vittadello F, Zulian F. Tonsillectomy efficacy in children with PFAPA syndrome is comparable to the standard medical treatment: a long-term observational study. Clin Exp Rheumatol. 2014; 32(Suppl 84):156–9.

44. Dytrych P, Krol P, Kotrova M, Kuzilkova D, Hubacek P, Krol L, et al. Polyclonal, newly derived T cells with low expression of inhibitory molecule PD-1 in tonsils define the phenotype of lymphocytes in children with periodic fever, Aphtous Stomatitis, Pharyngitis and adenitis (PFAPA) syndrome. Mol Immunol. 2015;65:139–47.

45. Forsvoll J, Janssen EA, Moller I, Wathne N, Skaland I, Klos J, et al. Reduced number of CD8+ cells in tonsillar germinal centers in children with the periodic fever, aphthous stomatitis, pharyngitis and cervical adenitis syndrome. Scand J Immunol. 2015;82:76–83.

46. Lantto U, Koivunen P, Tapiainen T, Glumoff V, Hirvikoski P, Uhari M, et al. Microbes of the tonsils in PFAPA (periodic fever, Aphtous stomatitis, Pharyngitis and adenitis) syndrome - a possible trigger of febrile episodes. APMIS. 2015;123:523–9.

47. Perko D, Debeljak M, Toplak N, Avcin T. Clinical features and genetic background of the periodic fever syndrome with aphthous stomatitis, pharyngitis, and adenitis: a single center longitudinal study of 81 patients. Mediat Inflamm. 2015; https://doi.org/10.1155/2015/293417.

48. Batu ED, Kara Eroglu F, Tsoukas P, Hausmann JS, Bilginer Y, Kenna MA, et al. Periodic fever, Aphthosis, Pharyngitis, and adenitis syndrome: analysis of patients from two geographic areas. Arthritis Care Res (Hoboken). 2016;68: 1859–65.

49. Dusser P, Hentgen V, Neven B, Kone-Paut I. Is colchicine an effective treatment in periodic fever, aphtous stomatitis, pharyngitis, cervical adenitis (PFAPA) syndrome? Joint Bone Spine. 2016;83:406–11.

50. Erdogan F, Kulak K, Ozturk O, Ipek IO, Ceran O, Seven H. Surgery vs medical treatment in the management of PFAPA syndrome: a comparative trial. Paediatr Int Child Health. 2016;36:270–4.

51. Rigante D, Vitale A, Natale MF, Lopalco G, Andreozzi L, Frediani B, et al. A comprehensive comparison between pediatric and adult patients with periodic fever, aphthous stomatitis, pharyngitis, and cervical adenopathy (PFAPA) syndrome. Clin Rheumatol. 2017;36:463–8.

52. Tejesvi MV, Uhari M, Tapiainen T, Pirttila AM, Suokas M, Lantto U, et al. Tonsillar microbiota in children with PFAPA (periodic fever, aphthous stomatitis, pharyngitis, and adenitis) syndrome. Eur J Clin Microbiol Infect Dis. 2016; https://doi.org/10.1007/s10096-016-2623-y.

53. Licameli G, Jeffrey J, Luz J, Jones D, Kenna M, Greg L, et al. Effect of adenotonsillectomy in PFAPA syndrome. Arch Otolaryngol Head Neck Surg. 2008;134:136–40.

25

The burden of chronic rhinosinusitis and its effect on quality of life among patients re-attending an otolaryngology clinic in south western Uganda

Victoria Nyaiteera[1]* ⓘ, Doreen Nakku[1], Esther Nakasagga[1], Evelyn Llovet[1], Elijah Kakande[2], Gladys Nakalema[3], Richard Byaruhanga[4] and Francis Bajunirwe[5]

Abstract

Background: Worldwide, the burden of chronic rhinosinusitis (CRS) is variable, but not known in Uganda. CRS has significant negative impact on quality of life (QOL) and as such QOL scores should guide adjustments in treatment strategies. However, most of these studies have been done in the west. Our hypothesis was that QOL scores of the majority of CRS patients in low- to- middle income countries are poorer than those among patients without CRS. The aim of this study was to determine the burden of CRS among patients re-attending the Otolaryngology clinic and whether CRS is related to poor QOL.

Methods: A cross sectional study was conducted at Mbarara Regional Referral Hospital Otolaryngology clinic. One hundred and twenty-six adult re-attendees were consecutively recruited. Data was collected using a structured questionnaire and the Sinonasal Outcome Test 22 (SNOT 22) questionnaire measured QOL.

Results: The proportion of re-attendees with CRS was 39.0% (95% CI 30–48%). Majority of CRS patients had poor quality of life scores compared to non-CRS (88% versus 20% $p < 01$). The poor quality of life scores on the SNOT 22 were almost solely as a result of the functional, physical and psychological aspects unique to CRS.

Conclusions: CRS is highly prevalent among re-attendees of an Otolaryngology clinic at a hospital in resource limited settings and has a significant negative impact on the QOL of these patients.

Keywords: Chronic rhinosinusitis, Quality of life, Sinonasal outcome test 22

Background

Chronic rhinosinusitis (CRS) is a condition characterized by the occurrence of two or more of the following signs and symptoms; nasal discharge or post-nasal drip, nasal obstruction, nasal congestion, facial pain, pressure or fullness and decreased sense of smell for a duration of 12 or more weeks with objective findings on either computed tomography or nasal endoscopy [1]. Globally, the prevalence of CRS is variable with occurrence above 10% in Europe and the United States but lower at 2% among populations in sub Saharan Africa [2–4]. In Uganda, anecdotal evidence suggests CRS is a common condition but no formal studies have been conducted to measure disease burden. Preliminary review of records at the otolaryngology Out Patients' Department (OPD) of Mbarara Regional Referral Hospital (MRRH) in western Uganda showed that 37% of the patients with sinonasal complaints had chronic symptoms evidenced by their re-attendances to the clinic.

Generally, symptoms of CRS interfere with work, leisure and sleep, disrupting the patient's day-to-day life [5]. This may significantly impact the health related quality of life (HRQoL) of these patients [6]. Moreover, the QoL scores of CRS patients are significantly lower in comparison with the quality of life scores in other common chronic diseases such as congestive heart failure, angina, chronic

* Correspondence: nyivicky@gmail.com
[1]Department of Ear, Nose and Throat, Mbarara University of Science and Technology, Mbarara, Uganda
Full list of author information is available at the end of the article

obstructive pulmonary disease and back pain [5]. Quality of life measures provide a reliable standard as a health outcome, most especially for chronic conditions [6] such as CRS and as such ought to be used routinely in clinical practice. It is therefore imperative that the degree to which a patient's day-to-day life is affected by CRS be measured and considered more than results of paranasal sinus CT scans or nasal endoscopy when planning or adjusting their management [7]. In order to make appropriate adjustments to the management strategies for CRS based on QoL results, it is necessary to know the factors that may contribute to the observed QoL scores. Documented factors associated with restrictions in HRQoL in CRS patients include; symptom type such as nasal obstruction and postnasal drip, nasal polyposis, comorbidities such as gastro-esophageal reflux disease (GERD), socio-demographic factors such as age and gender and behavioral factors such as smoking [8–10].

CRS patients in south western Uganda make repeated visits to the OPD clinics and consume significant health worker time. They are treated with various medications for prolonged time periods. While these medications are considered to provide relief, there are few studies done to assess the impact of the disease their QoL in Africa. It is also important to identify factors that are associated with poor HRQoL among these patients. This information may be used to make adjustments to CRS treatment in order to improve patient management and satisfaction.

Therefore, the aim of this study was to measure the disease burden of CRS among patients re-attending the Otolaryngology clinic at a tertiary health care facility in a resource limited setting, compare the proportion of patients with poor HRQoL among those with and without CRS and also determine the factors associated with poor HRQoL among these patients.

Methods

Study design and site

We conducted a cross sectional study at the otolaryngology clinic at Mbarara Regional Referral Hospital (MRRH) in south western Uganda for three months between June and August 2016. The otolaryngology clinic operates three days a week and attends to an average of three hundred patients per month and serves a catchment population of over 5 million people in the region. We consecutively enrolled study participants who met the eligibility criteria until the required sample size was achieved.

Eligibility criteria

Patients were recruited into the study if they were re-attending the Otolaryngology clinic at Mbarara Hospital with the recurring symptoms for twelve weeks or more despite previous appropriate treatment as per clinic protocols.

The protocols are based on the 2013 Canadian guidelines for management of CRS [11].. Only adult patients aged 18 years of age and over were enrolled. Patients were excluded from the study if they were pregnant because pregnancy related hormonal changes modify sino-nasal mucosal physiology and could therefore mimic CRS symptoms. Participants were also excluded if they could not tolerate the rigid nasal endoscopy (RNE) and there was no evidence of polyps on anterior rhinoscopy. We also excluded patients who were unable to give consent due to mental handicaps or declined participation in the study. Minors were generally excluded because majority of them come to the clinic unaccompanied, yet research guidelines require their caretakers to consent and the youth to provide assent.

Sample size determination

Sample size calculation was done based on sample size estimation formula for Cross-sectional studies [12]. Using a 95% confidence interval level, we made the assumption that prevalence of CRS among re-attending patients was 7.3%. With an error margin of 5%, the estimated sample size was 126 participants. These participants were then subjected to history and examination, including rigid nasal endoscopy to determine who had CRS and who did not have CRS.

Data collection procedures

Data was collected using a semi-structured questionnaire and the SNOT 22 tool [13]. The semi-structured questionnaire had two sections. The first part collected information on bio-demographics, presenting complaint, history of presenting complaint, treatment history, comorbidities and patient general health behavior. The second part collected data from physical examination of the sino-nasal region. The QoL assessment was done using the SNOT 22 tool. The SNOT 22 has four domains according to a psychometric analysis done on SNOT 22 responses from patients with CRS [14]. The four domains are rhinologic symptoms, ear and facial symptoms, sleep disturbance and psychological symptoms. Participants rated individual items on a six-point scale (0 - no problem, to 5 - most serious problem). Scores were summed up to obtain the individual domain scores and total scores for each participant. A total score of above 7 was considered an indicator of poor quality of life [15]. Participants were confirmed to be re-attendees by reviewing their previous medical records prior to enrollment.

After participants provided informed consent, the questionnaire was administered and physical examination carried out. The examination included anterior rhinoscopy and the three standard passes of rigid nasal endoscopy. If less than 3 passes were made on a participant with no visible polyps on anterior rhinoscopy, the participant was excluded from the quality of life assessment and therefore not enrolled as we could not then rule out any other endonasal abnormalities that would have been visible on endoscopy. The diagnosis of CRS was therefore based on symptoms and examination findings on rigid nasal endoscopy. Computed tomography was not used because it is an expensive investigation that is not readily available at our center, and Rigid nasal endoscopy is an acceptable objective measure for CRS [3].

Data analysis

Data were collected in coded form in the questionnaires, entered into Microsoft Excel, cleaned and exported to STATA 11.0 software (College Station, Texas) for analysis.

For the baseline characteristics of study participants such as demographics, summary statistics were generated while proportions were generated for categorical variables. The prevalence of CRS among patients re-attending the otolaryngology clinic at MRRH was determined using the formula; Prevalence = (n/N*100), where n was the total number of re-attendees with CRS and N was the total number of re-attendees enrolled.

The individual domain scores and total SNOT 22 score were obtained for each participant. A SNOT 22 score of above 7 was considered poor QoL and a score of 7 and below as considered normal [15]. The proportion of patients with a score of above 7 in each category of CRS was calculated. We conducted a chi square test to compare the proportion of patients with good QOL scores in the CRS and non- CRS categories. We also compared the mean SNOT 22 scores of patients with and without CRS, and using an independent samples t-test, determined whether the mean scores differed significantly. The same analysis was conducted to compare the mean scores derived within the domains, to determine whether the individual domain scores of SNOT 22 differed among patients with and without CRS.

To determine the association between poor quality of life and the clinical and non-clinical factors associated with the disease specific quality of life, we conducted a Univariate logistic regression analysis. The outcome variable was the total QOL score on SNOT 22 measured as a dichotomous variable. Variables with p values less than 0.05 and those of relevant clinical significance were entered into a multiple logistic regression model to build a predictive model for poor QOL. The crude odds ratios were calculated to eliminate confounders after which all statistically significant factors ($p < 0.05$) and those of biological significance were considered for multivariate analysis. We reported the adjusted odds ratios with 95% confidence intervals.

Ethical consideration

Ethical approval was given by the Mbarara University of Science and Technology Research and Ethics Committee (MUST-REC) study number 03/05–16. Signed informed consent was obtained from all study participants in English or the common local language (Runyankore) before enrollment into the study. Participants were informed that they were free to withdraw their consent at any point during the course of the study and that this would not affect their care in any way. All participants received appropriate management according to applied guidelines in the MRRH Otolaryngology clinic. Study participants were given unique identifiers to ensure confidentiality. Any information that could lead to identification of a participant was not collected.

Results

Prevalence of CRS and socio-demographic and behavioral characteristics of patients

One hundred and twenty six ($n = 126$) adult re-attendees at the MRRH Otolaryngology clinic were enrolled into this study. Overall 49 of the 126 patients or 38.8% had CRS. The median age of the group was 42 years with an inter quartile range (IQR) of 22–59, and 57% of respondents were female. The results of the baseline characteristics are shown in Table 1 below.

With data broken down by CRS status, there was no significant difference in terms of distribution of age, gender, education, smoking history and completion of treatment. The two groups of patients were similar on many baseline demographic characteristics. However, almost 20% of the study participants had a history of ever smoking and of these 44.0% had CRS. Patients with no CRS were more likely to be in the higher income categories compared to those without CRS and this difference was statistically significant.

In general, almost 40% of patients re-attending the ENT clinic at Mbarara Hospital had CRS and the two group patients were comparable regarding the distribution of most socio-demographic features.

Clinical characteristics of respondents stratified by CRS status

Overall, 46% ($n = 58$) of the respondents had a SNOT22 score of above 7, an indicator of poor quality of life. Among the patients with CRS, 43 (87.8%) had a poor quality of life while among those without CRS only 15 (19.4%) had a poor quality of life. Analysis of the clinical characteristics showed that 25.4% ($n = 32$) of all the respondents had symptoms of allergy and only 6.4% ($n = 8$) had symptoms of reflux for more than 12 weeks. This was taken to be indicative of gastroesophageal reflux disease (GERD). Patients with CRS were also more likely to have nasal polyps, nasal discharge, nasal mucosal edema and

Table 1 Socio-demographic and behavioral characteristics of patients stratified by CRS status among patients attending ENT clinic at Mbarara, Uganda

VARIABLE	CRS $n = 49$ Frequency (%)	No CRS $n = 77$ Frequency (%)	p value
Age categories in years			
18–35	17 (34.69)	30 (38.96)	0.86
36–59	24 (48.98)	34 (44.16)	
60–80	8 (16.33)	13 (16.88)	
Age (continuous)			
median, IQR	43 (30–53)	42 (29–54)	0.87
Gender			
Male	17 (34.69)	36 (46.75)	0.18
Female	32 (65.31)	41 (53.25)	
Formal Education			
None	14 (28.57)	13 (16.88)	0.32
Primary	12 (24.49)	27 (35.06)	
Secondary	19 (18.37)	18 (23.38)	
Tertiary	14 (28.57)	19 (24.68)	
Monthly income			
None	26 (53.06)	25 (32.47)	0.02
>/=USD 15	23 (46.94)	52 (67.53)	
History of ever smoking			
No	38 (77.50)	63 (81.82)	0.56
Yes	11 (22.45)	14 (18.18)	
Did not complete course of treatment			
No	43 (87.76)	72 (93.51)	0.27
Yes	6 (12.24)	5 (6.49)	

CRS Chronic rhinosinusitis, *IQR* Inter quartile range, *USD* United States Dollars

nasal crusts. In general, patients with CRS had a poorer quality of life and were more likely to have accompanying intra-nasal abnormalities.

Proportion of respondents with poor QOL scores on SNOT 22 among patients with CRS and those without CRS

Among patients with CRS, 43 (74.1%) had a poor QoL score on SNOT 22 compared to only 15 (25.9%) among those without CRS. Similarly, among the patients with CRS, only 6 (8.82%) had normal QoL scores while the majority ($n = 62$ or 91.2%) among patients that did not have CRS had normal QoL scores. The statistical test to compare the two groups showed a significant difference between these proportions (chi square test for independence, p value < 0.0001).

Overall, about two thirds of patients with CRS reported poor QOL compared to only one third of those without CRS indicating patients with CRS are significantly more likely to report poorer QOL.

Comparison of mean scores of SNOT 22 by CRS status

Overall, both the SNOT 22 and domain mean scores were higher in patients with CRS, signifying poorer quality of life among these patients, compared to those without CRS. These results are shown in Table 2 below. Among the respondents with CRS, the mean SNOT 22 score was 31.4 (95% CI 25.26–37.44) while that of patients without CRS was 4.10 (95% CI 2.35–5.86). The data on mean scores in each domain are shown in Fig. 1 below. The domains with the highest mean scores were nasal symptoms (14.1, 95% CI =11.68–16.61) among CRS patients and ear symptoms 1.44 (95% CI 0.92–1.96), among those without CRS. The domains with the lowest mean scores for patients with CRS and those without CRS were sleep disturbance (3.5, 95% CI = 1.96–5.0) and the psychological domain 0.79 (95% CI 0.10–1.48). The p values generated from this comparison of the mean quality of life scores were all significant ($p < 0.001$).

Table 2 Clinical characteristics of respondents stratified by CRS status, among patients attending ENT clinic, Mbarara, Uganda

VARIABLE	CRS n = 49 Frequency (%)	No CRS n = 77 Frequency (%)	p value
Quality of life on SNOT 22			
Good	6 (12.24)	62 (80.52)	< 0.01
Poor	43 (87.76)	15 (19.48)	
History of nasal trauma or nasal surgery			
No	40 (81.63)	70 (90.91)	0.13
Yes	9 (18.37)	7 (9.07)	
GERD			
No	45 (91.84)	73 (94.18)	0.51
Yes	4 (8.16)	4 (5.19)	
Nasal polyps			
No	37 (75.51)	76 (98.70)	< 0.01
Yes	12 (24.49)	1 (1.30)	
Nasal discharge			
No	14 (28.57)	73 (94.81)	< 0.01
Yes	35 (71.43)	4 (5.19)	
Nasal mucosal edema			
No	17 (34.69)	72 (97.40)	< 0.01
Yes	32 (65.31)	2 (2.60)	
Nasal crusts			
No	42 (85.71)	75 (97.40)	0.01
Yes	7 (14.29)	2 (2.60)	
Number of CRS symptoms:			
0	2 (4.08)	50 (64.94)	< 0.01
1	1 (2.04)	18 (23.38)	
>1	46 (93.88)	9 (11.69)	

SNOT 22 Sinonasal Outcome Test 22, *GERD* Gastroesophageal Reflux Disease

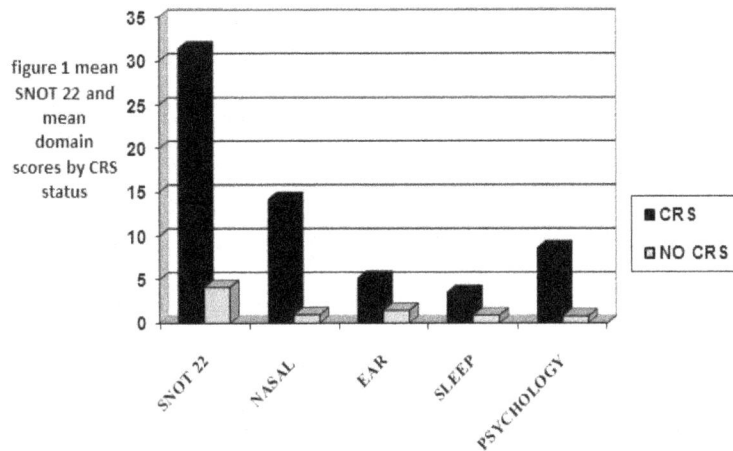

Fig. 1 Mean SNOT 22 scores and mean domain scores by CRS status

Overall, patients with CRS had higher mean SNOT22 scores suggesting significantly poorer QoL compared to those without CRS.

Factors associated with poor quality of life scores on SNOT 22 questionnaire

Table 3 shows the factors that were associated with a poor QoL in a crude analysis. Gender, age category, in-adherence to medication and presence of GERD symptoms, did not have a significant relationship with QoL. Patients with a monthly income over 50,000 Ugx were less likely to have poor QoL compared to patients that did not have a monthly income. A patient with a primary education was less likely to have a poor QoL compared to another with no formal education. Similarly, a secondary school and tertiary education made one times less likely to have a poor QoL. A history of smoking, whether past or current, was associated with a 2.5-fold increase in the odds of having a poor QoL compared to those that had never smoked before. Having allergies was associated with a 2.9 fold increased odds of having a poor quality of life compared to absence of allergies. Other variables associated with increased likelihood of poor quality of life were endo-nasal including nasal polyps (OR = 17.5, $p = 0.01$), nasal discharge (OR = 24.4, $p < 0.01$), and nasal mucosal edema (OR = 15.51, p < 0.01).

The main exposure variable, CRS, was significantly associated with poor quality of life, with a 29.6 fold increase in the odds of having a poor quality of life score (OR = 29.6, $p < 0.00$).

Socio-demographic and behavioral factors that were significantly associated with QoL ($p < 0.05$) from bivariate analysis included monthly income, in-adherence to treatment and a history of smoking. Clinical factors that were significantly associated with QoL were CRS status, allergies, nasal polyps, nasal discharge, mucosal edema, osteo-meatal complex abnormalities and number of

symptoms. These were included in the multivariate model together with GERD because it is of biological importance as modifier of disease specific quality of life in CRS.

The results of the multivariable regression are presented in Table 4. Here, patients with CRS had an 8.94-fold increase in the odds of having poor quality of life (OR = 8.94, $p < 0.01$), compared to those without CRS. Persons with nasal discharge had a 7.15 fold increase in the odds of having poor QoL compared to those without nasal discharge (OR = 7.15, $p = 0.01$).

Discussion

Prevalence of CRS among re-attendees at the MRRH ENT clinic

The prevalence of CRS among patients re-attending the ENT clinic in a resource limited setting was 39%. Our study results are generalizable to studies that have enrolled patients re-attending the ENT clinic in resource limited settings. However, very few studies have been done to measure CRS in this population, and not only in resource limited setting but globally. When compared to the prevalence of CRS in the general population surveys, the results are stunningly different. For instance a cross sectional survey of 19 European countries by the GA2LEN network of excellence showed variable prevalence of CRS ranging from 6.9% (95% CI 5.8–8.2%) to 27.1% (95% CI 25.0–29.3%) in Germany [2], the maximum prevalence measured was 27.1%which is still be lower than that in our study. In an African setting, Iseh and Makusidi recruited all new patients with the diagnosis of rhinosinusitis over a 2-year period and found a prevalence of CRS of 7.3% at a teaching hospital in north western Nigeria among patients attending an ENT clinic [16].

Clearly, the high prevalence in our study is because the respondents in our study were re-attendees, a high-risk

Table 3 Bivariate analysis for socio-demographic, behavioral and clinical factors associated with a poor quality of life (QoL) among patients attending ENT outpatients, Mbarara, Uganda

VARIABLE	Good QoL (%)	Poor QoL (%)	COR (95% CI)	p value
Age category in years				
18–35	28 (41.2)	19 (32.8)	1.0	
36–59	30 (44.1)	28 (48.3)	1.38 (0.6–4.6)	0.42
60–80	10 (14.7)	11 (19.0)	1.62 (0.6–4.6)	0.36
Gender				
female	40 (58.8)	33 (56.9)	1.0	
male	28 (41.2)	25 (43.1)	1.08 (0.5–2.2)	0.83
Monthly income				
< USD 15	20 (29.4)	31 (53.5)	1.0	
>/=USD 15	48 (70.6)	27 (46.6)	0.36 (0.2–0.8)	0.01*
Formal Education				
None	9 (13. 2)	18 (31.0)	1.0	
Primary	23 (33.8)	16 (27.6)	0.35 (0.1–1.0)	0.04*
Secondary	17 (25.0)	10 (17.2)	0.29 (0.1–1.0)	0.03*
Tertiary	19 (27.9)	14 (24.1)	0.37 (0.2–0.8)	0.06
History of ever smoking:				
No	59 (86.8)	42 (72.4)	1.0	
Yes	9 (13.2)	16 (27.6)	2.50 (1.0–6.2)	0.05
CRS				
No	62 (91.2)	15 (25.9)	1.0	
Yes	6 (8.8)	43 (74.1)	29.62(10.6–82.4)	0.01*
Allergy symptoms				
No	57 (83.3)	37 (63.8)	1.0	
Yes	11 (16.2)	21 (36.2)	2.94 (1.3–6.8)	0.01*
GERD				
No	64 (94.1)	54 (93.1)	1.0	
Yes	4 (5.9)	4 (6.9)	1.1 (0.3–5.0)	0.82
Nasal polyps:				
No	67 (98.5)	46 (79.3)	1.0	
Yes	1 9 1.5)	12 (20.7)	17.5(2.2–139.0)	0.01*
Nasal discharge:				
No	64 (94.1)	23 (37. 9)	1.0	
Yes	4 (5.9)	35 (60.3)	24.40 (7.8–76.1)	0.01*
Nasal mucosal edema				
No	63 (92.7)	26 (44.8)	1.0	
Yes	5 (7.4)	32 (55.2)	15.51 (5.5–44.2)	0.01*
Number of CRS symptoms:				
0	46 (67.7)	6 (10.3)	1.0	
1	12 (17.7)	7 (12.1)	4.47 (1.3–15.8)	0.02*
> 1	10 (14.7)	45 (77.6)	34.5(11.6–102.9)	0.01*

QoL Quality of life, *COR* Crude odds ratio
*p value =/< 0.05

Table 4 Factors associated with poor quality of life on SNOT 22 after controlling for confounders

VARIABLE	Crude odds ratio (95% CI)	Adjusted odds ratio (95% CI)	p value
CRS			
No			
Yes	29.62 (10.6–82.4)	8.94 (2.4–33.8)	0.00[a]
Polyps			
No			
Yes	17.5 (2.2–139.0)	2.14 (0.1–53.3)	0.64
Nasal discharge			
No			
Yes	24.40 (7.8–76.1)	7.15 (1.6–32.8)	0.01[a]
Allergy			
No			
symptoms			
Yes	2.94 (1.3–6.8)	1.94 (0.5–7.9)	0.35
GERD			
No			
Yes	1.1 (0.3–5.0)	0.69 (0.1–5.9)	0.74
History of smoking			
No			
Yes	2.50 (1.0–6.2)	3.65 (0.9–15.1)	0.07
Monthly income			
< USD 15			
>/=USD 15	0.36 (0.2–0.8)	0.48 (0.2–1.5)	0.20

CI Confidence interval, [a]significant at 0.05 level

group of patients with chronic ailments of which CRS is one. Secondly, we recruited patients at a large government health facility that attracts patients from a mostly low socioeconomic status because of free services. This category of patients is known to be at high risk for CRS [17] and our data also confirms this. The ENT clinic at our facility also serves a larger population than most Regional Referral Hospitals in Uganda. We serve patients from 10 districts of South Western Uganda and neighboring countries of Rwanda, Burundi, Southern Tanzania and The Democratic Republic of Congo. This might further explain the high prevalence we found in comparison to the studies reviewed [2–4].

Proportion of patients with poor HRQoL among those with and without CRS

Generally, CRS patients have poorer QoL compared to healthy individuals [18–20]. Our study showed the same as patients with CRS had poorer Health Related Quality of life, compared to those without CRS. The domain with the highest mean score among CRS patients was the nasal symptom domain. This might be because the aspects of QoL assessed in this domain relate to the mucosal inflammatory and ostial obstructive mechanisms within CRS. We found that the psychological domain had the second highest mean score among the CRS patients and attribute this to possibly unexplored sources of psychological stress such as financial struggles in this low socio-economic setting.. Browne et al., found the highest mean score in CRS patients in the nasal symptom domain, followed closely by the mean psychological score [14], a finding similar to that in our study.

Non-CRS patients scored highest in the ear/ facial symptom domain. We attribute this to the fact that the majority of patients seen in the MRRH otolaryngology clinic have ear related conditions from a review of the OPD records. This likely resulted in the majority of our non-CRS respondents having ear related complaints, thus reporting poorer quality of life scores in the ear symptom domain. Mean scores and trends in the SNOT 22 domains for non- CRS groups is variable across studies possibly because there is wide diversity in the non-CRS groups recruited [14, 21, 22].

Overall, both the total and mean domain scores were higher in the CRS patients compared to respondents without CRS and this is in keeping with results from studies done elsewhere. There is however little similarity in the scores from the non-CRS population between our study and studies done elsewhere.

Factors associated with poor quality of life scores

From the bivariate analysis, poor quality of life scores were generally significantly associated with the endonasal factors except septal deviation. Having a secondary education and a monthly income of over USD 15 appeared to confer protection from poor quality of life in CRS.

We expected to find a significant association between female gender and poor quality of life but this was not true. Males tend to seek health care when they have worse symptom scores compared to females and males were also more likely to be smokers. Although females tend to report poorer QoL [23], one may argue that male health seeking behavior and smoking may have wiped out the difference. However, this may not be entirely true since we adjusted for these differences. Ference et al., reviewed six studies on gender differences in self-reported quality of life among CRS patients. They concluded that the influence of gender on quality of life seems to be restricted primarily to the general aspects of quality of life, whereas the disease-specific health-related quality of life is not different between genders [23].

The lack of association between GERD symptoms and both CRS and quality of life on the SNOT 22 in our study is not supported by previous findings. Patients with GERD symptoms have been shown to have a reduced nose and sinus-related quality of life [24] and having GERD symptoms increases the mean SNOT-22

score in patients with CRS by 15.7 (95% CI, 6.5–24.9) [25]. We suspect that this discrepancy in findings may be because only 8 respondents in our study had GERD symptoms, with 4 of them having a poor quality of life.

Our study revealed that having a formal education was protective in CRS related quality of life. A study by Kilty et al., found that having a post-secondary education was significantly associated with low self-reported sinus symptom scores in CRS patients [26]. It is possible that for our population, patients with a formal education possibly understand prescription instructions better than those without a formal education and medical personnel find more ease in explaining disease processes to formally educated persons. This means that an educated patient might have realistic health expectations during the course of their treatment and are psychologically better equipped to manage their CRS symptoms.

Patients with a monthly income of over USD 15 were less likely to have poor quality of life. Also CRS occurred less frequently among patients with a monthly income. USD 15 is averagely sufficient to purchase a month's supply of CRS medication with some left over to cater to other basic needs of a patient in this population. Although we could not find studies that evaluated income level and quality of life in CRS patients, Pilan et al., found that CRS was significantly more prevalent in low-income groups [17]. The ability to purchase prescribed medication that would relieve CRS symptoms and thus result in better quality of sleep and psychological wellbeing may account for this relationship.

Because endonasal abnormalities result in persistent symptoms, they may have contributed greatly to increased nasal symptom and sleep disturbance scores for our patients. Nasal discharge is a major symptom of CRS, therefore it would seem imperative that it be associated with a poor Health Related Quality of Life in our patient sample.

In the multivariate analysis, only CRS and nasal discharge were found to be significantly associated with poor health related quality of life. Persons with CRS were almost nine times more likely to have poor quality of life compared to persons without CRS. The results agree with findings from other studies using SNOT22 among CRS patients [18–20].

Our study has some limitations. First, the SNOT-22 questionnaire has not been validated in any of the indigenous languages of Uganda, however, has been used elsewhere in Africa with similar cultural setting as Uganda. We used professional translation and hence language minimally affected the validity of the results obtained from the Quality of life assessment.

Second, the lack of CT scans limited our ability to accurately diagnose CRS. However we are confident that the symptoms and endoscopic findings were adequate to make a diagnosis of CRS as per the definition by Rosenfeld and Cornelius [3, 27].

Our study has some strength. Most quality of life studies have been done in regions that have significant seasonal variations compared to southwestern Uganda. The strength of our study is that it provides data from a region with less seasonal variation, such as sub Saharan Africa, for which information on quality of life in CRS is scarce.

Conclusions

In conclusion, the prevalence of chronic rhinosinusitis among our patients re-attending the ENT clinic is relatively high. Majority of patients with CRS in this resource limited settinghave significantly reduced disease specific QOL compared to those without CRS.

The poor quality of life scores on SNOT 22 appear to be almost solely as a result of the functional, physical and psychological aspects of chronic rhinosinusitis that the SNOT 22 evaluates.

Quality of life assessment should therefore be included in the routine evaluation of patients with CRS in low-to-middle income countries, and the quality of life scores used as one of the indices, alongside clinical findings to assess treatment strategies. This will ensure holistic care of these patients. Further studies need to be done to evaluate the impact of treatments available in low resource settings on the quality of life in CRS patients.

Abbreviations

CRS: Chronic Rhinosinusitis; FREC: Faculty of Medicine Research Ethical Committee; GERD: Gastroesophageal Reflux Disease; HRQoL: Health-related Quality of Life; IRB: Institutional Review Board; MRRH: Mbarara Regional Referral Hospital; MUST: Mbarara University of Science and Technology; QoL: Quality of Life; RNE: Rigid nasal endoscopy; SNOT-22: Sinonasal Outcome Test 22

Acknowledgements

Dr. Joseph Kiwanuka, and Dr. Imelda Tamwesigire reviewed and helped with editing of this work. Ms. Lillian Banura, Dr. Esther Nakasagga and residents in the otolaryngology clinic at MRRH assisted us in the enrollment and scheduling of patients for study procedures. Massachusetts General Hospital and Center for Global Health for funding this study.

Funding

This study was funded by the Massachusetts General Hospital and Center for Global Health as part of a masters scholarship. The funding body however took no active part in the writing, data collection and analysis of the work presented.

Authors' contributions

VN and FB conceived the idea. VN, DN, EL, EN and RB collected the data and assessed the patients. EK and VN analyzed the data. GN edited and interpreted the quality of life concepts. All authors reviewed the tables of results. VN wrote the first draft of the manuscript. All authors reviewed and approved the final draft of manuscript.

Competing interests

The authors declare that they have no competing interests.

Author details

[1]Department of Ear, Nose and Throat, Mbarara University of Science and Technology, Mbarara, Uganda. [2]Infectious Disease Research Collaboration, Mbarara, Uganda. [3]Department of Psychology, Mbarara University of Science and Technology, Mbarara, Uganda. [4]Department of Ear, Nose and Throat, Makerere University College of Health Sciences, Kampala, Uganda. [5]Department of Community Health, Mbarara University of Science and Technology, Mbarara, Uganda.

References

1. Fokkens WJ, Lund VJ, Mullol J, Bachert C, Alobid I, Baroody F, et al. EPOS 2012: European position paper on rhinosinusitis and nasal polyps 2012. A summary for otorhinolaryngologists. Rhinology. 2012;50(1):1–12.
2. Hastan D, Fokkens W, Bachert C, Newson R, Bislimovska J, Bockelbrink A, et al. Chronic rhinosinusitis in Europe–an underestimated disease. A GA2LEN study. Allergy. 2011;66(9):1216–23.
3. Cornelius RS, Martin J, Wippold FJ, Aiken AH, Angtuaco EJ, Berger KL, et al. ACR appropriateness criteria sinonasal disease. J Am Coll Radiol. 2013;10(4):241–6.
4. Mainasara MG, Labaran AS, Kirfi AM, Fufore MB, Fasunla AJ, Sambo GU. Clinical profile and management of chronic rhinosinusitis among adults in North-Western Nigeria. Magn Resonance Imaging (MRI). 2015; 9:11–2.
5. Metson RB, Gliklich RE. Clinical outcomes in patients with chronic sinusitis. Laryngoscope. 2000;110(S94):24–8.
6. Fitzpatrick R, Fletcher A, Gore S, Jones D, Spiegelhalter D, Cox D. Quality of life measures in health care. I: applications and issues in assessment. BMJ. 1992;305(6861):1074–7.
7. Schalek P. Rhinosinusitis-its impact on quality of life: INTECH open access Publisher; 2011.
8. Damm M, Quante G, Jungehuelsing M, Stennert E. Impact of functional endoscopic sinus surgery on symptoms and quality of life in chronic rhinosinusitis. Laryngoscope. 2002;112(2):310–5.
9. Alobid I, Benitez P, Bernal-Sprekelsen M, Roca J, Alonso J, Picado C, et al. Nasal polyposis and its impact on quality of life: comparison between the effects of medical and surgical treatments. Allergy. 2005;60(4):452–8.
10. Baumann I, Blumenstock G. Impact of gender on general health-related quality of life in patients with chronic sinusitis. Am J Rhinol. 2005;19(3):282–7.
11. Kaplan A. Canadian guidelines for chronic rhinosinusitis: clinical summary. Can Fam Physician. 2013;59(12):1275–81.
12. Kelsey J, Whittemore A, Evans A, Thompson W. Methods of sampling and estimation of sample size. Methods Observational Epidemiol. 1996;311:340.
13. Piccirillo JF, Merritt MG, Richards ML. Psychometric and clinimetric validity of the 20-item Sino-nasal outcome test (SNOT-20). Otolaryngol Head Neck Surg. 2002;126(1):41–7.
14. Hopkins C, Gillett S, Slack R, Lund V, Browne J. Psychometric validity of the 22-item Sinonasal outcome test. Clin Otolaryngol. 2009;34(5):447–54.
15. Gillett S, Hopkins C, Slack R, Browne J. A pilot study of the SNOT 22 score in adults with no sinonasal disease. Clin Otolaryngol. 2009;34(5):467–9.
16. Iseh K, Makusidi M. Rhinosinusitis: a retrospective analysis of clinical pattern and outcome in north western Nigeria. Ann Afr Med. 2010;9(1)22–26
17. Pilan RR, FdR P, Bezerra TF, Mori RL, Padua FG, Bento RF, et al. Prevalence of chronic rhinosinusitis in Sao Paulo. Rhinology. 2012;50(2):129–38.
18. Browne JP, Hopkins C, Slack R, Cano SJ. The Sino-nasal outcome test (SNOT): can we make it more clinically meaningful? Otolaryngol Head Neck Surg. 2007;136(5):736–41.
19. Lange B, Holst R, Thilsing T, Baelum J, Kjeldsen A. Quality of life and associated factors in persons with chronic rhinosinusitis in the general population: a prospective questionnaire and clinical cross-sectional study. Clin Otolaryngol. 2013;38(6):474–80.
20. Kosugi EM, Chen VG, da Fonseca VMG, Cursino MMP, Neto JAM, Gregório LC. Translation, cross-cultural adaptation and validation of SinoNasal outcome test (SNOT)-22 to Brazilian Portuguese. Braz J Otorhinolaryngol. 2011;77(5):663–9.
21. Jalessi M, Farhadi M, Kamrava SK, Amintehran E, Asghari A, Hemami MR, Mobasseri A, Masroorchehr M. The reliability and validity of the persian version of sinonasal outcome test 22 (snot 22) questionnaires. Iran Red Crescent Med J. 2013;15(5):404–8.

22. Mascarenhas JG, VMGd F, Chen VG, Itamoto CH, CAPd S, Gregório LC, et al. Results in longo prazo da cirurgia endoscópica nasossinusal no tratamento da rinossinusite crônica com e sem polipos nasais. Braz J Otorhinolaryngol. 2013; 79 (3): 306–11.

23. Ference EH, Tan BK, Hulse KE, Chandra RK, Smith SB, Kern RC, et al. Commentary on gender differences in prevalence, treatment, and quality of life of patients with chronic rhinosinusitis. Allergy & Rhinology. 2015;6(2):e82.

24. Katle E-J, Hart H, Kjærgaard T, Kvaløy JT, Steinsvåg SK. Nose-and sinus-related quality of life and GERD. Eur Arch Otorhinolaryngol. 2012;269(1):121–5.

25. Bohnhorst I, Jawad S, Lange B, Kjeldsen J, Hansen JM, Kjeldsen AD. Prevalence of chronic rhinosinusitis in a population of patients with gastroesophageal reflux disease. Am J Rhinol Allergy. 2015;29(3):e70–e4.

26. Kilty SJ, McDonald JT, Johnson S, Al-Mutairi D. Socioeconomic status: a disease modifier of chronic rhinosinusitis? Rhinology. 2011;49(5):533.

27. Rosenfeld RM, Piccirillo JF, Chandrasekhar SS, Brook I, Kumar KA, Kramper M, et al. Clinical Practice Guideline (Update) Adult Sinusitis. Otolaryngol Head Neck Surg. 2015;152(2 suppl):S1–S39.

26

Glomangiomyoma of the neck in a child in Nepal

Bishow Tulachan* and Buddha Nath Borgohain

Abstract

Background: Glomangiomyoma is a rare histological variant of glomus tumour. Clinically, it mimicks as a haemangioma and is challenging to diagnose. Its occurrence in the neck of a child has not been previously described.

Case presentation: A 3 year old girl presented with the complaints of painless progressive neck swelling in the right side for one and half year. Sonography, computed tomography (CT), magnetic resonance imaging (MRI), CT neck angiography and fine needle aspiration cytology (FNAC) were suggestive of vacular malformation i.e. giant haemangioma or arteriovenous malformation. The mass was removed in toto under general anaesthesia without postoperative complications. The histopathology confirmed it to be glomangiomyoma with haemangiopericytoma like features.

Conclusion: It's an extremely rare variant of glomus tumour and may be the first report of a glomangiomyoma in the neck of a child. Despite a rare entity, it should be borne in mind during differential diagnosis.

Keywords: Glomangiomyoma, Glomus tumour, Angiography, Postoperative

Background

Glomus tumour, an uncommon neoplasm, arises from the glomus bodies, cells having resemblance of the modified smooth muscle cells of the normal glomus body. Glomangiomyoma is a rare variant of it. Glomus bodies possess peculiar fibrous perivascular structures and regulate body temperature by functioning as arteriovenous shunts [1]. These are located in the reticular dermis throughout the body, especially in the sub ungual region, distal digits, and more acral portions of the body, but may occur wherever arteriovenous anastomoses are found [1–3]. However, these lesion are different from head and neck paragangliomas, which are also referred to as glomus tumours. Paragangliomas are tumours of the autonomic system arising from chromaffin cells of the parasympathetic paraganglia of the skull base and neck e.g. carotid body tumour [4].

In 1924, the first description about glomangiomyoma was given by Mason. It rarely occurs extradigitally particulary the neck region. And other extradigital sites where normal glomus bodies may be sparse or even absent, such as the patella, chest wall, bone, stomach, colon, nerve, eyelid, nose, mediastinum, small bowel, rectum, urinary tract, lung, cervix, vagina, oral cavity, mesentery, heart, lymph nodes, larynx, back and trachea have been reported [5–10]. Here, we report a case of glomangiomyoma of the neck in a 3 year old child. The histological and imaging findings are described.

* Correspondence: tulachanbishow@hotmail.com; drbtulachan@gmail.com
Department of ENT - Head and Neck Studies, Universal College of Medical Sciences, Tribhuvan University Teaching Hospital, Bhairahawa, Nepal

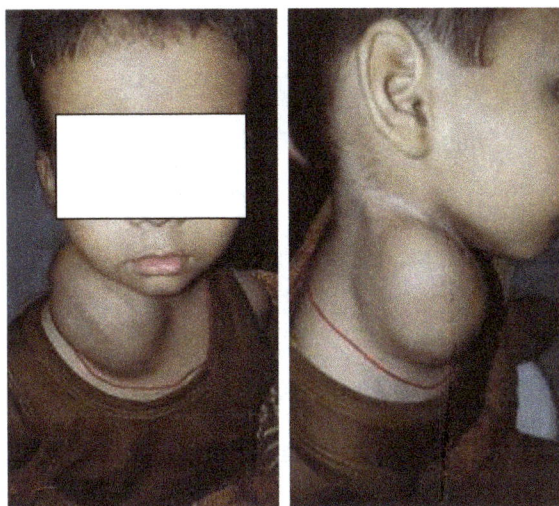

Fig. 1 Anterior and lateral view of neck mass

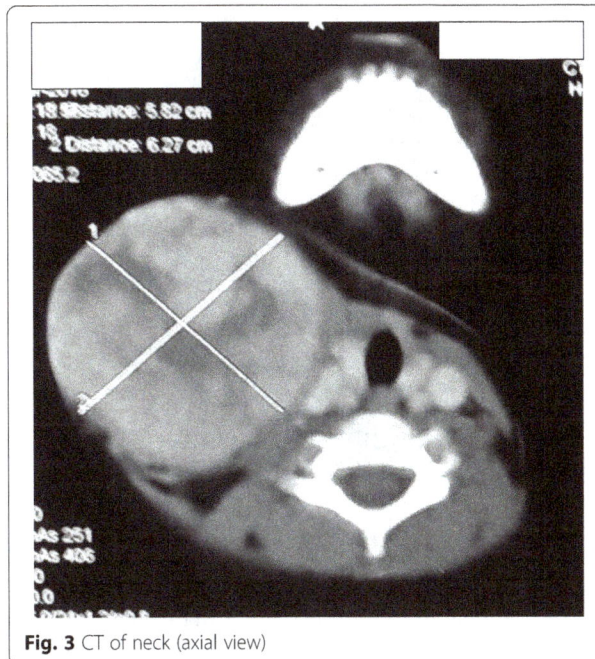

Fig. 3 CT of neck (axial view)

Case presentation

This is a case report of a 3 year old female child presented with chief complaints of swelling in the right side of neck for around 1 ½ years in ENT OPD of Universal College of Medical Sciences, Bhairahawa, Lumbini zone. The onset was insidious and gradually progressive, painless and without aggravating and relieving factors. On examination, there was a 8 X 6 cm, ovoid, nontender, soft swelling, nonpulsatile, mobile in all directions, not fixed to overlying skin, smooth surface and prominent superficial neck veins and the transillumination test was positive. The swelling was extending superiorly at level of right angle of mandible, inferiorly 2 cm below the suprasternal notch, laterally 1 cm behind the posterior border of right sternocleidomastoid muscle and medially in the midline of neck (Fig. 1).

The oral cavity, oropharynx and larynx examination were unremarkable. Hence, a provisional diagnosis of

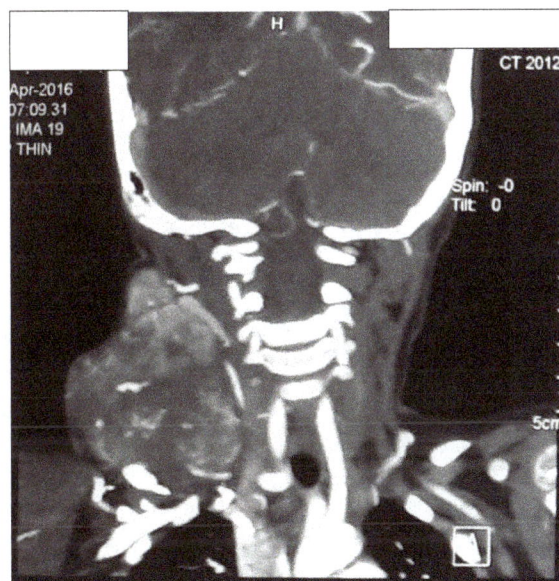

Fig. 2 CT of neck (coronal view)

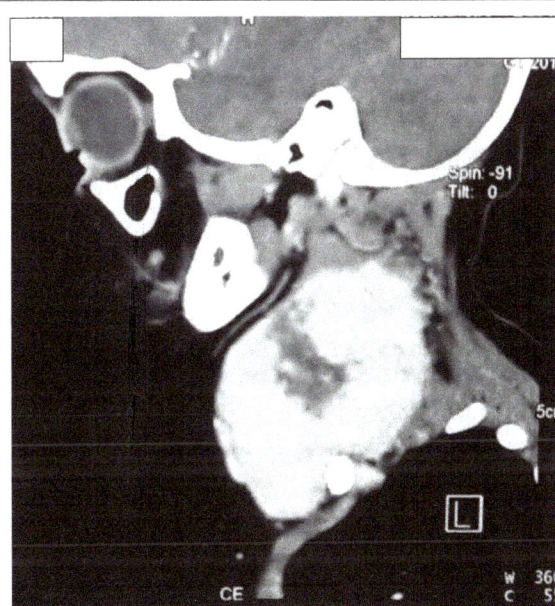

Fig. 4 CT of neck (sagittal view)

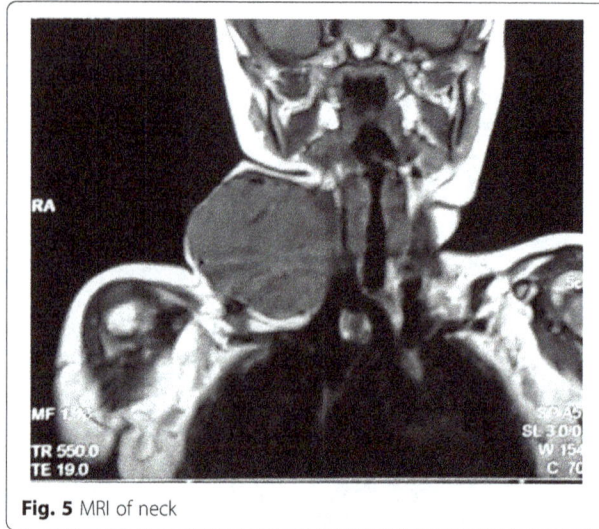

Fig. 5 MRI of neck

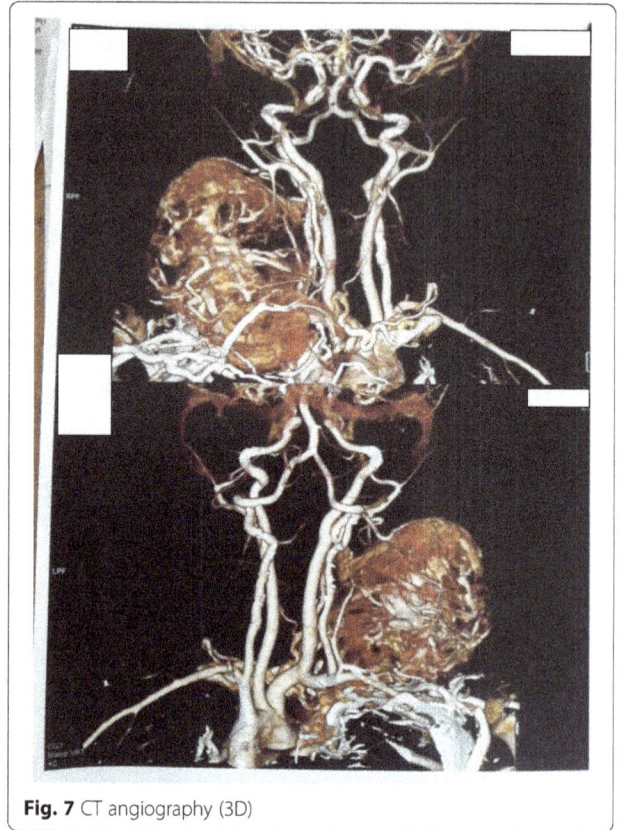

Fig. 7 CT angiography (3D)

neck haemangioma/arteriovenous malformation was made. Ultrasonography with 9 MHz probe showed a large globular swelling nearly 10X8 cm filling right half of neck, multiple circumscribed primarily an-echoic structures with appreciable fine internal echoes size varying from 0.87 to 3.67 cm, well marginated and the loculations are separated by thick intervening septa containing various sized vessels. Doppler couldn't show flow in the swelling but the intervening tissue show larger blood vessels. Feeding vessel was not found and the whole large swelling was placed over the carotid sheath. FNAC showed only polymorphs, lymphocytes and macrophages in a background of RBCs suggestive of vascular lesion

(Haemangioma). It was negative for malignancy. Plain and contrast enhanced CT was suggestive of high flow vascular malformation (Figs. 2, 3, 4). MRI was suggestive of high flow vascular malformation or neoplastic mass having high vascularity in it (Fig. 5).

CT neck angiography was also suggestive of vascular malformation- giant haemangioma or arteriovenous malformation (AVM) (Figs. 6, 7).

She underwent excision of the mass under general anaesthesia. Preoperative endovascular embolisation

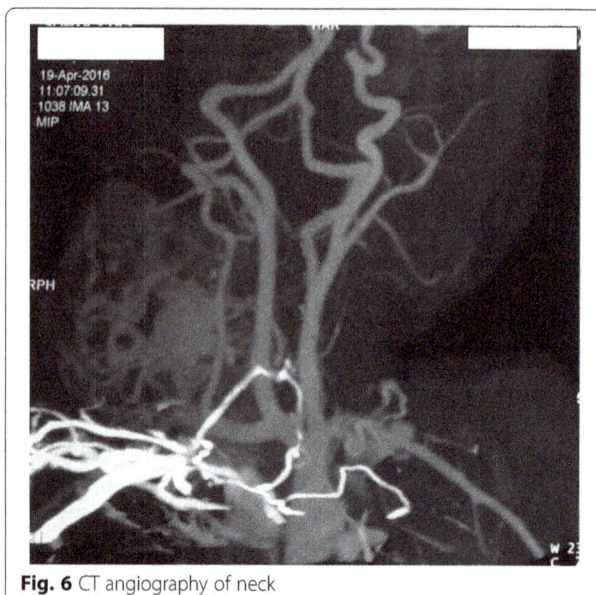

Fig. 6 CT angiography of neck

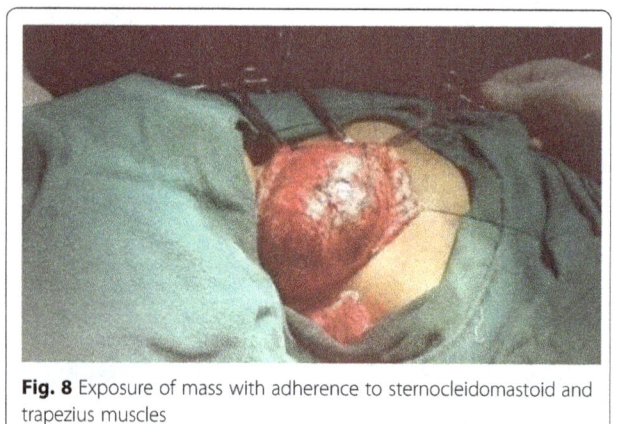

Fig. 8 Exposure of mass with adherence to sternocleidomastoid and trapezius muscles

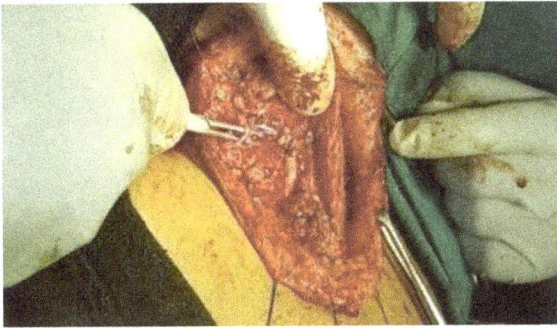

Fig. 9 Accessory nerve

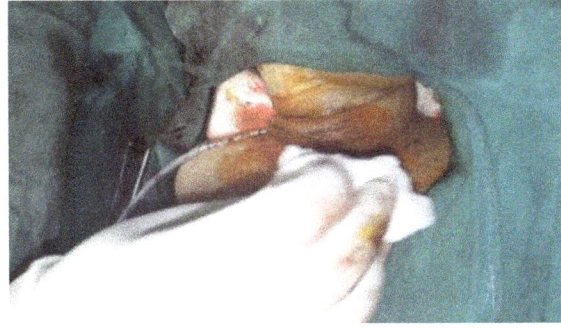

Fig. 11 Skin closure with Prolene cutting body suture 4.0 and number 10 Romovac drain in situ

would have been better anticipating the blood loss during surgery but it's not available locally. Hence, we solely depended upon the ligatures and electrocautery. Intraoperatively, the mass was adhered to sternocleidomastoid muscle extending upto hyoid bone level superiorly and extended inferiorly upto the supraclavicular fossa, feeding vessels from right subclavian, external carotid, common carotid artery, thyrocervical trunk were ligated and also the draining vessels towards internal jugular vein were also ligated and the entire mass was removed in toto (Figs. 8, 9, 10). Haemostasis was secured and closed with Romovac drain number 10 (Fig. 11).

Postoperatively she was free of complications and also at her subsequent follow ups (Fig. 12). Histopathology showed capsulated structure comprising of tumour cells arranged predominantly in solid sheets and nodules interrupted by variable sized vessels; many of which show staghorn like appearance. Few of the areas showed tumour cells arranged in nests and cords. Individual tumour cells revealed round to oval nuclei, bland dispersed nuclear chromatin, discernible nucleoli and moderate amount of cytoplasm. At the periphery of the sheets and nodules, many cells were spindled with elongated nuclei and bipolar eosinophilic cytoplasm resembling smooth muscle differentiation blended into tumour cells. Areas of necrosis were also evident. However, no overt atypia/atypical mitosis evident (Fig. 13). It was suggestive of perivascular tumour; glomangiomyoma with haemangiopericytoma like features.

Discussion and conclusions

Glomus tumours are rare neoplasms, found typically in soft tissue of the extremities, notably in the subungual region of the finger tip. However, extradigital identification have been done in different parts of the body [5, 6].Histologically, the tumour cells consists of varying proportions of glomus cells, vascular structures, and smooth muscle tissue. These are well-circumscribed lesions with tight convolutes of capillaries entangled by uniform glomus cells in a hyalinized or myxoid stromal background. Round and somewhat cohesive nature of the cells give them an epithelioid appearance. The histologic appearance of

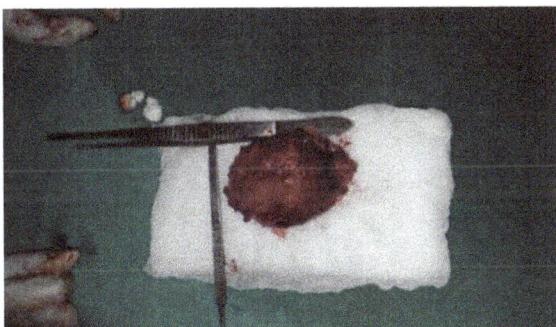

Fig. 10 Excised mass 8 × 7 cm

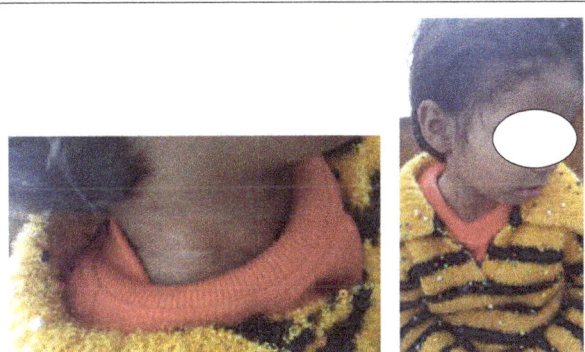

Fig. 12 7 months follow up

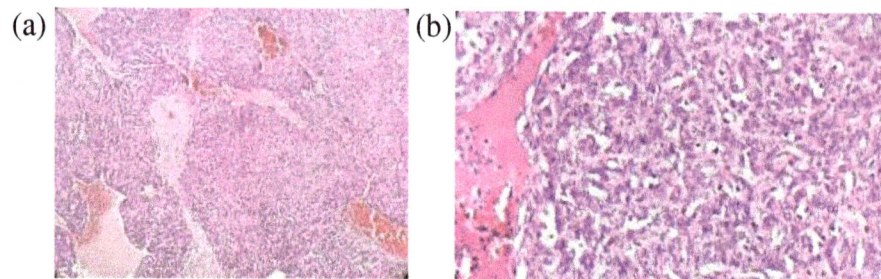

Fig. 13 (a) low power view (×100) prominent thin walled blood vessels with proliferation of tumor cells around it along with variable proportion of smooth muscle and, (b) high power view (×400) individual tumor cells are small, uniform, round with central nucleus, discernible nucleoli and eosinophilic cytoplasm

the tumors depends on the different factors like vascular cell–glomus cell ratio, their differentiation, and the amount and composition of the stroma. Solid glomus tumour (25%), glomangioma (60%) and glomangiomyoma are the recognized histological variants (15%) [7, 11]. Glomangiomyomas may have resemblance to that of an ordinary glomus tumour or a glomangioma. However, there's a gradual trasition from glomus cells to elongated, mature smooth muscle cells. Immunohistochemically, glomus tumours show positive reactions for smooth muscle actin and CD34, and negative reactions for S-100 and cytokeratin [5]. Recently, glomuvenous malformations term was given to glomangiomas or glomangiomyomas. Glomuvenous malformations may either be acquired or congenital, and heterogenous germline mutations in the glomulin gene (GLMN) [12].

In our centre, it was diagnosed with the help of imaging like USG, contrast enhanced CT, CT angiography, MRI, FNAC and the histopathological evaluation.

The treatment of choice for glomus tumour is surgical excision. Several sclerosants like sodium tetradecyl sulphate, polidocanol and hypertonic saline has been reported to be effective. Ablative therapy with Argon and Carbon dioxide laser is of potential benefit for small, superficial lesions [12]. Here, we've described the clinical, radiological and the histopathological findings of a case of glomangiomyoma of the neck in a child. It can make the diagnosis difficult to other soft tissue tumours like haemangioma and av. malformations. However, it can be treated successfully with complete excision. To our knowledge, this may be the first report of a glomangiomyoma of the neck in a child.

Abbreviations
AVM: Arteriovenous malformation; CT: Computed tomography; FNAC: Fine needle aspiration cytology; GLMN: Germline mutations in the glomulin gene; MRI: Magnetic resonance imaging

Acknowledgements
No acknowledgement.

Funding
No fund received.

Authors' contributions
T. B wrote the the entire article and did much of the literature review. B.N.B completed most of the edits as the main editor. Both authors read and approved the final manuscript.

Competing interests
The authors declare that they have no competing interests.

References
1. Pepper MC, Laubcnhcimcr R, Cripps DJ. Multiple glomus tumors. J Cutan Pathol. 1977;4(5):244–57.
2. Appelman HD, Helwig EB. Glomus tumors of the stomach. Cancer. 1969;23: 203–13.
3. Provcnzn DV, Biddix JC. Cheng TC. Studies on the etiology of periodontosis 11. Glomera as vascular components in the periodontal membrane. Oral Surg. 1960;13:157–64.
4. Offergeld C, Brase C, Yaremchuk S, et al. Head and neck paragangliomas: clinical and molecular genetic classification. Clinics. 2012;67(1):19–28.
5. Weiss SW, Goldblum JR. Perivascular tumors. In: Weiss SW, editor. Enzinger and Weiss's soft tissue tumors. 4th ed. St. Louis: Mosby Inc; 2001. p. 985–93.
6. Baek SH, Huh DM, Park JH, Kwak EK, Kim BH, Han WK. Glomangiomyoma of the trachea. Korean J Thorac Cardiovasc Surg. 2011;44(6):440–3.
7. Imane H, Lakjiri S, Harmouch T, et al. Glomangiomyoma of back : a case report and literature review. Research. 2014;1:923.
8. Shek T, Hui Y. Glomangiomyoma of the nasal cavity. Am J Otolaryngol. 2001;22:282–5.
9. Lo AWI, Chow LTC, To KF, et al. Gastric glomangiomyoma. A pedunculated extramural mass with a florid angiomyomatous pattern. Histopathology. 2004;44:297–8.
10. Usuda K, Gildea T, Lorenz R. Laryngeal Glomangiomyoma. Journal of Bronchology. 2005;12(2):102–3.
11. Fletcher C.D., Unni K.K., Mertens F (Eds). World Health Organisation Classification of Tumors. Pathology and Genetics of Tumors of Soft Tissue and Bone (3rd edition). Lyon: IARC Press, International Agency for Research on Cancer; 2002.
12. Brauer JA, Analik R, Tzu J, Meehan S, Lieber CD, Geronemus RG. Glomuvenous malformations (familial generalized multiple glomangiomas). Dermatology Online J. 2011;17(10):9.

27

A retrospective study of long-term treatment outcomes for reduced vocal intensity in hypokinetic dysarthria

Christopher R. Watts

Abstract

Background: Reduced vocal intensity is a core impairment of hypokinetic dysarthria in Parkinson's disease (PD). Speech treatments have been developed to rehabilitate the vocal subsystems underlying this impairment. Intensive treatment programs requiring high-intensity voice and speech exercises with clinician-guided prompting and feedback have been established as effective for improving vocal function. Less is known, however, regarding long-term outcomes of clinical benefit in speakers with PD who receive these treatments.

Methods: A retrospective cohort design was utilized. Data from 78 patient files across a three year period were analyzed. All patients received a structured, intensive program of voice therapy focusing on speaking intent and loudness. The dependent variable for all analyses was vocal intensity in decibels (dBSPL). Vocal intensity during sustained vowel production, reading, and novel conversational speech was compared at pre-treatment, post-treatment, six month follow-up, and twelve month follow-up periods.

Results: Statistically significant increases in vocal intensity were found at post-treatment, 6 months, and 12 month follow-up periods with intensity gains ranging from 5 to 17 dB depending on speaking condition and measurement period. Significant treatment effects were found in all three speaking conditions. Effect sizes for all outcome measures were large, suggesting a strong degree of practical significance.

Conclusions: Significant increases in vocal intensity measured at 6 and 12 moth follow-up periods suggested that the sample of patients maintained treatment benefit for up to a year. These findings are supported by outcome studies reporting treatment outcomes within a few months post-treatment, in addition to prior studies that have reported long-term outcome results. The positive treatment outcomes experienced by the PD cohort in this study are consistent with treatment responses subsequent to other treatment approaches which focus on high-intensity, clinician guided motor learning for voice and speech production in PD. Theories regarding the underlying neurophysiological response to treatment will be discussed.

Keywords: Voice, Voice disorders, Parkinson's disease, Speech and language therapy

Background

Among the physiological impairments resulting from Parkinson's disease (PD) include the onset and progression of hypokinetic dysarthria. Hypokinetic dysarthria in PD is characterized by deviations in the rate, range, force, and tone of neuromuscular function in the muscles underlying speech production [1]. These deviations translate to effects on speech that include abnormalities in articulation and phonation. The classic clinical presentation of speech impairment in PD is characterized by a perceptually salient low volume and breathy voice quality, short rushes of speech, and imprecise articulation [2]. These vocal abnormalities result from impairments to neuromuscular control of respiratory and laryngeal muscles which numerous treatments, both medical and behavioral, have aimed to improve.

The pathophysiology of PD is linked to basal ganglia dysfunction and/or neural networks tied to this system. Unlike the limb effects of PD, however, evidence for

Correspondence: c.watts@tcu.edu
Davies School of Communication Sciences & Disorders, Texas Christian University, TCU Box 297450, Fort Worth, TX 76129, USA

pharmaceutical and surgical treatments improving hypokinetic dysarthria has been equivocal, suggesting that speech and voice manifestations of PD are influenced by pathways related to, but outside, the basal ganglia nuclei [3]. The model of PD progression proposed by Braak et al. (2004) suggested that early stage PD is characterized by neuronal impairment in the medulla and pons, including nuclei of the vagus and glossopharyngeal nerves [4]. Sapir (2014) has suggested that this model could explain why hypokinetic dysarthria is not sensitive to dopamine replacement therapy (cranial nerves are influenced by dopaminergic pathways, but do not directly utilize dopamine for neuronal communication) [3]. The muted effect of medication for treating the voice manifestations of PD, specifically the glottal incompetence resulting in low volume which progresses along with the disease, lends support to that position.

The laryngeal dysfunction resulting from hypokinetic dysarthria in PD is manifested by glottal incompetence due to bowing of the vocal folds, in some cases with accompanying atrophy [5]. The perceptual and physiological consequences of this impairment are reduced speech volume and vocal sound intensity, respectively. In theory these changes result from rigidity (Hypertonicity) in respiratory and laryngeal muscles due to the extrapyramidal dysfunction underlying the disease, although alternative theories of hypotonicity have also been presented [6–9]. In addition, alternative explanations for hypokinetic dysarthria tying voice and speech effects to factors other than rigidity have been proposed. Among these include impaired scaling of vocal effort resulting in the reduced vocal amplitude that is characteristic of speakers with PD [3]. This theory links the basal ganglia mediation of physical effort sense to the reduced vocal effort and subsequent low volume characterizing speech patterns of speakers with PD.

Bowed vocal folds are a characteristic of some speakers with PD, and surgical correction for the glottal incompetence has primarily involved injection laryngoplasty [10, 11]. Injectable substances are temporary, however, and repeated injections would be required for continuing improvement of glottal closure. Alternatively, a number of voice therapy approaches have demonstrated effective short and long-term outcomes for improving vocal amplitude and perceptual voice quality in populations with PD. A ubiquitous characteristic of voice therapy treatments for glottal incompetence, including those associated with PD, is a focus on high intensity (e.g., large number of repetitions) clinician guided exercise to promote adaptation in muscles and neurological pathways, and increased muscular effort to increase motor unit recruitment and the resulting amplitude of motor activity. These treatments target the issue of underscaling of vocal effort which is ubiquitous in speakers with PD [3].

A well-known evidence-based approach for treating the respiratory and laryngeal impairments in PD is the Lee-Silverman Voice Treatment (LSVT), now known as LSVT LOUD®. This structured intervention targets vocal effort scaling through increased vocal loudness via intensive, high effort vocalization and speech exercises designed to transfer to activities of daily living by improving neuromotor abilities and recalibrating the patients' perception of effort during speech production [12]. LSVT utilizes a singular target and cueing strategy of "think loud" with the aim of facilitating neuromotor adaptation during speech production so that the elevated level of effort and resulting increased amplitude of motor activity becomes automatic and is perceived as natural by the patient. A number of modifications to the traditional LSVT method (16 treatment sessions over 4 consecutive weeks) have been described, including the employment of distance technologies and reduced frequency of sessions (e.g., 2× per week over 8 weeks), with similar reported treatment outcomes [13, 14]. Interestingly, the focus on increasing the amplitude of motor activity during LSVT has also been shown to improve articulation and swallowing abilities in some patients, reportedly due to carry-over effects in neuromotor abilities associated with structures and pathways tangentially trained in the LSVT exercises [15–17].

Vocal effort scaling and the underlying glottal incompetence in some speakers with PD has also been treated with other voice therapy approaches whose clinical goals relate to a similar focus on increased motor amplitude. A recent report described Phonation Resistance Training Exercise (PhoRTE) therapy applied to 60 individuals with glottal incompetence due to presbyphonia. The therapy tasks required of patients receiving PhoRTE were adapted from LSVT but differed in the frequency of treatments (1× per week instead of 4×), the incorporation of high pitch and low pitch productions of functional phrases, and a less rigorous home practice schedule. The authors reported significant improvements in participants' perceptions of quality of life and perceived effort of voice production. These outcomes were similar to a comparison treatment, Vocal Function Exercises, and both experimental treatments resulted in greater clinical improvement compared to a control group who received no intervention [18].

Another related treatment focusing on vocal scaling, called "SPEAK OUT!®", targets vocal effort by prompting patients to speak with "intent", defined and modeled as a purposeful cognitive focus on increasing vocal loudness and intonation variability during speech [19]. Similar to LSVT, this treatment requires an intensive program although the number of treatment sessions is based on patient progress (e.g., 16 sessions are not required, as were in the original method for LSVT) and sessions last approximately 45 min. Each treatment session is structured with a hierarchy of speech, voice, and cognitive exercises progressing in the following manner: warm-up vocalizations → sustained vowel production → pitch glides → counting → reading → cognitive exercises. In the published literature, outcome data from only six patients receiving this treatment has been reported [20]. Reports which document clinical outcomes from larger samples, both in retrospective and prospective designs, will better inform clinical practice and evidence-based application of treatment approaches. The purpose of the present study was to investigate clinical outcomes in a large case series of patients who have received the SPEAK OUT! treatment in an effort to determine if measures of vocal function in patients with PD are positively or negatively impacted by this approach, and to compare results with the previously reported case reports.

Methods
Study design
This study used a retrospective design analyzing existing data from a consecutive case series of patients meeting inclusion criteria over a 3 year period. The primary outcome variable was vocal intensity (dBSPL) measured in three different speaking conditions: sustained vowel, reading, and conversation. Available data from records of patients within the cohort who were measured at 6 months and 1 year post-treatment was also collected. The methodology for this study was approved by a university Institutional Review Board (IRB# 1501–012–1501). The author has no competing interests to declare.

Study population
Data for this study was collected from patient records of the clinical population at Parkinson Voice Project in Richardson, TX, who were treated between March 2011 and October 2014, who completed at least 12 treatment sessions and for whom pre-treatment and post-treatment data were recorded. All data came from patients diagnosed with idiopathic PD and who were experiencing vocal impairments. Of 100 consecutive patient files, 78 completed at least 12 treatment sessions before post-treatment measures were collected. Of the 22 who did not complete 12 treatments, reasons included (a) meeting treatment goals prior to 12 treatments or (b) illness or other life situations requiring withdrawal from treatment. When available, data was also recorded from post-treatment follow-up periods at approximately six months and twelve months.

Description of the SPEAK OUT! therapy program
Data was recorded from patient files that underwent at least 12 treatment sessions. Each treatment was

organized around a hierarchical framework through which a patient progressed during the course of a 45-minute (approximate) session and during home practice (once daily on treatment days, twice daily on non-treatment days). Clinicians administering treatment attended a training workshop specific to the intervention protocol which was administered by experienced clinicians, and each had more than two years of clinical experience. Each patient whose file was included in this study received three treatment sessions per week and completed homework exercises for which they returned homework logs at the subsequent treatment session. Each treatment and homework session followed the exact organizational framework, with stimuli printed in a therapy workbook provided to the patient who placed it open and in front of them during each session. The treatment hierarchy was as follows:

1. Warm-up vocalizations on nasal words (e.g., "may", "me", "my")
2. Sustained vowel productions
3. Vowel pitch glides
4. Counting
5. Reading (phrases, sentences, and paragraphs)
6. Cognitive exercises (conversational speech) – these exercises provided written prompts to the patient in the form of carrier phrases which required the patient to complete in sentence form and then extend in conversation by providing the clinician with additional novel information about the topic. The cognitive exercises focused on improving word retrieval and processing speed. These responses required each patient to generate novel information while focusing on the treatment goal of speaking with intent.

The primary treatment goal and cueing strategy for treatment sessions was for each patient to speak with "intent". Prior to the initiation of treatment, each participant was seen for a "Parkinson's Information Session" in which the concept of "intent" was explained to them and treatment only began after a patient indicated understanding of the concept. "Intent" was defined as a purposeful cognitive focus in which the patient would direct attentional capacities on speech production. Cues such as "speak with authority," "use your CEO voice," and "say it with gusto" were associated with the concept of "intent" and utilized during treatment sessions. Confirmation of speaking intent included an increase in vocal loudness combined with variation of intonation which approximated more natural speech prosody during connected speech utterances. Patients were asked to speak with "intent" for every production throughout the treatment hierarchy. During treatment sessions, patients

were cued by asking them to determine if prior utterances were produced with "intent" or not, and where appropriate "intent" was modeled for them by the
clinician.

Measures
Data for this study was collected from daily treatment
logs of each patient, as recorded by the treating clinician.
The Parkinson Voice Project has standardized their
method of data collection during each treatment session,
as follows:

- Patients were seated in front of a desk, behind
  which the clinician sat.
- A digital sound level meter (Radio Shack model 33–
  2055) was placed via a stand on the desktop in front
  of the patient, with the microphone head placed at
  arm's length specific to each patient (determined by
  the patient extending their arm while seated
  comfortably, and the clinician placing the
  microphone head of the sound level meter at the
  patient's wrist). This resulted in varied mouth-to-
  microphone distances between patients, but exact
  mouth-to-microphone distances within patients so
  that valid measures of vocal intensity could be compared across sessions. The interpatient variation in
  mouth-to-microphone distance was considered minimal, and the background noise in treatment rooms
  was less than 45dBSPL. The response rate of the
  sound level meter was set to fast.
- Patients were asked to produce any utterance while
  facing the clinician (with mouth directed toward
  microphone head of sound level meter).
- For each production within the hierarchical stages,
  the clinician recorded the minimum decibel level
  across the utterance duration (in dBSPL) on a daily
  record sheet.
- Dependent variables for this study included dB from
  three speaking conditions in the treatment
  hierarchy: sustained vowels, reading and
  conversation during the cognitive exercises. Mean
  minimum dB averaged across the respective
  utterance types at pre-treatment stages and post-
  treatment stages (e.g., data collected on the 12th

treatment session, at 6-months post-treatment
follow-up and 12-months post-treatment follow-up)
were analyzed.

Statistical analysis
To compare treatment outcomes separate one-way
multivariate analyses of variance (MANOVA) with repeated measures were applied to the pre-treatment and
post-treatment data. Three separate MANOVA's were
used to compare pre-treatment to initial post-treatment
measures, post-treatment at 6-months, and post-
treatment at 12-months. In these statistical models,
treatment time (pre vs. post) was the primary independent variable with decibel level in the three different
speaking contexts (vowel, reading, conversation) as additional factors.

Results
The mean age of the full sample was 71.3 years, which
comprised 52 males (mean age = 72.9 years) and 26 females (mean age = 67.2 years). Mean years post-diagnosis
onset at which treatment first began was 7.0 years. Table 1
presents group descriptive statistics across the dependent
variables at the four measurement periods. Mean intensity
increased across all three dependent variables after 12
treatment sessions by approximately 17dB, 9dB, and 6 dB
for sustained vowels, reading, and conversation, respectively. These increases represented large effect sizes of $d =$
3.56 for sustained vowel, $d = 3.09$ for reading, and $d = 2.58$
for conversation.

From among this cohort 55 patients were measured at
the 6-month follow-up period and 30 were measured
again at the 12-month follow-up. Figure 1 illustrates
mean intensity across the three speaking conditions at
pre-treatment ($n = 78$), post-treatment ($n = 78$), the first
follow-up ($n = 55$), and the second follow-up measurement periods ($n = 30$). At both follow-up periods speaking intensity remained above pre-treatment baseline
levels. Effect sizes for mean intensity change comparing
pre-treatment to the 6-month follow-up period
remained large at $d = 3.46$, $d = 0.75$, and $d = 1.87$ for
vowel, reading, and conversation, respectively. At the
12-month follow-up period effect sizes remained large at

Table 1 Descriptive statistics (mean and standard deviation in parentheses) from for the dependent variables (in dB) at the different
measurement periods

Condition	Pre-Treatment	Post-Treatment	Follow-up 1	Follow-up 2
	$n = 78$	$n = 78$	$n = 55$	$n = 30$
Sustained Vowel	71.16 (6.01)	88.34 (3.23)	88.54 (4.91)	87.43 (6.39)
Reading	67.57 (3.18)	76.54 (2.58)	73.26 (10.67)	75.00 (3.70)
Conversation	66.64 (2.85)	72.89 (1.90)	71.32 (2.33)	71.33 (2.62)

Pre- and post-treatment measures reflect data from 78 patients, Follow-up 1 (at 6 months) reflect data from 55 patients, and Follow-up 2 (at 12 months) reflect
data from 30 participants

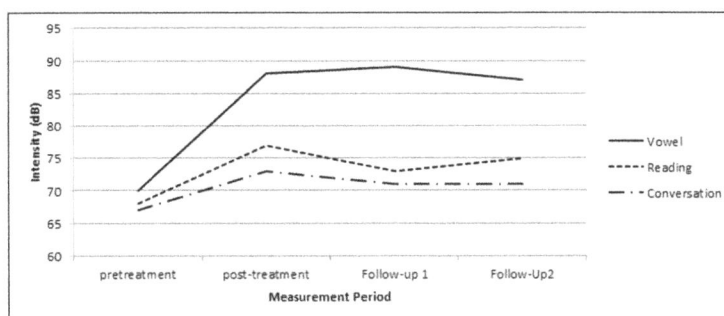

Fig. 1 Mean minimum intensity (in dB) levels across the three speaking condition at four measurement timeframes: pre-treatment ($n = 78$), post-treatment ($n = 78$), Follow-up 1 @ 6-months ($n = 55$), and Follow-up 2 @ 12-months ($n = 30$)

$d = 2.90$, $d = 2.21$, and $d = 1.64$ for vowel, reading, and conversation, respectively.

Three separate MANOVA's were applied to the data to compare pre-treatment intensity levels to those at post-treatment, 6-month follow-up, and 12-month follow-up periods, respectively. For the pre-treatment vs. post-treatment analysis, there was a significant main effect for measurement period (Pillai's Trace = 0.793, F[3,152] = 193.7, $p < 0.001$) with a corresponding large effect size as calculated by partial eta squared ($\eta^2 = 0.793$), which reflects the error variance between the three speaking conditions as a percent variance explained. In this analysis there were significant treatment effects for sustained vowel (F[1,154] = 494.64, $p < 0.001$), reading (F[1,154] = 373.12, $p < 0.001$), and conversation (F[1,154] = 259.72, $p < 0.001$). For the pre-treatment vs. 6-month follow-up analysis there was a significant main effect for measurement period (Pillai's Trace = 0.755, F[3,106] = 108.66, $p < 0.001$) with a corresponding large effect size ($\eta^2 = 0.755$). In this analysis there were significant treatment effects for sustained vowel (F[1,108] = 329.06, $p < 0.001$), reading (F[1,108] = 15.27, $p < 0.001$), and conversation (F[1,108] = 95.72, $p < 0.001$). In the pre-treatment vs. 12-month follow-up analysis there was a significant main effect for measurement period (Pillai's Trace = 0.692, F[3,56] = 42.03, $p < 0.001$) with a corresponding large effect size ($\eta^2 = 0.685$). In this analysis there were significant treatment effects for sustained vowel (F[1,58] = 126.34, $p < 0.001$), reading (F[1,58] = 73.27, $p < 0.001$), and conversation (F[1,58] = 40.55, $p < 0.001$).

Collectively the statistical analyses revealed a significant treatment effect on vocal intensity measured at post-treatment, 6-month follow-up, and 12-month follow-up when compared to pre-treatment vocal intensity. In all comparisons vocal intensity increased as a result of treatment. In addition, the results revealed that intensity increased for all three speaking conditions (sustained vowel, reading, conversation) at post-treatment, 6-month follow-up, and 12-month follow-up, respectively, when compared to pre-treatment measurements. For all comparisons

effect sizes were large, suggesting a strong degree of practical significance.

Discussion

The purpose of this study was to investigate clinical outcomes in a large case series of patients who received an intensive program of speech therapy by measuring vocal intensity during sustained vowel, reading, and conversation at pre-treatment, post-treatment, and two follow-up periods. Findings revealed a significant treatment effect of on all measurements when compared to pre-treatment levels. These treatment effects were associated with large effect sizes. Collectively, the results of this study further support the notion that intensive speech and voice treatments focusing on vocal effort scaling are effective for increasing speaking intensity secondary to Parkinson's disease. Additionally, results from this study suggested that treatment effects remained up to one-year post-treatment.

The largest treatment effect in this study was found on sustained vowel production. This was expected as both reading and conversation required connected speech with its variable intonation patterns resulting in a lower mean intensity across the utterances. The influence of speaking task on sound intensity and the differential influence of speaking task on response to treatment in patients with PD has also been demonstrated in prior studies [21]. Although long-term treatment effects across all speaking conditions are not unequivocal among previously reported investigations, the significant 6-month and 12-month follow-up effects found in this study are consistent with prior studies investigating long-term treatment effects secondary to LSVT [21, 22].

The significant post-treatment and long-term gains in vocal intensity subsequent to treatment are in line with outcomes from other evidence-based approaches which target reduced vocal intensity subsequent to glottal incompetence in PD or ageing. Interventions such as SPEAK OUT!, LSVT, and PhoRTE share methodological characteristics including high-intensity exercise protocols with clinician guided instruction and feedback to promote sustained motor learning. Theories explaining the neurophysiological changes subsequent to high-intensity vocal and speech exercises in PD have included improvement in glottal closure and/or vocal tension for increased sound pressure levels in speech, changes to extrapyramidal motor functions, and changes in limbic system pathways regulating goal-directed behavior [22]. A unique element of the treatment employed in the current study was the requirement for novel productions during conversational speech as a core element of the approach. The focus on "intent" is a method, similar to LSVT's prompting of "think loud", which helps the patient to rescale vocal effort during speech. In theory this may recruit and align cognitive pathways with the direct activation pyramidal pathways to facilitate increases in the number of motor units recruited in respiratory and laryngeal musculature during speech production. This hypothesis will need to be tested in future studies.

Study limitations

This investigation was a retrospective study, which presents limitations on interpretation due to the nature of the research design. Important among these limitations were the inability to control for confounding factors that may have influenced within-subject responses to treatment (i.e., clinician differences, medication types/levels/schedule). Related to this, there was no comparison with a control group, so any improvement measured in this study may be the result of separate factors other than or in addition to the intervention. Due to the retrospective nature of the design treatment fidelity could not be assessed. Additionally, data from 22 patients among the initial cohort of 100 was not included in the final analysis due to lack of meeting full inclusion criteria, and subsequent intention-to-treat analysis was not performed. The patient cohort in this study also included males and females, although sex was not a factor in the study design. The degree to which sex influences outcomes will need to be addressed in subsequent experiments. This study did not include a rigid control over mouth-to-microphone distance, which is known to influence measurements of acoustic intensity. Prospective studies controlling for this factor are needed to further validate the results of this study. The outcome measures were not blinded to treatment or time point and were conducted by the treating clinicians, which could have led to measurement bias. The findings from this investigation will require validation from future prospective studies with designs controlling for the above mentioned limitations.

Conclusion

This study investigated the effect of an intensive speech treatment focusing on rescaling of vocal effort to treat reduced vocal intensity due to hypokinetic dysarthria in PD. Retrospective data from 78 patients was analyzed to determine treatment effects after 12 therapy sessions (post-treatment), at a 6 month follow-up period, and at a 12 month follow-up period. Statistical analyses revealed significant treatment effects in the form of increased vocal intensity in sustained vowels, reading, and conversation at all three post-treatment measurement periods. These findings support the need for future prospective studies which control for additional factors as part of the scientific design. The positive treatment outcomes experienced by the PD cohort in this study are consistent with treatment responses subsequent to other treatment approaches which focus on high-intensity, clinician guided motor learning for voice and speech production in PD.

Abbreviations

dBSPL: decibels in sound pressure level; IRB: Institutional Review Board; LSVT: Lee Silverman Voice Treatment; MANOVA: Multivariate Analysis of Variance; PD: Parkinson's disease; PhoRTE: Phonation Resistance Training Exercise.

Competing interests

The author declares that he has no competing interests.

Acknowledgments

The author would like to thank Samantha Elandary and the clinicians at the Parkinson Voice Project in Richardson, TX for allowing IRB approved access to historical data.

Financial disclosures

The author has no financial disclosures to report associated with this research.

References

1. Duffy JR. Motor speech disorders: Substrates, differential diagnosis, and management. Philadelphia: Elsevier; 2005.
2. Darley FL, Aronson AE, Brown JR. Motor speech disorders. Philadelphia: W.B. Saunders; 1975.
3. Sapir S. Multiple factors are involved in the dysarthria associated with Parkinson's disease: a review with implications for clinical practice and research. J Speech Lang Hear Res. 2014;57(5):1330–43.
4. Braak H, Ghebremedhin E, Rub U, Bratzke H, Del Tredici K. Stages in the development of Parkinson's disease-related pathology. Cell Tissue Res. 2004; 318:121–34.
5. Sinclair CF, Gurey LE, Brin MF, Stewart C, Blitzer A. Surgical management of airway dysfunction in Parkinson's disease compared with Parkinson-plus syndromes. Ann Otol Rhinol Laryngol. 2013;122(5):294–8.
6. Blumin JH, Pcolinsky DE, Atkins JP. Laryngeal findings in advanced Parkinson's disease. Ann Otol Rhinol Laryngol. 2004;113(4):253–8.
7. Baker KK, Ramig LO, Luschei ES, Smith ME. Thyroarytenoid muscle activity associated with hypophonia in Parkinson disease and aging. Neurology. 1998;51(6):1592–8.
8. Gracco C, Marek K. Laryngeal eledromyographic findings in Parkinson's disease. Neurology. 1996;46 suppl 1:378.
9. Zarzur AP, Duprat AC, Shinzato G, Eckley CA. Laryngeal electromyography in adults with Parkinson's disease and voice complaints. Laryngoscope. 2007; 117(5):831–4.

10. Remacle M, Lawson G. Results with collagen injection into the vocal folds for medialization. Curr Opin Otolaryngol Head Neck Surg. 2007;15(3):148–52.
11. Seino Y, Allen JE. Treatment of aging vocal folds: surgical approaches. Curr Opin Otolaryngol Head Neck Surg. 2014;22(6):466–71.
12. Ramig LO, Fox C, Sapir S. Speech treatment for Parkinson's disease Expert Rev. Neurotherapeutics. 2008;8(2):299–311.
13. Halpern AE, Ramig LO, Matos CE, Petska-Cable JA, Spielman JL, Pogoda JM, et al. Innovative technology for the assisted delivery of intensive voice treatment (LSVT®LOUD) for Parkinson disease. Am J Speech Lang Pathol. 2012;21(4):354–67.
14. Spielman J, Ramig LO, Mahler L, Halpern A, Gavin WJ. Effects of an extended version of the lee silverman voice treatment on voice and speech in Parkinson's disease. Am J Speech Lang Pathol. 2007;16(2):95–107.
15. Dromey C, Ramig LO, Johnson AB. Phonatory and articulatory changes associated with increased vocal intensity in Parkinson disease: a case study. J Speech Hear Res. 1995;38(4):751–64.
16. Sapir S, Spielman JL, Ramig LO, Story BH, Fox C. Effects of intensive voice treatment (the Lee Silverman Voice Treatment [LSVT]) on vowel articulation in dysarthric individuals with idiopathic Parkinson disease: acoustic and perceptual findings. J Speech Lang Hear Res. 2007;50(4):899–912.
17. El Sharkawi A, Ramig L, Logemann JA, Pauloski BR, Rademaker AW, Smith CH, et al. Swallowing and voice effects of Lee Silverman Voice Treatment (LSVT): a pilot study. J Neurol Neurosurg Psychiatry. 1996; 72(1):31–6.
18. Ziegler A, Verdolini Abbott K, Johns M, Klein A, Hapner ER. Preliminary data on two voice therapy interventions in the treatment of presbyphonia. Laryngoscope. 2014;124(8):1869–76.
19. Wiley K, Elandary S. SPEAK OUT!® a practical approach to treating Parkinson's. San Antonio: Texas Speech and Hearing Association Annual Convention; 2014.
20. Levitt JA. Case study: The effects of the "SPEAK OUT! ®" voice program for Parkinson's disease. Int J Appl Sci Technol. 2014;4(2):20–8.
21. Wight S, Miller N. Lee Silverman voice treatment for people with Parkinson's: audit of outcomes in a routine clinic. Int J Lang Commun Disord. 2015;50(2):215–25.
22. Ramig LO, Sapir S, Countryman S, Pawlas AA, O'Brien C, Hoehn M, et al. Intensive voice treatment (LSVT) for patients with Parkinson's disease: a 2 year follow up. J Neurol Neurosurg Psychiatry. 2001;71(4):493–8.

28

Survival in sinonasal and middle ear malignancies: a population-based study using the SEER 1973–2015 database

Mitchell R. Gore (ID)

Abstract

Background: The sinuses, nasal cavity, and middle ear represent a rarer location of head and neck malignancy than more common sites such as the larynx and oral cavity. Population-based studies are a useful tool to study the demographic and treatment factors affecting survival in these malignancies.

Methods: Population-based database search of the Survival, Epidemiology, and End Results (SEER) database from 1973 to 2015 for malignancies involving the nasal cavity, paranasal sinuses, and middle ear. Data were analyzed for demographics, treatment type, stage, primary site and histopathologic type. Kaplan-Meier analysis was used to assess and compare survival.

Results: A total of 13,992 cases of sinonasal or middle ear malignancy were identified and analyzed. The majority of patients were between ages 50 and 80 at the time of diagnosis. Overall 5-, 10-, and 20-year survival was 45.7%, 32.2%, and 16.4%, respectively. Lymph node metastasis was reported in 4.4% of patients, while distant metastasis was present in 1.5% of cases. On univariate analysis surgical vs. nonsurgical treatment, sex, race, age at diagnosis, T stage, N stage, M stage, AJCC overall stage, primary site, tumor grade, and histopathologic subtype significantly affected survival. On multivariate analysis age, race, sex, primary site, overall AJCC stage, surgical vs. nonsurgical treatment, and T, N, and M stage remained significant predictors of overall survival.

Conclusions: Malignancies of the nasal cavity, paranasal sinuses, and middle ear account for a minority of overall head and neck cancers. The overall 5-, 10-, and 20-year survival for these malignancies is relatively low. Higher T, N, M, and overall stage and higher tumor grade is associated with lower survival. Patients treated with surgery as part of the treatment regimen had higher overall survival. Demographics and primary site also significantly affect survival. Certain histopathologic subtypes were associated with poorer survival.

Keywords: Head and neck Cancer, SEER, Survival, Kaplan-Meier, Sinonasal Cancer, Middle ear Cancer

Background

Malignancies of the head and neck comprise a diverse group of histopathological subtypes and tumor subsites. The majority of head and neck cancers are found in the oral cavity, oropharynx, and larynx. Malignancies of the nasal cavity, paranasal sinuses, and middle ear are far less common, with an incidence of less than 1 per 100,000 people and less than 20% of total head and neck malignancies [1, 2]. Symptoms in patients with sinonasal

or middle ear cancer may be relatively innocuous, gradual in onset, and may mimic other more benign conditions, and these cancers may be discovered at a later stage relative to oral or laryngeal cancers. These factors and the relative proximity to important anterior and lateral skull base structures and neural and vascular structures may make surgical treatment more difficult, and these tumors tend to have a relatively poor survival rate.

Given the relative rarity of nasal cavity, sinus, and middle ear malignancies, this study aimed to update the population-based literature and to report the demographics, effects of treatment modality, and survival outcomes of patients treated for nasal cavity, paranasal

Correspondence: mgoremdphd@gmail.com
Department of Otolaryngology, State University of New York Upstate Medical University, Physicians Office Building North, Suite 4P, 4900 Broad Road, Syracuse, NY 13215, USA

sinus, and middle ear malignancy from the updated 1973–2015 Survival, Epidemiology, and End Results (SEER) database. The study examined the correlation between survival outcomes and the AJCC (American Joint Committee on Cancer) stage, tumor grade, tumor type, treatment type, tumor (T), nodal (N), and distant metastasis (M) stage, patient age at diagnosis, patient sex, and patient race.

Methods

The most recent SEER database contains patient data from 1973 to 2015. Maintained by the National Cancer Institute, SEER collects data on cancer cases from various locations and sources throughout the United States, including various hospitals across many different states. The database, available at https://seer.cancer.gov/, was queried for malignant neoplasm, nose, nasal cavity, and middle

ear, any subsite, any age, and was extracted using SEER*-Stat version 8.3.5 (National Cancer Institute, Bethesda, Maryland) and exported into Microsoft Excel 2016 (Microsoft Corporation, Redmond, Washington) for analysis. XLstat Biomed (Addinsoft, New York City, NY/Paris, France) was used for Kaplan-Meier overall survival analysis and log-rank analysis. Statistical significance was set at 0.05. SEER data was analyzed for overall survival, patient age, sex, and race, and overall AJCC (American Joint Committee on Cancer), tumor (T), nodal (N), and distant metastasis (M) stage, surgical treatment, histopathological type, and primary tumor site.

Results

A total of 13,992 patients with malignancies of the nasal cavity, paranasal sinuses, and middle ear were identified from the 1973–2015 SEER database. Patient demographics

Table 1 Patient demographics

Demographics	n	%
Total	13,992	100%
Female	5751	41.1%
Male	8242	58.9%
Black	1311	9.4%
Other (American Indian/AK Native, Asian/Pacific Islander)	1188	8.5%
Unknown	99	0.7%
White	11,395	81.4%
Age at diagnosis		
00 years	7	0.05%
01–04 years	51	0.4%
05–09 years	57	0.4%
10–14 years	64	0.5%
15–19 years	112	0.8%
20–24 years	128	0.9%
25–29 years	178	1.3%
30–34 years	280	2.0%
35–39 years	421	3.0%
40–44 years	626	4.5%
45–49 years	891	6.4%
50–54 years	1228	8.8%
55–59 years	1459	10.4%
60–64 years	1650	11.8%
65–69 years	1633	11.7%
70–74 years	1537	11.0%
75–79 years	1444	10.3%
80–84 years	1162	8.3%
85+ years	1065	7.6%

Table 2 Tumor histopathological types

Histopathological subtype	n	%
unspecified neoplasms	247	1.8%
epithelial neoplasms, NOS	1202	8.6%
squamous cell neoplasms	7116	50.9%
basal cell neoplasms	76	0.5%
transitional cell papillomas and carcinomas	128	0.9%
adenomas and adenocarcinomas	1768	12.6%
adnexal and skin appendage neoplasms	15	0.1%
mucoepidermoid neoplasms	190	1.4%
cystic, mucinous and serous neoplasms	94	0.7%
ductal and lobular neoplasms	27	0.2%
acinar cell neoplasms	24	0.2%
complex epithelial neoplasms	93	0.7%
paragangliomas and glomus tumors	3	0.02%
nevi and melanomas	1062	0.8%
soft tissue tumors and sarcomas, NOS	125	0.9%
fibromatous neoplasms	91	0.7%
myomatous neoplasms	388	2.8%
complex mixed and stromal neoplasms	78	0.6%
synovial-like neoplasms	9	0.06%
germ cell neoplasms	29	0.2%
trophoblastic neoplasms	1	0.007%
blood vessel tumors	52	0.4%
osseous and chondromatous neoplasms	97	0.7%
miscellaneous tumors	48	0.3%
gliomas	13	0.1
neuroepitheliomatous neoplasms	972	7.0%
meningiomas	2	0.01%
nerve sheath tumors	42	0.3%
granular cell tumors & alveolar soft part sarcoma	1	0.007%

Table 3 Tumor primary sites

Primary site	n	%
Nasal cavity	6455	46.1%
Middle ear	439	3.1%
Maxillary sinus	4449	31.8%
Ethmoid sinus	1205	8.6%
Frontal sinus	152	1.1%
Sphenoid sinus	442	3.2%
Overlapping lesion of accessory sinuses	281	2.0%
Accessory sinus, NOS	570	4.1%

are summarized in Table 1. The majority of patients were > 50 years old, with age 60–64 years representing the largest group (1650/13992; 11.8%). There was a male predominance, with a 8242:5751 M:F ratio (1.4:1). Patients were 81.4% white (11,395/13992), with black patients representing 9.4% (1311/13992), other (American Indian/ Alaska (AK) Native, Asian/Pacific Islander) representing 8.5% (1188/13992), and 0.7% (99/13992) unknown. Table 2 summarizes the histopathological data from the cohort. Squamous cell neoplasms (7116, 50.9%) and adenomas and adenocarcinomas (1768, 12.6%) were the most common tumor types. Table 3 summarizes the primary site

data from the cohort. Nasal cavity (6455, 46.1%), maxillary sinus (4449, 31.8%), and ethmoid sinus (1205, 8.6%) were the most common primary sites.

Figure 1 shows the Kaplan-Meier actuarial overall survival for the entire cohort. Five-year, 10-year, and 20-year overall survival was 45.7%, 32.2%, and 16.4%, respectively. Figure 2 shows the Kaplan-Meier overall survival by primary site. Five-, 10-, and 20-year survival was highest for nasal cavity and middle ear tumors and lowest for maxillary sinus and frontal sinus tumors ($p < 0.001$). Figure 3 illustrates the Kaplan-Meier overall survival by overall AJCC (American Joint Committee on Cancer) stage. Survival was significantly lower for Stage III and IV tumors than Stage I and II tumors ($p < 0.0001$). Figure 4 shows the Kaplan-Meier overall survival by tumor (T) stage. Survival decreased with increasing T stage ($p < 0.0001$). Figure 5 shows the Kaplan-Meier overall survival by nodal (N) stage. Survival decreased with increasing N stage ($p < 0.0001$). Figure 6 illustrates the Kaplan-Meier overall survival by M stage. Survival was significantly lower for M1 patients than M0 patients ($p < 0.0001$). Figure 7 illustrates the Kaplan-Meier overall survival for patients treated with surgery as part of their treatment regimen vs. patients for whom surgery was not recommended. Overall survival was lower for patients for whom surgery

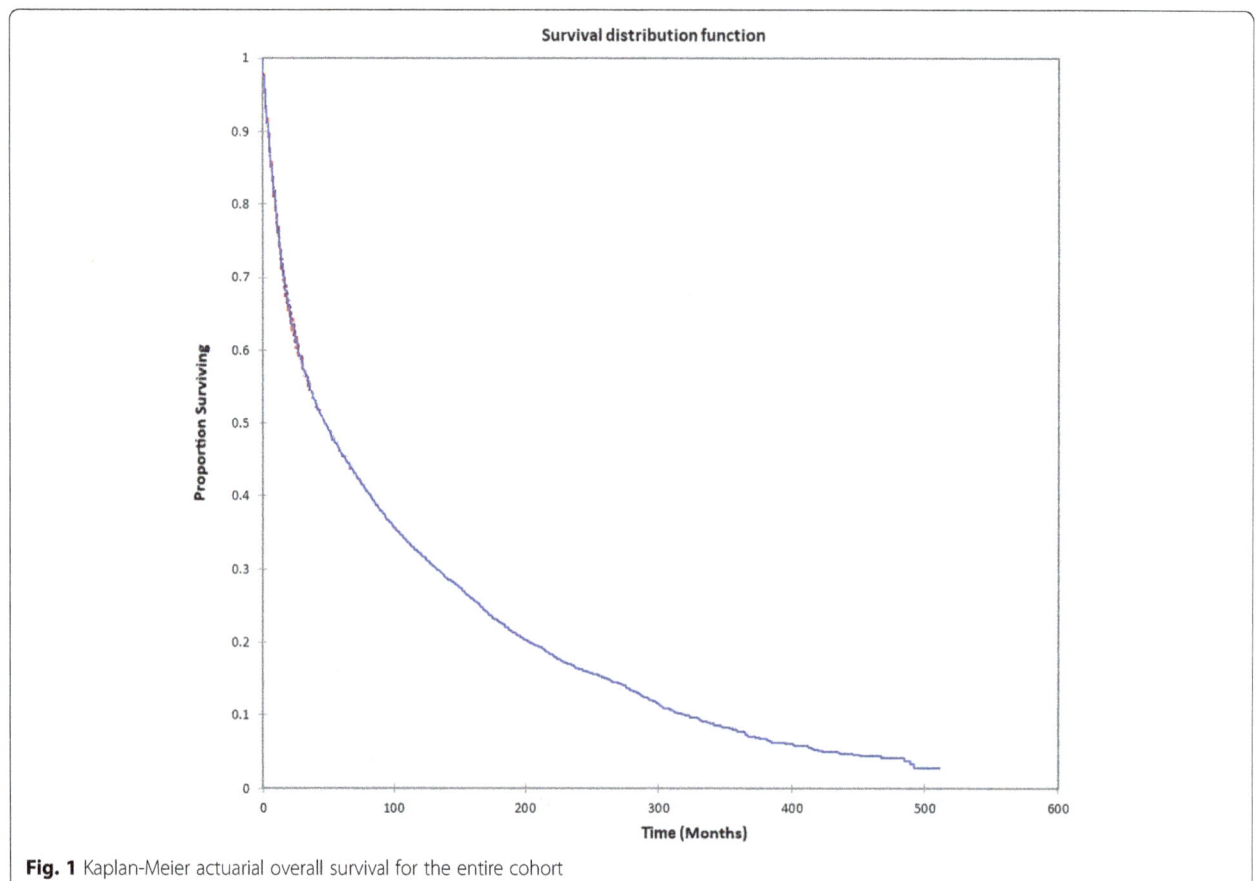

Fig. 1 Kaplan-Meier actuarial overall survival for the entire cohort

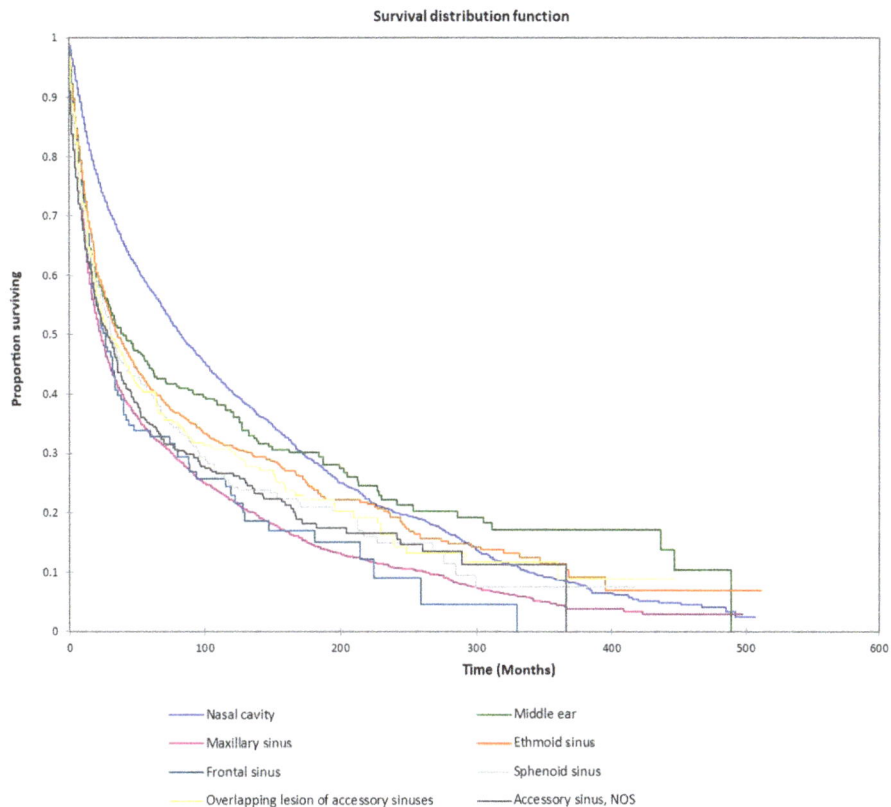

Fig. 2 Kaplan-Meier actuarial overall survival by primary site

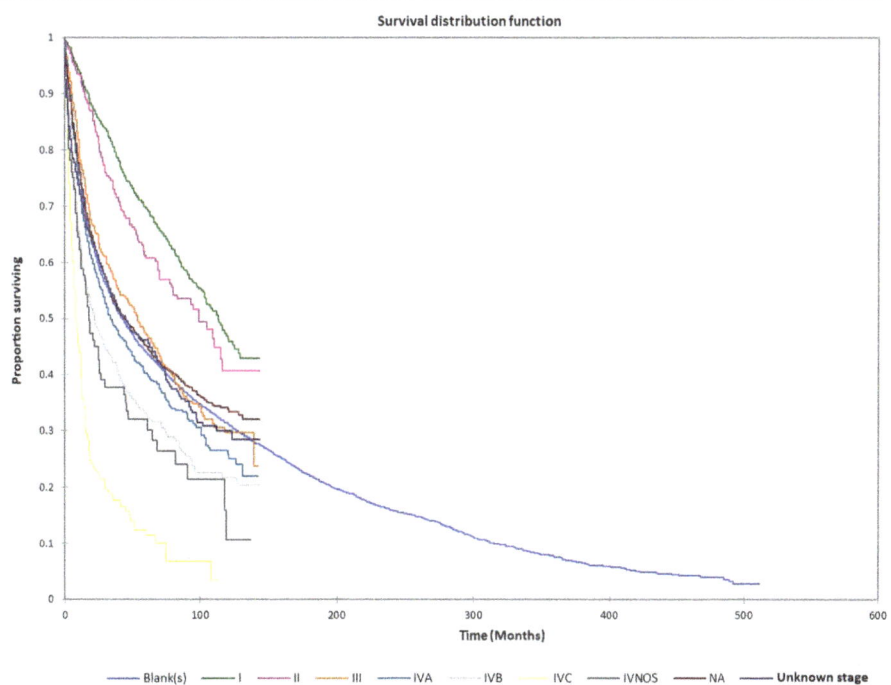

Fig. 3 Kaplan-Meier actuarial overall survival by AJCC stage

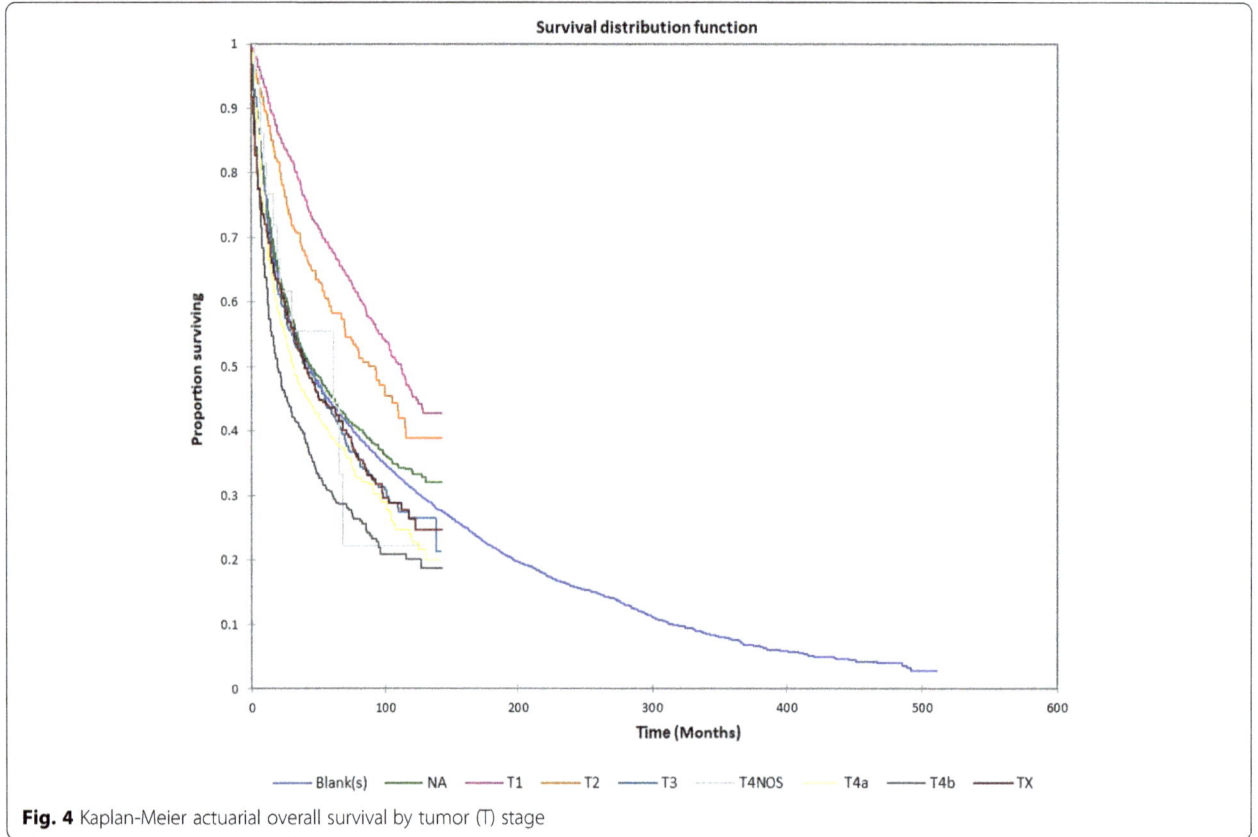

Fig. 4 Kaplan-Meier actuarial overall survival by tumor (T) stage

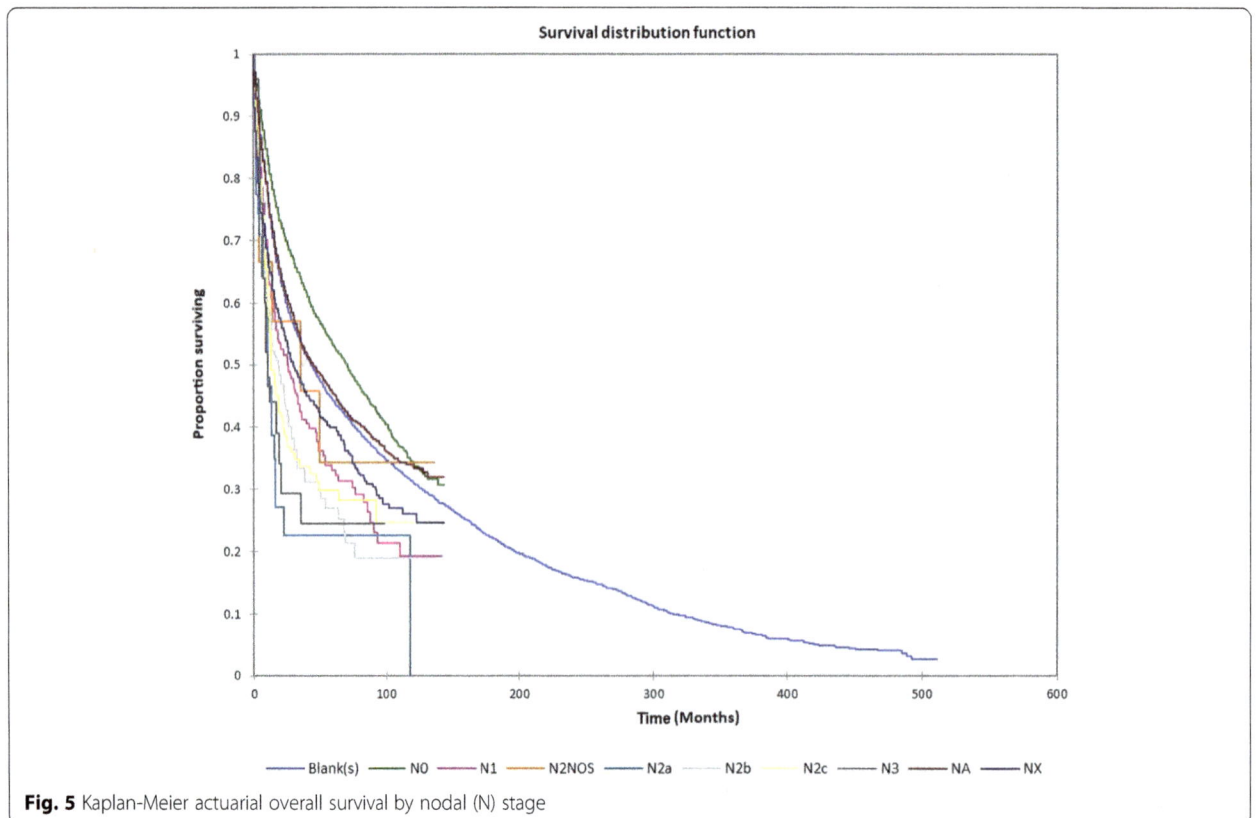

Fig. 5 Kaplan-Meier actuarial overall survival by nodal (N) stage

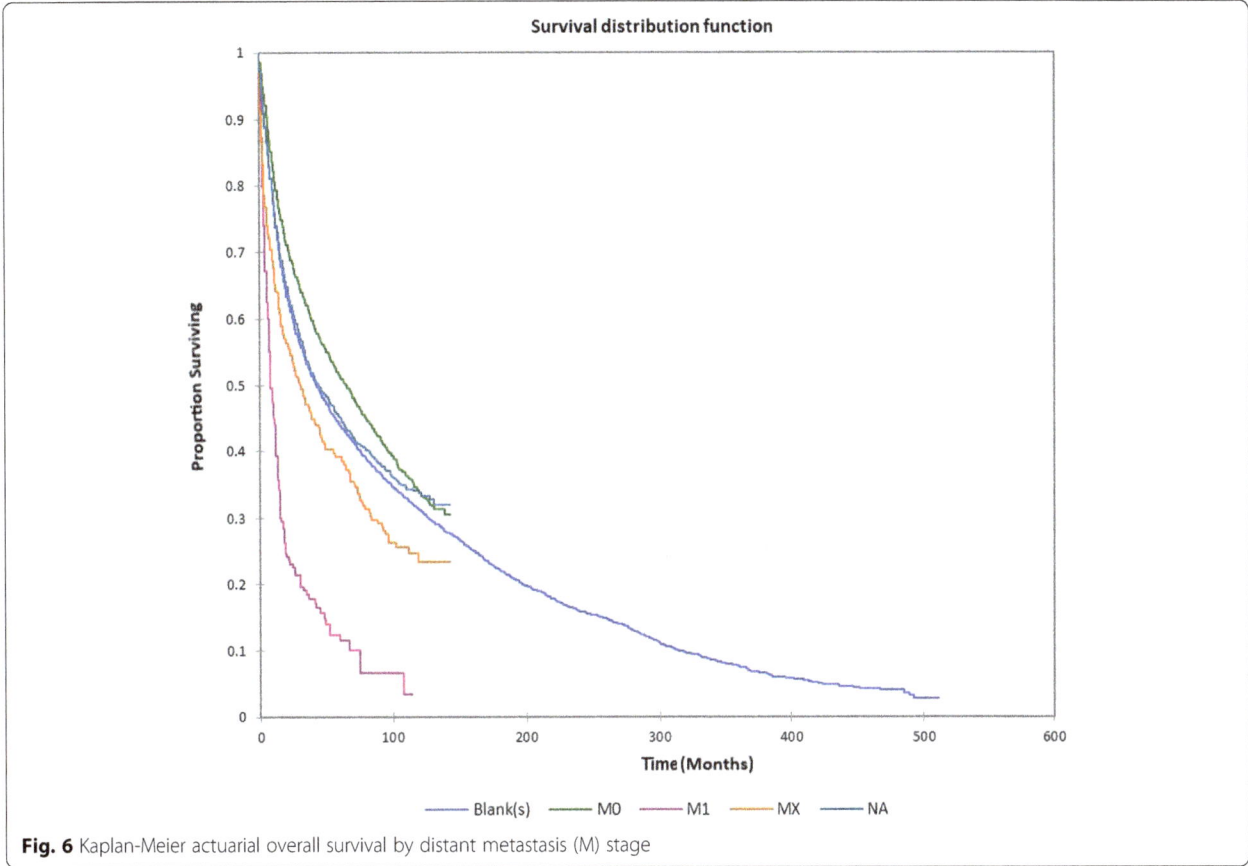

Fig. 6 Kaplan-Meier actuarial overall survival by distant metastasis (M) stage

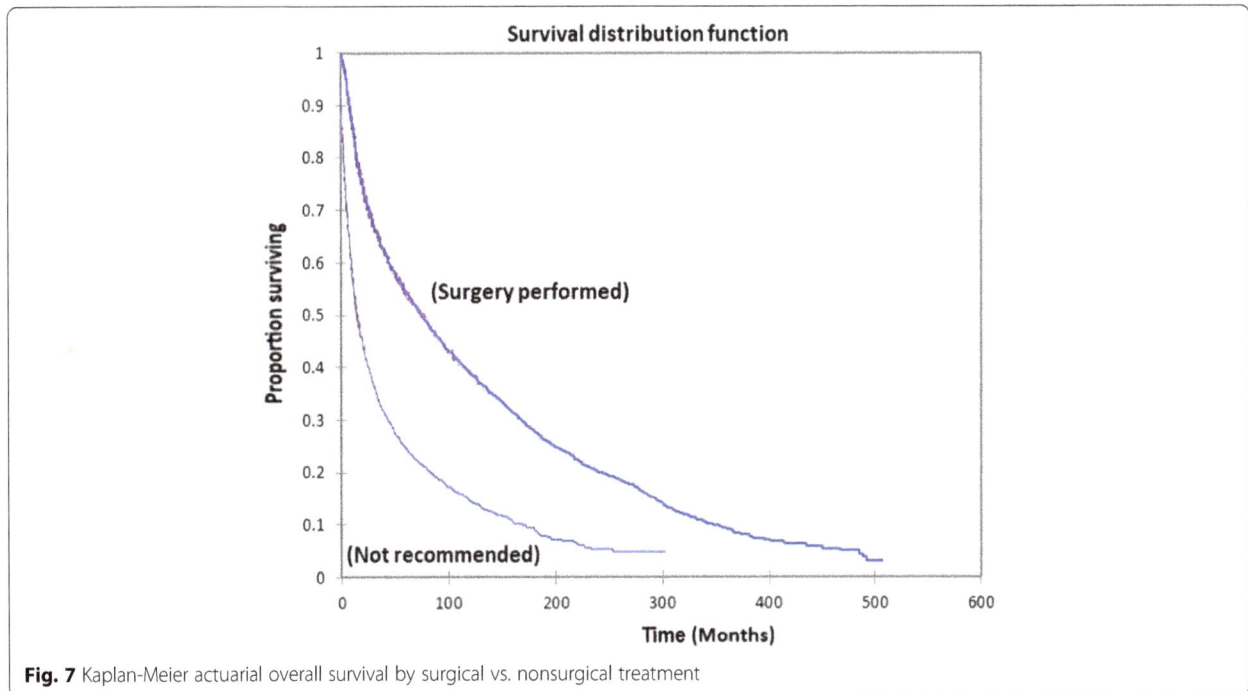

Fig. 7 Kaplan-Meier actuarial overall survival by surgical vs. nonsurgical treatment

was not recommended vs. patients on whom surgery was performed ($p < 0.0001$). Figure 8 illustrates the Kaplan-Meier overall survival for patients by age at diagnosis. Survival decreased with increasing age at diagnosis ($p < 0.0001$). Figure 9 illustrates the Kaplan-Meier overall survival by sex. Survival was significantly lower for males than for females ($p = 0.01$). Figure 10 illustrates the Kaplan-Meier overall survival by patient race. Survival was significantly lower for black patients than white or other (Native American/Alaska Native/Asian/Pacific Islander) patient ($p < 0.0001$). Figure 11 illustrates the Kaplan-Meier overall survival by tumor grade. Survival decreased with increasing tumor grade ($p < 0.0001$). Figure 12 illustrates the Kaplan-Meier overall survival by tumor histopathological subtype. Survival was highest for nerve sheath tumors, gliomas, osseous and chondromatous neoplasms, germ cell neoplasms, synovial-like neoplasms, acinar cell neoplasms, adnexal and skin appendage neoplasms, and ductal and lobular neoplasms and lowest for nevi and melanomas ($p < 0.0001$). Multivariate analysis using linear regression demonstrated that age at diagnosis, race, sex, primary site, AJCC stage, surgical treatment vs. nonsurgical treatment, tumor grade, and T, N, and M stage all significantly affected survival ($p < 0.0001$, Table 4).

Discussion

Sinonasal and middle ear malignancies account for a minority of head and neck cancers. The relative rarity of these tumors makes population-based studies a favorable method for analyzing variables and factors affecting survival in these uncommon malignancies. Dutta et al. [1] noted an incidence of sinonasal malignancy of 0.83 per 100,000 people in their SEER 1973–2011-based study. They noted a male predominance (58.6% of cases), and found that white patients comprised 81.5% of cases, while black patients accounted for 8.7%. The present study using the 1973–2015 SEER database noted a similar proportion of male patients (58.9%) and white patients (81.4%), with a slightly larger proportion of black patients (9.4%). They noted that squamous cell carcinoma was the most common sinonasal malignancy (41.9%), and that the nasal cavity was the most common primary site (45.7%). The present study found that squamous cell cancers comprised 50.9% of the cohort, and nasal cavity tumors accounted for 46.1% of patients. The Dutta study found an overall 5-year disease specific survival for all sinonasal malignancies of 53.7%, while in the present study the 5-year overall survival was only 45.7%. It is unclear what accounts for the lower overall survival in the present study

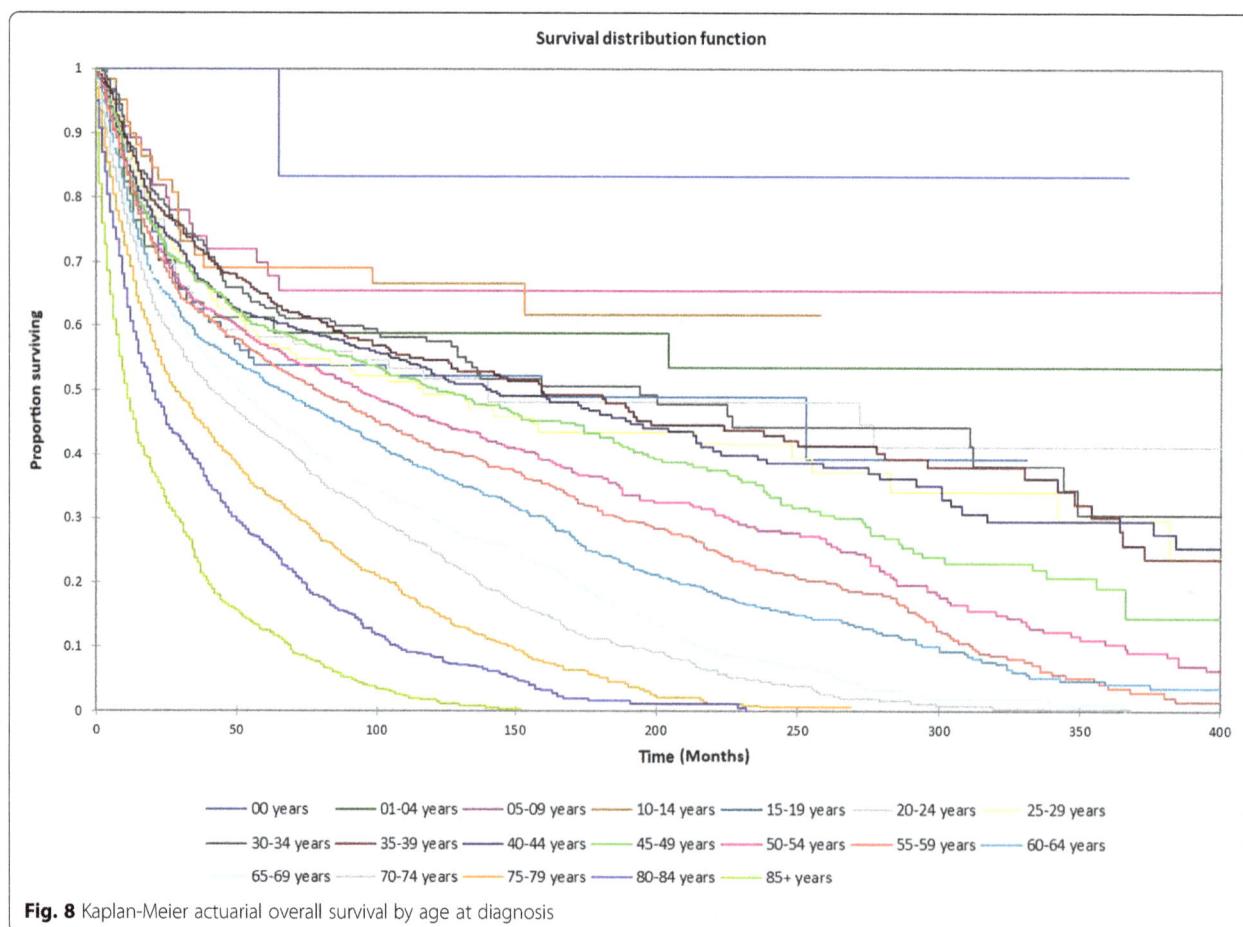

Fig. 8 Kaplan-Meier actuarial overall survival by age at diagnosis

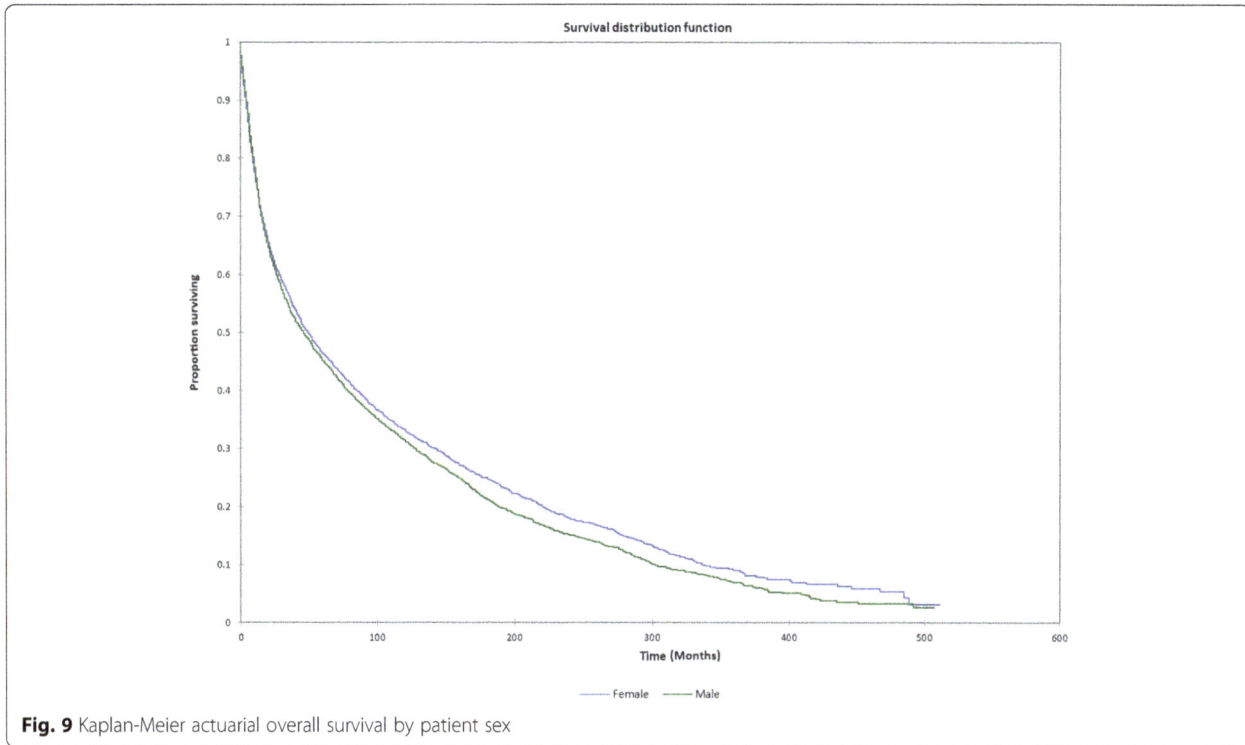

Fig. 9 Kaplan-Meier actuarial overall survival by patient sex

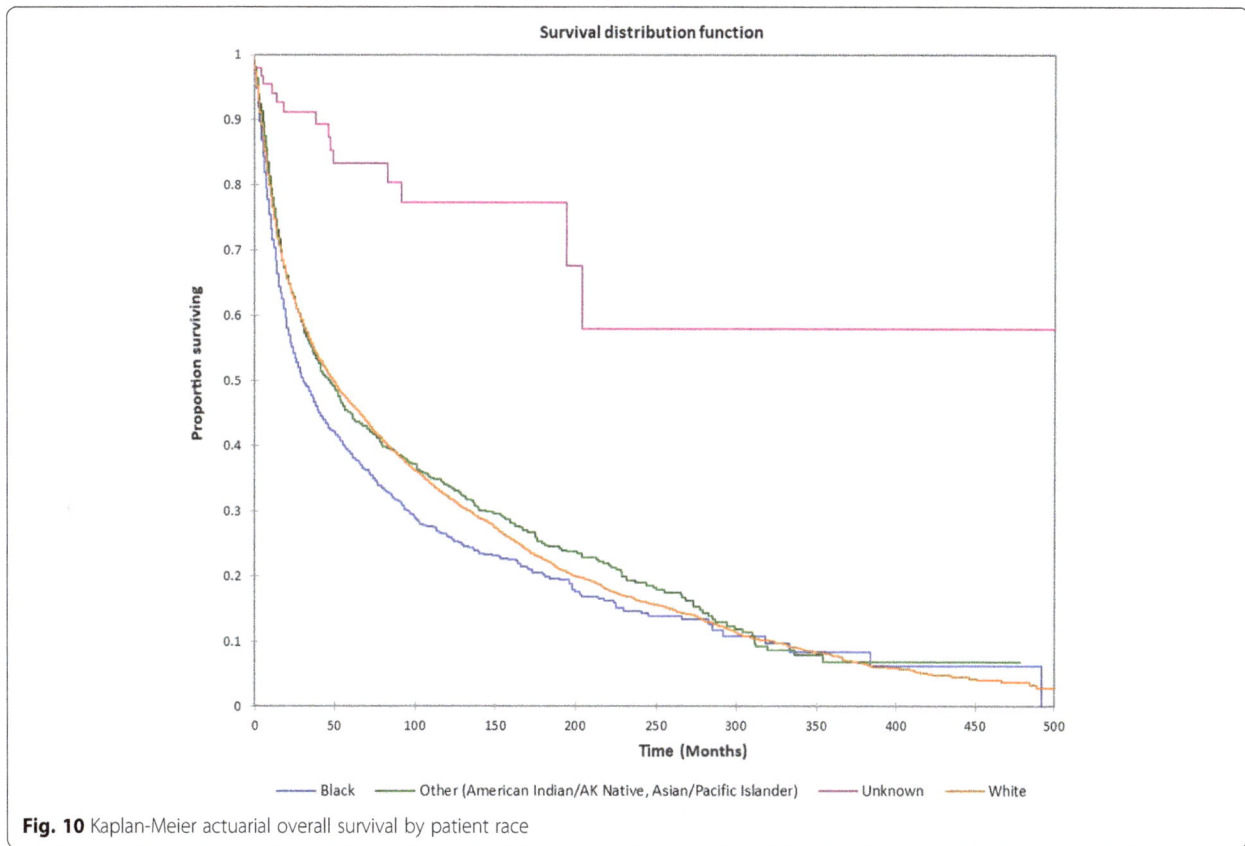

Fig. 10 Kaplan-Meier actuarial overall survival by patient race

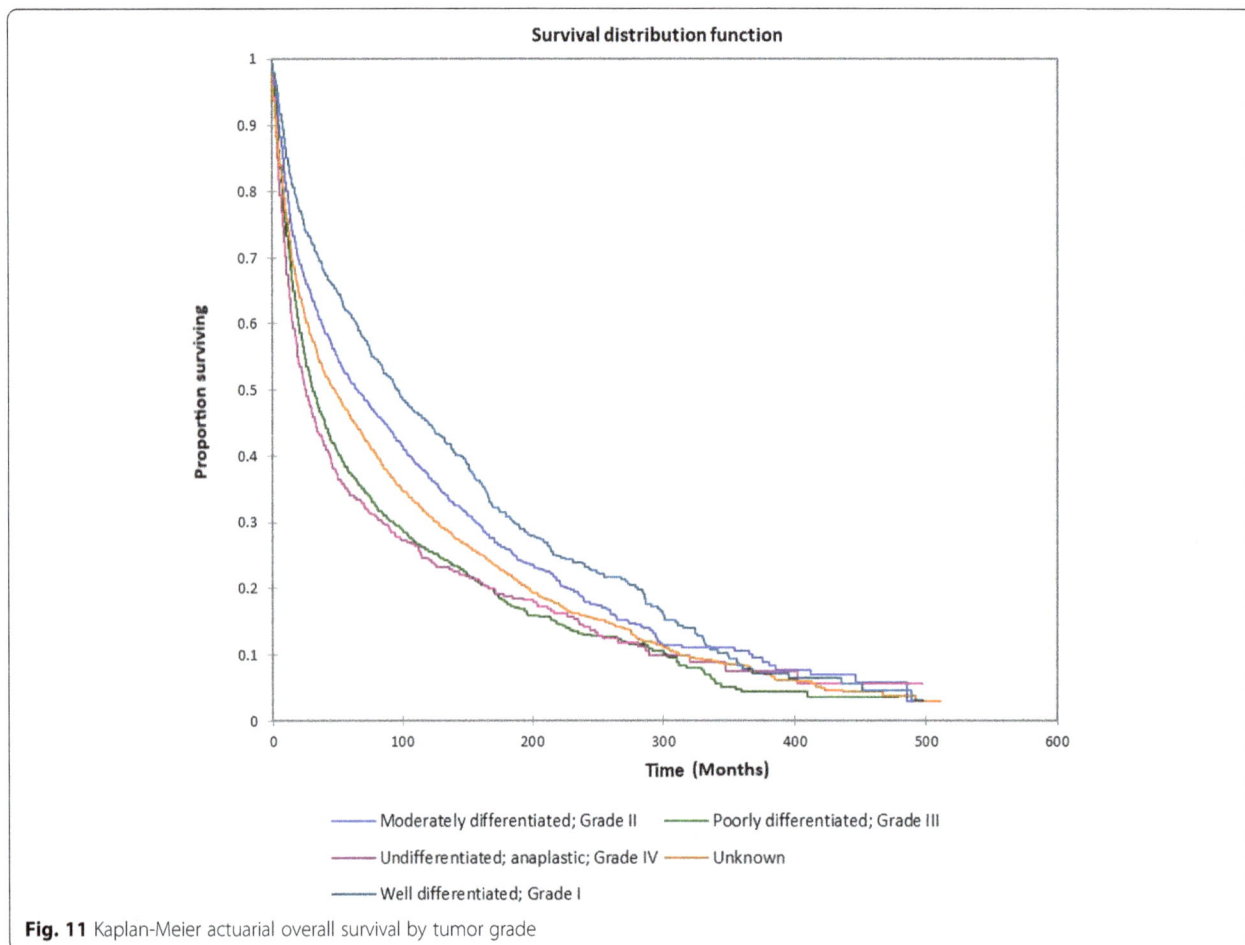

Fig. 11 Kaplan-Meier actuarial overall survival by tumor grade

relative to the Dutta study. The difference may be partially accounted for by the lower overall survival for middle ear malignancies. In their study of the 1973–2004 SEER database for middle ear malignancies Gurgel et al. [2] noted a 5-year observed survival rate of only 36.4%. In the present study the 5-year overall survival for the middle ear group was 44.4%, somewhat higher than that found in the Gurgel study but similar to the overall 5-year survival for the entire cohort in the present study (45.7%). Additionally, in the present study survival for middle ear tumors was significantly lower than that of nasal cavity tumors, but similar to or higher than paranasal sinus subsites. The higher proportion of squamous cell carcinomas in the present study relative to the Dutta study may also partially account for this difference, as the 50.9% of squamous cell neoplasms in the present study had a 5-year overall survival (45%) that was similar to that of the cohort as a whole (45.7%). Of the patients with known N and M staging in the present study, the rates of nodal metastasis (4.4%) and distant metastasis (1.5%) were relatively low. Survival rates were particularly low for patients with melanoma in the present study (5-year survival 25.1%, median survival time 51.3 months). This is consistent with

previous studies [3] showing relatively dismal survival for sinonasal melanoma, with average survival on the order of 24 to 27 months.

The present study showed that on univariate analysis age at diagnosis, race, sex, primary site, histopathological subtype, AJCC overall stage, T, N, and M stage, surgical treatment vs. nonsurgical treatment, and tumor grade significantly affected survival, with all variables except histopathological subtype remaining significant on multivariate analysis. It is interesting that black patients showed significantly lower 5-, 10-, and 20-year overall survival (38.1%, 26.6%, and 14.8%, respectively) than white patients (46.4%, 32.0%, and 16.0%, respectively) and patients identified as other (46.1%, 32.5%, and 19.0%, respectively). In their 2007 study using the 1988–2002 SEER database [4] Nichols and Bhattacharyya found a similar result, noting that black patients with oral tongue and glottic squamous cell carcinoma presented with higher T and N stage, and had shorter mean overall survival. Even after controlling for stage and treatment they noted that black patients demonstrated worse survival, implying that other factors influenced survival such as extrinsic socioeconomic factors or intrinsic genetic factors, etc. In the present study

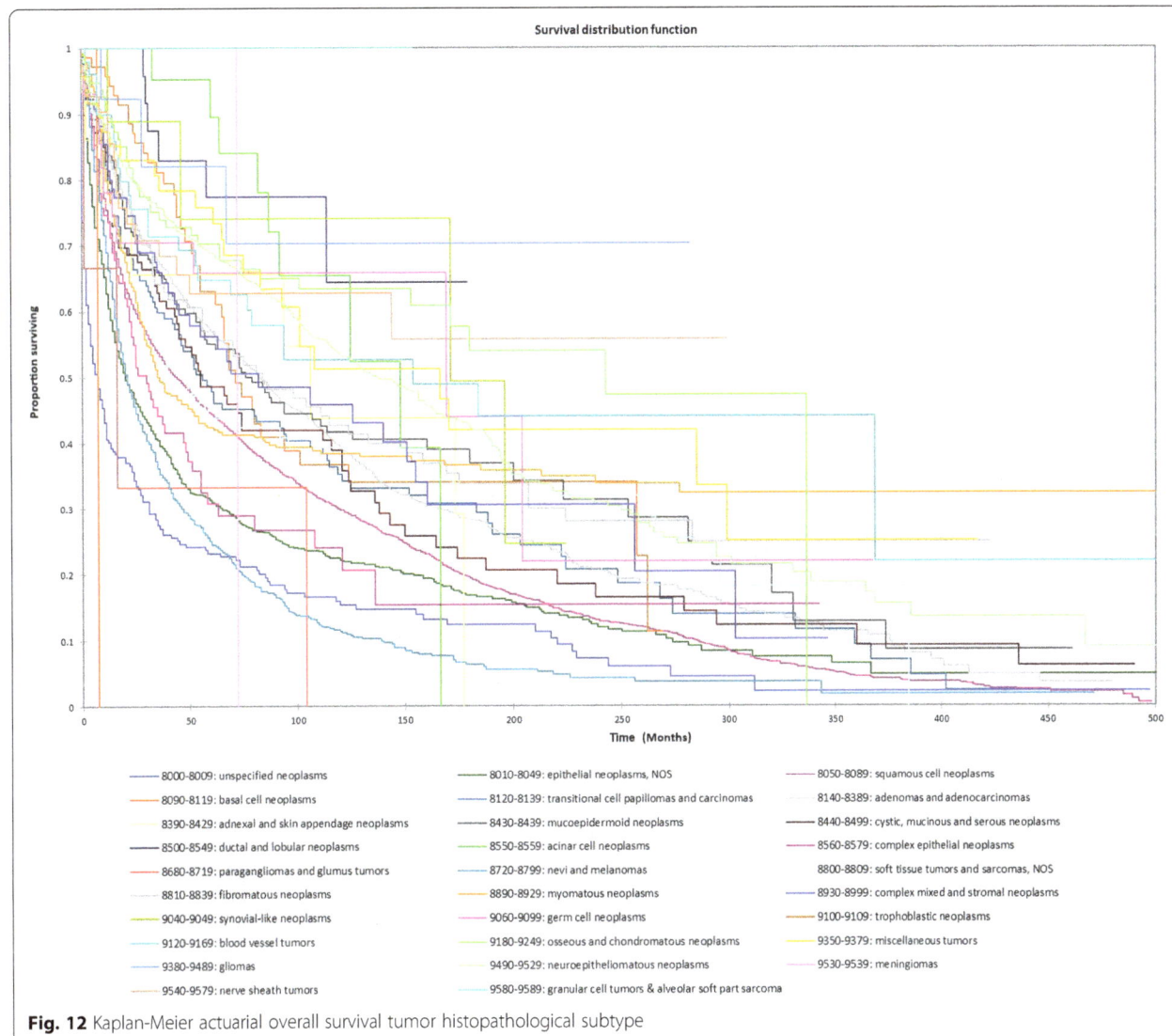

Fig. 12 Kaplan-Meier actuarial overall survival tumor histopathological subtype

Table 4 Multivariate analysis results

Multivariate analysis variable	p-value
Age at diagnosis	$p < 0.0001$
Race	$p < 0.0001$
Sex	$p < 0.0001$
Primary site	$p < 0.0001$
Histological subtype	$p = 0.2$
AJCC overall stage	$p < 0.0001$
Surgical vs. nonsurgical treatment	$p < 0.0001$
T stage	$p < 0.0001$
N stage	$p < 0.0001$
M stage	$p < 0.0001$
Tumor grade	$p < 0.0001$

race remained significant even on multivariate analysis, implying a similar effect as that seen in the Nichols study. Patel et al. [5] found a similarly lower 5-year survival for Hispanic whites and blacks (52%) vs. non-Hispanic whites (64%) in patients with sinonasal cancer in the 2000–2008 SEER database. They noted after multivariate analysis factors significantly affecting survival in addition to race were age, stage, histology, grade, comorbidity status, and standard of care, with lower stage and receiving standard of care multimodality treatment appropriate to stage being the most important prognostic factors.

The present study has limitations, including the retrospective nature of the data in the SEER database, the wide range of centers and states from which the data is compiled, and the presence of missing/unknown data for some variables such as T, N, and M stage. This makes recall and selection bias a possibility. Additionally, the inclusion of middle ear cancers (which are grouped with paranasal sinus and nasal cavity cancers in the SEER database) has the potential to add heterogeneity to the data. The fact that middle ear cancers account for only 3.1% of the cohort, and that the actuarial overall survival for the middle ear cohort is similar to the overall cohort is similar makes this less of a concern. The large number of patients in this 1973–2015 SEER cohort increases the reliability of the data, and the highly significant nature of the p-values noted on univariate and multivariate analysis, and the multiple studies demonstrating the utility of SEER-derived studies, makes the conclusions noted in the present study more reliable.

Conclusions

Malignancies of the nasal cavity, paranasal sinuses, and middle ear are relatively uncommon relative to more prevalent sites such as oral cavity and larynx. The present study demonstrated that patient race, sex, and age at diagnosis all significantly affected survival, with black patients, males, and patients older than 50 demonstrating worse survival. Additionally, tumor histopathological type, primary site, grade, surgical vs. nonsurgical treatment, and AJCC, T, N, and M stage all significantly affected survival. Overall 5-, 10-, and 20-year survival is relatively low, and surgical resection when possible combined with adjuvant therapy when indicated appears to provide the best chance for survival in patients with these rare malignancies.

Abbreviations
AJCC: American Joint Committee on Cancer; AK: Alaska; DFS: Disease-free survival; DSS: Disease-specific survival; G: Grade; M: Metastasis; N: Nodal; NA: Not available; OS: Overall survival; SEER: Surveillance, Epidemiology, and End Results; T: Tumor

Authors' contributions
MRG designed the study, performed the SEER database search, performedliterature, and wrote and edited the manuscript. The author read and approved the final manuscript.

Competing interests
The author declares that he has no competing interests.

References
1. Dutta R, Dubal PM, Svider PF, Liu JK. Baredes S1, Eloy JA. Sinonasal malignancies: a population-based analysis of site-specific incidence and survival. Laryngoscope. 2015 Nov;125(11):2491–7.
2. Gurgel RK, Karnell LH, Hansen MR. Middle ear cancer: a population-based study. Laryngoscope. 2009 Oct;119(10):1913–7.
3. Gore MR, Zanation AM. Survival in Sinonasal Melanoma: A Meta-analysis. J Neurol Surg B Skull Base. 2012 Jun;73(3):157–62. https://doi.org/10.1055/s-0032-1301400.
4. Nichols AC, Bhattacharyya N. Racial differences in stage and survival in head and neck squamous cell carcinoma. Laryngoscope. 2007 May;117(5):770–5.
5. Patel ZM, Li J, Chen AY, Ward KC. Determinants of racial differences in survival for sinonasal cancer. Laryngoscope. 2016 Sep;126(9):2022–8.

29

An abrupt bleeding of the anteriorly-displaced sigmoid sinus: a rare complication of myringoplasty

Sarah Zaher Addeen[1*] [iD] and Mohammad Al- Mohammad[2]

Abstract

Background: The location of the sigmoid sinus within the mastoid cavity is quite variable. An anteriorly- displaced vertical segment of the sigmoid sinus constitutes an uncommon but dangerous anatomical variation that surgeons rarely encounter during surgery. In this variation, the sigmoid sinus lays underneath a very thin bony flap, which makes it easily damaged. Thus, an abrupt fatal bleeding might occur. Despite the many hypotheses about its origin (Chronic otitis media, hypopneumatization, etc.), the pathogenesis of this variation is still not completely understood.

Case presentation: We present a case where the vertical segment of the left sigmoid sinus was encountered just underneath a one- millimeter bony flap in the posterior wall of the external auditory canal during an attempted myringoplasty.

Conclusion: Anatomical variations of the sigmoid sinus are not uncommon, and the otolaryngologist should be aware of such variations to prevent unpleasant, intra- operative surprises.

Keywords: Sigmoid sinus, Myringoplasty, Abnormally displaced, Anterior course, Anatomical variation

Background

The location of the sigmoid sinus within the mastoid cavity is quite variable, and thus impacts surgical planning and execution profoundly [1]. An anteriorly- displaced vertical segment of the sigmoid sinus is an important anatomical variation that triggered a debate about its causality [1–4]. Some studies showed that the distance between the sigmoid sinus and the posterior wall of the external auditory canal is significantly smaller in patients with sclerotic mastoids due to chronic otitis media (COM) in childhood, or genetic factors that provoke mastoid hypopneumatization [2], while other studies refuted this claim [3], and hypothesized that volume reduction may result from the sclerotic change in the air cell system, rather than from shrinkage of the mastoid bone [5], and even suggested that the sinus location is responsible for decreasing the mastoid pneumatization [6]. This variation has been scarcely reported during surgery nevertheless, it might easily provoke a massive bleeding if the surgeon didn't take caution to the abnormal sinus that

lies underneath a millimeter- thin bony flap. [7–9]. The anteriorly- displaced sinus is a well-defined anomaly in high-resolution computed tomography imaging (HRCT) [10]. We report a case where the sigmoid sinus was encountered just underneath a one- millimeter bony flap in the posterior wall of the external auditory canal during an attempted myringoplasty.

Case presentation

A 40- year- old female patient presented to Al Mouwassat Universityhospital outpatients' clinics with hearing loss, and tinnitus in her left ear.

She had a history of acoustic trauma 3 years earlier. On physical examination, the external ear canal was normal. A sclerotic –edged perforation was found to involve the whole antero- inferior quadrant of the tympanic membrane. Her thorough otorhinolaryngolgical examination was otherwise normal. The pure tone audiogram (PTA) demonstrated a conductive hearing loss with 32 dB gap in the left ear; hearing on the right side was within normal. Left myringoplasty was scheduled. Entry was via the post- auricular approach. Then the temporalis fascia superficialis was harvested. After that, the triangular musculoperiosteal flap was anteriorly

* Correspondence: sarah.zaheraddeen@gmail.com
[1]Faculty of Medicine, Damascus University, Damascus, Syria
Full list of author information is available at the end of the article

elevated to the level of the meatus. A sudden venous profuse bleeding from the posterior wall of the external bony canal was encountered as soon as the tympanosquamous suture was reached. It seemed like there is a millimeter- thin bony shell covering this wall that fractured with a slight touch from the knife. The bleeding was controlled by gauze followed by gelfoam packing successfully, and the operation was completed thereafter. The middle ear was inspected, the ossicles were intact and mobile. No abnormal vascular structure was seen. The packing was removed at the end of the operation. The patient received antibiotic treatment with Ceftriaxone 500 mg twice daily for 10 days. A postoperative high-resolution computed tomography (HRCT) of the temporal bone showed that the vertical segment of the left sigmoid sinus was abnormally anteriorly- displaced; dehiscent to the posterior wall of the external auditory canal (Fig. 1). The posterior wall of the lateral part of the bony external auditory meatus was defective and thinned by the sigmoid sinus that lays just underneath a 1- mm flap of bone. A PTA was obtained 2 months after the surgery, and revealed that the conductive hearing loss gap improved to 22 dB (Fig. 2).

Discussion

The Sigmoid sinus originates at the junction of the transverse and the superior petrosal sinuses at the superior border of the petrous bone, from this point on goes medially in the vertical plane toward the medial portion of the mastoid cavity, sculpturing a deep, S- shaped canal and terminates anteriorly at the jugular bulb that descends from the jugular foramen as a jugular vein [11].

An anterior course of the sigmoid sinus is a rare anatomical variation that has been reported in the medical literature. Gangopadhyay et al. reported a similar case to ours, as they came upon the sigmoid sinus underneath the skin of the posterior wall of the external auditory canal during an attempted myringoplasty [7], while Ulug and colleagues confronted massive bleeding from an anteriorly- displaced sigmoid sinus during stapedectomy [9]. Moreover, Puraviappan and colleagues discovered the abnormal anterior course of a ruptured sigmoid sinus in a referral case of middle ear and mastoid exploration via post- auricular approach [8]. There has been a controversy on whether the abnormally- located sigmoid sinus in the mastoid cavity plays a role in otologic pathologies, or the variation itself is a consequence of pathology. Some studies showed that the distance between the sigmoid sinus and the posterior wall of the external auditory canal is significantly smaller in patients with sclerotic mastoids due to chronic otitis media (COM) in childhood, or genetic factors that provoke mastoid hypopneumatization [2], while other studies refuted this claim [3], and hypothesized that volume reduction may result from the sclerotic change

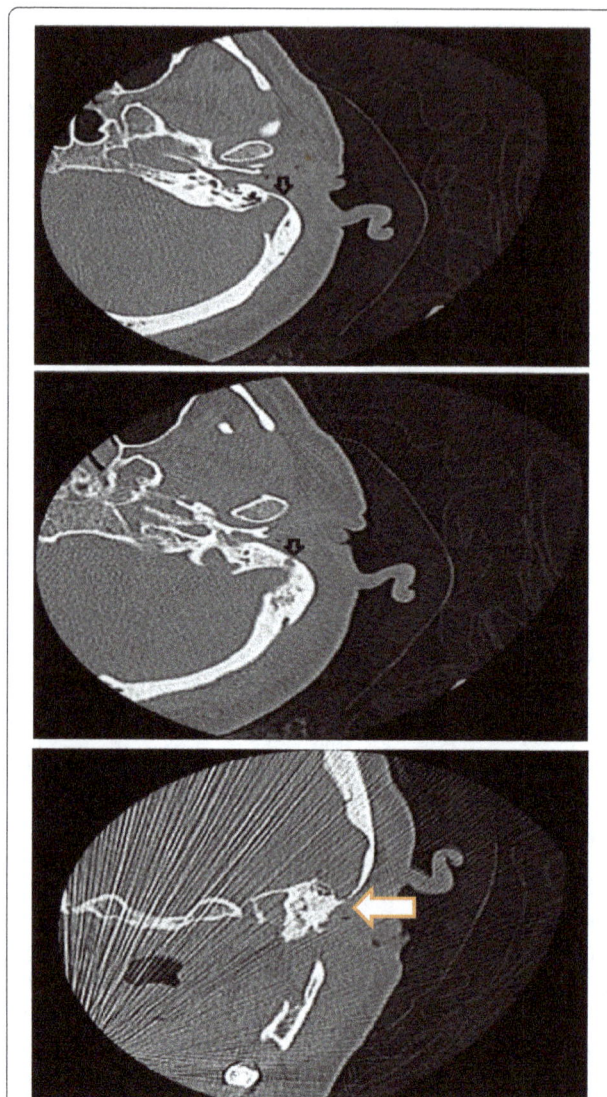

Fig. 1 A postoperative high-resolution computed tomography (HRCT) of the temporal bone shows that the vertical segment of the left sigmoid sinus (arrow) is abnormally forward- displaced

in the air cell system, rather than from shrinkage of the mastoid bone [5], and even suggested that the sinus location is responsible for decreasing the mastoid pneumatization [6]. From an embryologic aspect, The degree of pneumatization of the mastoid varies greatly in normal temporal bones [12]. The age at which the gas cells develop is subject to huge individual variation, as well as the number, size and volume of the mastoidian cells which are considered as individual characteristics. In fact, many factors impact the growth and pneumatization of the mastoid, especially heredity, environment, nutrition, gas exchanges and frequency of infections. In addition, anatomic variability of adjacent structures affect the development of the mastoid pneumatization and vice versa [13].

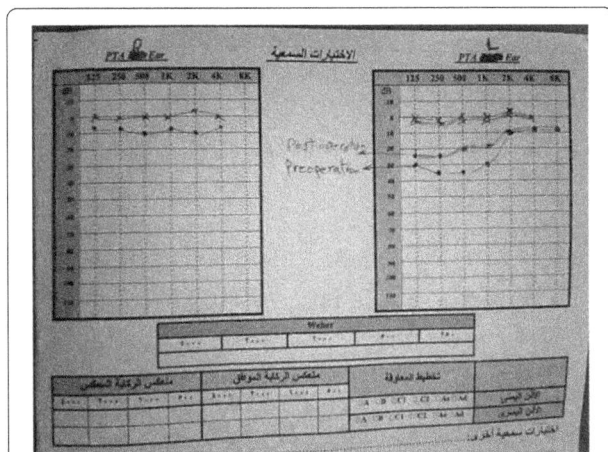

Fig. 2 Pre and postoperative PTA (pure tone audiogram) of the patient that shows the decrease of air - bone gap to 22 db

An antero- medially displaced sinus has been described in patients with Ménière's disease, the researchers justified this finding as a result of tightened Trautmann's triangle in these patients [4]. Nevertheless, it's not infrequent to catch this same variation in disease- free temporal bone as stated by Sarmiento and colleagues [1], Ulug and colleagues [9], and as we suggest in our case.

In our patient, we stopped the sinusoidal bleeding by gauze and gelfoam packing. This method was applied by other authors to control anomalous jugular bulb hemorrhage during middle ear surgery [14]. This method, however, implicates the risk of intracranial venous hypertension, especially when the dominant sinus is occluded (usually the right sinus), the sinus was previously healthy, and no patent connection exists between the two sigmoid sinuses via transverse sinuses [15]. Yet, we didn't face this complication in our patient, regarding that we packed the left -non dominant- sinus and that the two sigmoid sinuses were normally connected. After 2 months of follow- up, the patient is still doing well, and no evidence of intracranial hypertension showed up. In this case, we used the temporalis fascia to close the tympanic membrane perforation. The temporalis fascia is widely used in myringoplasty [16]. Some studies suggest that the hearing results of the temporalis fascia graft are comparable to those of the cartilage palisades, especially in large perforations [16, 17]. In contrary, other studies suggest that the anatomical success rate for a cartilage myringoplasty is higher than for a fascia one, with no significant difference on the functional results [18].

Although high-resolution computed tomography imaging (HRCT) was not performed to our patient preoperatively since it's not routinely performed in our hospital, it is still a crucial investigation in temporal bone disorders management and anatomical variations detection [10]. It's an accurate tool to evaluate mastoid pneumatization and aditus ad antrum blockage (which play a role in failure of myringoplasty) [19].

However, this imaging technique has its limitations in regard to detecting the dehiscence of some anatomic structures such as facial canal, lateral semicircular canal, and tegmen [20]. In addition, we noticed that there is a scarce in studies that investigate HRCT importance in first attempt myringoplasty whereas most of them focused on revision myringoplasty.

A study compared the intraoperative data and computed tomography measures of 30 patients and concluded that the a tomographic distance between the sigmoid sinus and the external ear canal measuring less than 9 mm complicated the procedure, their lowest distance was 4.7 mm [21].

Another study measured the same distance as 13.2 mm [22]. In this report, the distance was about 1 mm, which exposed the sinus to hemorrhage jeopardy.

Conclusion

Anatomical variations of the sigmoid sinus are not uncommon. The otolaryngologist should be aware of such variations to prevent unpleasant, intra- operative surprises. In addition, if HRCT was performed before surgery for any reason, the sigmoid sinus should be carefully inspected.

Abbreviations
COM: Chronic otitis media; dB: Decibles; HRCT: High- resolution computed tomography imaging; PTA: Pure tone audiogram

Acknowledgements
Not applicable.

Funding
None.

Authors' contributions
SZ: Wrote the first draft as a whole, and helped in finalizing the paper. MA: Finalized, revised the paper, and approved the final version.

Competing interests
The authors declare that they have no competing interests.

Author details
[1]Faculty of Medicine, Damascus University, Damascus, Syria.
[2]Otorhinolaryngology Department, Al- Mouwassat University Hospital,
Damascus, Syria.

References
1. Sarmiento PB, Eslait FG. Surgical classification of variations in the anatomy
    of the sigmoid sinus. Otolaryngol Head Neck Surg. 2004;131(3):192–9.
2. Shatz A, Sade J. Correlation between mastoid pneumatization and position
    of the lateral sinus. Ann Otol Rhinol laryngol. 1990;99(2 Pt 1):142–5.
3. Orr JB, Wendell Todd N. Jugular bulb position and shape are unrelated to
    temporal bone pneumatization. Laryngoscope. 1988;98(2):136–8.
4. Paparella M, Sajjadi H: The lateral sinus and Trautmann's triangle in
    Meniere's disease: considerations of pathogenesis. In: Proceedings of the
    Second International Symposium on Menieres's Disease Amsterdam: Kugler
    Publications: 1988; 1988.
5. Lee D-H, Jung M-K, Yoo Y-H, Seo J-H. Analysis of unilateral sclerotic
    temporal bone: how does the sclerosis change the mastoid pneumatization
    morphologically in the temporal bone? Surg Radiol Anat. 2008;30(3):221–7.
6. Çam OH, Karatas M. A life threatening pitfall in ear surgery: extracranial
    sigmoid sinus. J Craniofac Surg. 2015;26(7):e619–20.
7. Gangopadhyay K, McArthur P, Larsson S. Unusual anterior course of the
    sigmoid sinus: report of a case and review of the literature. J Laryngol Otol.
    1996;110(10):984–6.
8. Puraviappan P, Prepageran N, Ong CA, Abd KR, Lingham OR, Raman R. An
    abnormal sigmoid sinus with a dire clinical implication. Ear Nose Throat J.
    2014;93(6):E55.
9. Ulug T, Basaran B, Minareci O, Aydin K. An unusual complication of stapes
    surgery: profuse bleeding from the anteriorly located sigmoid sinus. Eur
    Arch Otorhinolaryngol. 2004;261(7):397–9.
10. Visvanathan V. Anatomical variations of the temporal bone on high-
    resolution computed tomography imaging: how common are they? J
    Laryngol Otol. 2015;129(07):634–7.
11. Cummings CW, et al. Otolaryngology Head & Neck Surgery, Vol-5. Elsevier;
    1998:3700.
12. Ars B, Dirckx J, Ars-Piret N, Buytaert J. Insights in the physiology of the
    human mastoid: message to the surgeon. Int Adv Otol. 2012;8(2):296–310.
13. Ars B, Ars-Piret N. Morpho-functional partition of the middle ear cleft. Acta
    Otorhinolaryngol Belg. 1997;51(3):181–4.
14. Moore PJ. The high jugular bulb in ear surgery: three case reports and a
    review of the literature. J Laryngol Otol. 1994;108(09):772–5.
15. Sekhar LN, Tzortzidis FN, Bejjani GK, Schessel DA. Saphenous vein graft
    bypass of the sigmoid sinus and jugular bulb during the removal of glomus
    jugulare tumors: report of two cases. J Neurosurg. 1997;86(6):1036–41.
16. Kalcioglu M, Tan M, Croo A. Comparison between cartilage and fascia grafts
    in type 1 tympanoplasty. B-ENT. 2013;9(3):235–9.
17. Arun K, Shakya D. Comparison of outcomes of Myringoplasty with cartilage
    palisades and Temporalis fascia in large perforations. Otolaryngol Head
    Neck Surg. 2014;151(1_suppl):199.
18. Yegin Y, Çelik M, Koç AK, Küfeciler L, Elbistanlı MS, Kayhan FT. Comparison
    of temporalis fascia muscle and full-thickness cartilage grafts in type 1
    pediatric tympanoplasties. Braz J Otorhinolaryngol. 2016;82(6):695–701.
19. El-kady AS, Haroun Y, Kassem KM, Galal O. The value of computed
    tomography scanning in assessment of Aditus ad Antrum patency and
    choice of treatment line in revision Myringoplasty. Med J Cairo Univ.
    2009;77(2):53–7.
20. Tatlipinar A, Tuncel A, Öğredik EA, Gökçeer T, Uslu C. The role of computed
    tomography scanning in chronic otitis media. Eur Arch Otorhinolaryngol.
    2012;269(1):33–8.
21. Pereira AR, Pinheiro SD, de Castro JDV, Ximenes Filho JA, de Freitas MR.
    Mastoidectomy: anatomical parameters x surgical difficulty. Arquivos
    Internacionais de Otorrinolaringologia. 2012;16(01):057–61.
22. Fkinci G, Ko A, Baltaciğlu F, Veyseller B, Altintaş O, Han T. Temporal
    bone measurements on high-resolution computed tomography. J
    Otolaryngol. 2004;33(6):33–6.

Permissions

List of Contributors

Hisham S Khalil and Ahmed Z Eweiss
Department of Otolaryngology, Derriford Hospital, Plymouth, U.K. and Faculty of Medicine, University of Alexandria, Egypt

Nicholas Clifton
Department of Otolaryngology, Derriford Hospital, Plymouth, UK

Julia Wittig and Orlando Guntinas-Lichius
Department of Otorhinolaryngology, Jena University Hospital, Lessingstrasse 2, Jena D-07740, Germany

Claus Wittekindt
Department of Otorhinolaryngology, Jena University Hospital, Lessingstrasse 2, Jena D-07740, Germany
Present address: Department of Otorhinolaryngology, University Giessen, Giessen, Germany

Michael Kiehntopf
Institute of Clinical Chemistry and Laboratory Diagnostics, Jena University Hospital, Jena, Germany

Chris Ladefoged Jacobsen, Mikkel Attermann Bruhn and Michael L Gaihede
Department of Otolaryngology, Head and Neck Surgery, Aalborg Hospital - Aarhus University Hospital, Aalborg, Denmark

Yousef Yavarian
Department of Radiology, Aalborg Hospital - Aarhus University Hospital, Aalborg, Denmark

Ada Hiu Chong Lo and Bradley McPherson
Division of Speech and Hearing Sciences, Faculty of Education, University of Hong Kong, Pokfulam Road, Pokfulam, Hong Kong

Dagnachew Muluye, Yitayih Wondimeneh, Getachew Ferede and Feleke Moges
School of Biomedical and Laboratory Sciences, College of Medicine and Health Sciences, University of Gondar, Gondar, Ethiopia

Tesfaye Nega
Unit of Bacteriology, Gondar University Hospital, P.O. Box 196, Gondar, Ethiopia

Japhet M Gilyoma and Phillipo L Chalya
Department of Surgery, Weill- Bugando University College of Health Sciences, Mwanza, Tanzania

Mads Henrik Strand Moxness
Center for Endoscopic Nasal and Sinus surgery, Aleris Hospital Trondheim, Trondheim, Norway

Ståle Nordgård
The department of Otorhinolaryngology, Head and Neck Surgery, St Olav University Hospital, Trondheim, Norway
The Institute of Neuroscience, The Norwegian University of Science and Technology (NTNU), Trondheim, Norway
Post: Department of Neuroscience, NTNU, The Medical Faculty, N-7489 Trondheim, Norway

Andreas Keller
Laboratory of Neurogenetics and Behavior, Rockefeller University, New York, NY, USA

Dolores Malaspina
Department of Psychiatry, New York University School of Medicine, New York, NY, USA
Creedmoor Psychiatric Center, New York State Office of Mental Health, New York, NY, USA

Bernd Lütkenhöner and Türker Basel
ENT Clinic, Münster University Hospital, Münster, Germany

Said A Said, Phillipo L Chalya and Japhet M Gilyoma
Department of Surgery, Catholic University of Health and Allied Sciences Bugando, Mwanza, Tanzania

Mabula D Mchembe
Department of Surgery, Muhimbili University of Health and Allied Sciences, Dar Es Salaam, Tanzania

Peter Rambau
Department of Pathology, Catholic University of Health and Allied Sciences Bugando, Mwanza, Tanzania

Thomas Forkmann, Thomas Vehren, Eftychia Volz-Sidiropoulou, Siegfried Gauggel and Maren Boecker
Institute of Medical Psychology and Medical Sociology, University Hospital of RWTH Aachen, Pauwelsstraße 30, 52074 Aachen, Germany

Christine Norra
Dept. of Psychiatry and Psychotherapy, LWL-University-Clinic, Ruhr-University Bochum, Alexandrinenstr. 1-3, 44791 Bochum, Germany

Markus Wirtz
Institute of Psychology, University of Education Freiburg, Kartäuserstr. 61b, 79117 Freiburg, Germany

Martin Westhofen
Clinic for Otorhinolaryngology, University Hospital of RWTH Aachen, Pauwelsstraße 30, 52074 Aachen, Germany

Anne-Sofie Helvik
Department of Ear, Nose and Throat, Head and Neck Surgery, St. Olavs Hospital NTNU, Trondheim, Norway
Department of Public Health and General Practice, NTNU, Trondheim, Norway

Aleksander Grande Hansen, Ståle Nordgård and Vegard Bugten
Department of Ear, Nose and Throat, Head and Neck Surgery, St. Olavs Hospital NTNU, Trondheim, Norway
Department of Neuroscience, St. Olavs hospital NTNU, Trondheim, Norway

Lars Jacob Stovner and Asta K Håberg
Department of Neuroscience, St. Olavs hospital NTNU, Trondheim, Norway

Mari Gårseth
Department of Diagnostic Imaging, Levanger Hospital, Levanger, Norway

Heidi Beate Eggesbø
Department of Radiology and Nuclear Medicine, Oslo University Hospital, Oslo, Norway

Japhet M Gilyoma
Otorhinolaryngology unit, Bugando Medical Centre, Mwanza, Tanzania
Department of Surgery, Catholic University of Health and Allied Sciences, Mwanza, Tanzania

Phillipo L Chalya
Department of Surgery, Catholic University of Health and Allied Sciences, Mwanza, Tanzania

Veerle L Simoens
Cognitive Brain Research Unit, Cognitive Science, Department of Behavioural Sciences, University of Helsinki, Helsinki, Finland
Finnish Centre of Excellence in Interdisciplinary Music Research, Department of Music, University of Jyväskylä, Jyväskylä, Finland
BRAMS, International Laboratory for Brain, Music, and Sound research, Montreal, Canada

Sylvie Hébert
BRAMS, International Laboratory for Brain, Music, and Sound research, Montreal, Canada
École d'orthophonie et d'audiologie, Faculté de médecine, Université de Montréal, Canada, and Centre de recherche de l'Institut universitaire de gériatrie de Montréal, Montréal, Canada
Université de Montréal BRAMS, Pavillon 1420, Mont-Royal C.P. 6128, succ. Centre-ville, Montréal, QC H3C 3J7, Canada

Magnus Jannert
Department of Clinical Sciences, Division of Oto-Rhino-Laryngology, Skåne University Hospital, Malmö, Lund University, Lund, Sweden

Hillevi Pendleton
Department of Clinical Sciences, Division of Oto-Rhino-Laryngology, Skåne University Hospital, Malmö, Lund University, Lund, Sweden
Department of Oto-Rhino-Laryngology, Lasaretts gatan 21, Skåne University Hospital, SE-22185 Lund, Sweden

Marianne Ahlner-Elmqvist
Department of Health Sciences, Lund University, Lund, Sweden

Rolf Olsson
Divison of Medical Radiology, Diagnostic Centre of Imaging and Functional Medicine, Skåne University Hospital, Malmö, Lund University, Lund, Sweden

Ola Thorsson
Division of Nuclear Medicine, Diagnsotic Centre of Imaging and Functional Medicine, Skåne University Hospital, Malmö, Lund University, Lund, Sweden

Bodil Ohlsson Oskar Hammar
Department of Clinical Sciences, Divison of Internal Medicine, Skåne University Hospital, Malmö, Lund University, Lund, Sweden

Haimei Chen, Il Soo Kim, Chio Yokose, Joseph Kang and David Cho
Division of Allergy-Immunology, Department of Medicine, Northwestern University Feinberg School of Medicine, 676 N. St Clair street #14028, Chicago, IL 60611, USA

Seong Ho Cho
Division of Allergy-Immunology, Department of Medicine, Northwestern University Feinberg School of Medicine, 676 N. St Clair street #14028, Chicago, IL 60611, USA

Kyung Hee University, College of Medicine, Seoul, Korea

Tae J Yoo and Chun Cai
University of Tennessee, College of Medicine, Memphis, TN, USA

Silvia Palma
University of Modena, Modena, Italy

Micol Busi and Alessandro Martini
University of Ferrara, Ferrara, Italy

Nikolaos Spantideas
Athens Speech Language and Swallowing Institute, 10 Lontou Street, Glyfada, Athens 16675, Greece

Eirini Drosou
Athens Speech Language and Swallowing Institute, 37 Oinois Street, Glyfada, Athens 16674, Greece

Anastasia Bougea
Athens Speech and Language Institute, 1 Griva Digeni Street, Agios Dimitrios, Athens 17342, Greece

Dimitrios Assimakopoulos
Department of Otorhinolaryngology, University Hospital of Ioannina, Medical School of Ioannina University, 51 Napoleontos Zerva Street, Ioannina 45332, Greece

Hazem Kaheel, Andreas Breß and Marlies Kniper
University, HNO – universities Klink-Tubingen, Tubingen, Germany

Mohamed A. Hassan
University, HNO – universities Klink-Tubingen, Tubingen, Germany
Department of Bioinformatics, Africa city of technology, Khartoum, Sudan
Division of Molecular Genetics, Institute of Human Genetics, University of Tübingen, Tübingen, Germany, African city of Technology, Khartoum, Sudan

Aftab Ali Shah
Faculty of Biotechnology, University of Malakand, Khyber Pakhtunkhwa, Pakistan

Mutaz Amin
Department of Biochemistry, Faculty of Medicine, University of Khartoum, Khartoum, Sudan

Yousuf H. Y. Bakhit
Department of Basic Medical Sciences, Faculty of Dentistry-University of Khartoum, Khartoum, Sudan

Kaitesi Batamuliza Mukara
ENT department, College of medicine and health Sciences, University of Rwanda, and Health Policy, Planning and Management, Makerere University School of Public Health, Kampala, Uganda

Peter Waiswa
Department of Health Policy, Planning and Management, Makerere University School of Public Health, Uganda and Global Health Division, Karolinska Institutet, Stockholm, Sweden

Richard Lilford
Warwick Medical School, University of Warwick, Coventry, UK

Debara Lyn Tucci
Head and Neck Surgery and Communication Sciences, Duke University, Durham, USA

Alexandra Rodriguez Ruiz and Thibaut Demaesschalck
Department of Otolaryngology - Head and Neck Surgery, CHU Saint Pierre, Free University of Brussels, rue Haute 322, B1000 Brussels, Belgium

Jérôme R. Lechien and Sven Saussez
Department of Otolaryngology - Head and Neck Surgery, CHU Saint Pierre, Free University of Brussels, rue Haute 322, B1000 Brussels, Belgium
Laboratory of Anatomy and Cell Biology, Faculty of Medicine, UMONS Research Institute for Health Sciences and Technology, University of Mons (UMons), Mons, Belgium

Peder O. Laugen Heggdal, Flemming Vassbotn and Hans Jørgen Aarstad
Department of Otolaryngology/Head and Neck Surgery, Haukeland University Hospital, Bergen, Norway Department of Clinical Medicine, Faculty of Medicine and Dentistry, University of Bergen, Bergen, Norway

Anne Kari Aarstad
Department of Otolaryngology/Head and Neck Surgery, Haukeland University Hospital, Bergen, Norway
Department of Health Science, Faculty of Health Sciences, University of Stavanger, Stavanger, Norway

Øyvind Nordvik
Faculty of Health and Social Sciences, Bergen University College, Bergen, Norway

Jonas Brännström
Department of Clinical Science, Section of Logopedics, Phoniatrics and Audiology, Lund University, Lund, Sweden

Panagiotis A. Dimitriadis, Matthew R. Farr and Jaydip Ray
Department of Otolaryngology, Sheffield Teaching Hospitals, Sheffield, UK

Ahmed Allam
Department of Otolaryngology, Sheffield Teaching Hospitals, Sheffield, UK
Department of Otolaryngology, Mansoura University Hospitals, Mansoura, Egypt

Aleksander Grande Hansen, Jens Øyvind Loven, Hanne Berdal-Sørensen and Magnus TarAngen
Department of Ear, Nose and Throat, Head and Neck Surgery, Lovisenberg Diaconal Hospital, Oslo, Norway

Rolf Haye
Department of Ear, Nose and Throat, Head and Neck Surgery, Lovisenberg Diaconal Hospital, Oslo, Norway
Institute of Clinical Medicine, Faculty of Medicine, University of Oslo, Oslo, Norway

Chi Zhang
Institute of Basic Medical Sciences, Faculty of Medicine, University of Oslo, Oslo, Norway
Jostein Førsvoll and Knut Øymar
Department of Paediatrics, Stavanger University Hospital, 4068 Stavanger, Norway
Department of Clinical Science, University of Bergen, Bergen, Norway

Victoria Nyaiteera, Doreen Nakku, Esther Nakasagga and Evelyn Llovet
Department of Ear, Nose and Throat, Mbarara University of Science and Technology, Mbarara, Uganda

Elijah Kakande
Infectious Disease Research Collaboration, Mbarara, Uganda

Gladys Nakalema
Department of Psychology, Mbarara University of Science and Technology, Mbarara, Uganda

Richard Byaruhanga
Department of Ear, Nose and Throat, Makerere University College of Health Sciences, Kampala, Uganda

Francis Bajunirwe
Department of Community Health, Mbarara University of Science and Technology, Mbarara, Uganda

Bishow Tulachan and Buddha Nath Borgohain
Department of ENT - Head and Neck Studies, Universal College of Medical Sciences, Tribhuvan University Teaching Hospital, Bhairahawa, Nepal

Christopher R. Watts
Davies School of Communication Sciences and Disorders, Texas Christian University, TCU Box 297450, Fort Worth, TX 76129, USA

Mitchell R. Gore
Department of Otolaryngology, State University of New York Upstate Medical University, Physicians Office Building North, Suite 4P, 4900 Broad Road, Syracuse, NY 13215, USA

Sarah Zaher Addeen
Faculty of Medicine, Damascus University, Damascus, Syria

Mohammad Al-Mohammad
Otorhinolaryngology Department, Al- Mouwassat University Hospital, Damascus, Syria

Index

A
Abducens Palsy, 14-15
Acute Mastoiditis, 14-15, 18
Acute Otitis Media (AOM), 14
Adenoid Hypertrophy, 78-79, 81-83
Adenotonsillectomy, 82, 84, 182-183, 185-188
Angiography, 17, 152, 198, 200, 202
Anhedonia, 45, 47, 54-55, 61, 63
Anosmia, 45-46, 52-55, 60-63, 79, 104
Aphthous Stomatitis, 182-183, 185-188
Apical Petrositis, 14-15
Atherosclerosis, 8

B
Baha Attract, 167-173

C
C-reactive Protein (CRP), 8
Cardiac Infarction, 8
Cardiovascular Disease, 7, 13
Chronic Otitis Media (COM), 221
Chronic Rhinosinusitis (CRS), 189
Chronic Sinusitis, 1, 63, 81, 84, 117, 196
Computed Tomography (CT), 14, 198
Concha Bullosa, 4, 41
Conductive Hearing Loss (CHL), 168
Cortisol, 107-116

D
Depressive Disorder, 90-92
Drug Susceptibility, 29, 33
Dysphagia, 102, 117-118, 120

E
Ent Injuries, 101-106
Epistaxis, 34-39, 101, 104-106

F
Fine Needle Aspiration Cytology (FNAC), 198
Functional Endoscopic Sinus Surgery (FESS), 1
Functional Gastrointestinal Disorder, 117-118
Fusobacterium Necrophorum, 14-15, 17-18

G
Gastroesophageal Reflux, 124, 131, 133, 135-137, 191-192, 196-197
Gastrointestinal Disorders, 122-123

Glomangiomyoma, 198, 201-202
Glomus Tumour, 198, 202

H
Haemangioma, 198, 200, 202
Hearing Impairments (HI), 138
Hearing Threshold, 21, 107, 111, 113
Hibernoma, 150-153
Hyperemic Tympanic Membrane, 15
Hyperfibrinogenemia, 7, 10-13
Hyperlipidemia, 8
Hypokinetic Dysarthria, 203-204, 208

I
Idiopathic Sudden Sensorineural Hearing Loss (SSNHL), 7
Intranasal Tumor, 34

L
Laryngo-pharyngeal Reflux, 117, 122-123, 137
Laryngology, 117-118, 123, 175
Laryngopharyngeal Reflux, 124, 131, 136-137

M
Magnetic Resonance Imaging (MRI), 94, 198
Mann-whitney U-test, 9, 122
Mean Threshold Reduction (MTR), 65, 67
Metabolic Syndrome, 8, 10
Mucosal Thickening, 94, 96-99
Myringoplasty, 221-224

N
Nasal Endoscopy, 38, 189-191, 196

O
Obstructive Pulmonary Disease, 133, 136, 190
Obstructive Sleep Apnea (OSA), 40
Oesophago-gastro-duodenoscopy, 117
Olfactory Dysfunction, 45-52, 60-63
Opacification, 2-3, 5, 94, 96-98
Otorhinolaryngology, 7-8, 13, 36, 40, 44, 78, 84-85, 87-88, 92, 136

P
Paranasal Sinuses, 2-3, 5, 45, 89, 94-100, 210-211, 220
Parosmia, 45, 62-63
Pathopsychology, 87
Phantosmia, 45, 47, 55, 59-60, 63

Phonosurgery, 175, 178, 180
Posterior Laryngitis (PL), 117, 120-121
Prognostic Marker, 7, 13

R
Radioimmunoassay (RIA), 119
Retention Cysts, 94, 96-99

S
Septoplasty, 40-44, 62
Serology, 7, 10

Sinonasal Cancer, 210, 219-220
Sinus Thrombosis, 14-15, 17-18, 143
Speech Therapy, 177-178, 207

T
Tonsillectomy, 79, 81-82, 84, 86, 182-183, 185-187
Transcutaneous Bone Conduction Device, 167, 174
Turbinate, 1-6, 40-44, 78-81, 84
Tympanic Membrane Perforation, 102, 142-143, 223

www.ingramcontent.com/pod-product-compliance
Lightning Source LLC
Chambersburg PA
CBHW080523200326
41458CB00012B/4318